Cambridge Guides to the Psychological Therapies

Series Editor

Patricia Graham
Consultant Clinical Psychologist, NHS Lanarkshire, UK

The go-to resource for up-to-date, scientifically rigorous, and practical information on the key, evidence-based psychological interventions.

This series of clinical handbooks provides clear and concise guides to understanding and delivering therapy, and offers clinicians a handy reference for matching a specific therapy to a particular patient. Each book follows a consistent style, with chapters on theory, technique, indications and efficacy, so that healthcare professionals can move seamlessly between different volumes to learn about various therapies in a consistent, familiar and trusted format. The books also provide guidance on relevant adaptations for each therapy, such as for children, adolescents and older people, as well as different methods of delivery, such as group interventions and digital therapy.

Books available in the series

Cambridge Guide to Cognitive Behavioural Therapy (CBT)
Jessica Davies, Kenneth Laidlaw and Paul Salkovskis

Cambridge Guide to Cognitive Behavioral Analysis System of Psychotherapy (CBASP)
Massimo Tarsia, Todd Favorite and James McCullough Jr.

Cambridge Guide to Dialectical Behaviour Therapy (DBT)
Jim Lyng, Christine Dunkley, Janet Feigenbaum, Amy Gaglia and Michaela Swales

Cambridge Guide to Interpersonal Psychotherapy (IPT)
Laura Dietz, Fiona Duffy and Patricia Graham

Cambridge Guide to Mentalization-Based Treatment (MBT)
Anthony Bateman, Peter Fonagy, Chloe Campbell, Patrick Luyten and Martin Debbané

Cambridge Guide to Psychodynamic Psychotherapy
Adam Polnay, Rhiannon Pugh, Victoria Barker, David Bell, Allan Beveridge, Adam Burley, Allyson Lumsden, C. Susan Mizen and Lauren Wilson

Cambridge Guide to Schema Therapy
Robert N. Brockman, Susan Simpson, Christopher Hayes, Remco van der Wijngaart and Matthew Smout

"This handbook has some 'unique selling points': An updated and critical view of the model, a comprehensive overview of the latest research, and a detailed description of over-controlling coping modes. Definitely worth reading!"

Eckhard Roediger, MD
Director, Frankfurt Schema Therapy Institute

"This book, based on a comprehensive and up-to-date review of research on schema therapy, offers practical guidance and suggestions about the subtleties of the assessment and therapy process. The book reflects recent developments in understanding and differentiating schema modes and the chapter on case conceptualisation draws on new developments in the approach to case conceptualisation used in training by the ISST. Useful clinical examples in the form of short vignettes and longer summaries bring the details of the practice to life. This is well illustrated by the comprehensive chapter on assessment which includes valuable discussion of the complexities involved in integrating a range of sources of information. These include the client's verbal and non-verbal responses to interview questions, behaviours that result in avoidance of straightforward answers, and responses to schema therapy inventories, where the authors emphasize the importance of a qualitative perspective and the exercise of clinical judgment. The book's approach, at the same time practical, and reflective of the complexities involved, is continued in the comprehensive coverage of the range of interventions that are central to schema therapy in practice. Because of its depth and sophistication, this is a book that will be valuable not only for those at the early stages of development as schema therapists but also for experienced schema therapists, supervisors, and trainers."

David Edwards, PhD
Professor of Psychology, Rhodes University

"I am delighted to endorse this extraordinary book offered by Robert Brockman, Susan Simpson, Christopher Hayes, Remco van der Wijngaart, and Matthew Smout.

Complete with the classic theoretical concepts, guiding principles, and effective strategies founded in schema therapy, Cambridge Guide to Schema Therapy is a comprehensive and practical resource, that also offers the most up-to-date, beautifully nuanced, and thoughtfully illustrated elements of this science-supported model in theory and practice.

This book provides the wisdom, the data, and the guiding navigational tools – making it one of the most valuable contributions to clinical practitioners, across the globe. Informed by the work of Dr. Jeffrey Young (founder of schema therapy) and presented by some of the most talented and experienced schema therapy practitioners and educators, Cambridge Guide to Schema Therapy offers a robust and relevant understanding of schema theory, supported science, and applications of schema therapy strategies with some of the most challenging treatment populations. Hats off to my esteemed colleagues!

I am so pleased to confidently recommend this essential resource for your clinical library."

Wendy Behary, Past-President
International Society of Schema Therapy (ISST)
Author, *Disarming the Narcissist*

Cambridge Guide to Schema Therapy

Robert N. Brockman
Schema Therapy Training Australia, University of Technology Sydney

Susan Simpson
Schema Therapy Training Scotland

NHS Forth Valley, Scotland

Christopher Hayes
Schema Therapy Training Australia

Remco Van Der Wijngaart
Dutch Institute for Schema Therapy

Matthew Smout
University of South Australia

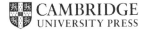

CAMBRIDGE
UNIVERSITY PRESS

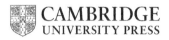

Shaftesbury Road, Cambridge CB2 8EA, United Kingdom

One Liberty Plaza, 20th Floor, New York, NY 10006, USA

477 Williamstown Road, Port Melbourne, VIC 3207, Australia

314–321, 3rd Floor, Plot 3, Splendor Forum, Jasola District Centre, New Delhi – 110025, India

103 Penang Road, #05–06/07, Visioncrest Commercial, Singapore 238467

Cambridge University Press is part of Cambridge University Press & Assessment, a department of the University of Cambridge.

We share the University's mission to contribute to society through the pursuit of education, learning and research at the highest international levels of excellence.

www.cambridge.org
Information on this title: www.cambridge.org/9781108927475

DOI: 10.1017/9781108918145

© Cambridge University Press & Assessment 2023

First published 2023 (version 2, July 2023)

Printed in Great Britain by CPI Group (UK) Ltd, Croydon CR0 4YY

A catalogue record for this publication is available from the British Library.

ISBN 978-1-108-92747-5 Paperback

Contents

Foreword

Over recent decades, schema therapy has gained increased popularity around the world as a treatment for chronic difficulties associated with characterological problems. Several reasons for this can be offered. First, the theory underlying schema therapy – that frustration of core emotional needs early in childhood and adolescence increases the risk of the development of maladaptive schemas, which in turn underlie personality disorders and other forms of character-related psychopathology – makes sense to most people. Moreover, despite empirical evidence, such early factors relevant for the development and maintenance of these forms of psychopathology have been relatively neglected in traditional cognitive-behavioural therapy models. It is therefore understandable that therapists confronted in their clinical practice with clients with these types of problems are interested in and even need such a theory. Second, the use of schema modes as a central construct in understanding and treating severe forms of psychopathology is extremely helpful for both clients and therapists. Case conceptualisations based on schema modes give clients a metacognitive understanding of their problems and how they link to early childhood experiences. Likewise, they help therapists to understand complex problems as well as sudden and often extreme changes in their clients' emotional states. Moreover, understanding the relevant schema modes of a specific patient provides guidance for the therapist, who can then choose from a range of appropriate techniques as the techniques are directly linked to working with specific schema modes. Third, the intelligent way in which the founder of schema therapy integrated methods and techniques of various therapy schools in an overarching cognitive schema model is extremely attractive as it offers different channels of change (cognitive, experiential, and behavioural) in different domains (therapeutic relationship, past, and present world outside the therapy room). Integrating these within one coherent model undoubtedly contributed to the high acceptability and effectiveness of schema therapy. Fourth, effectiveness and cost-effectiveness of schema therapy is supported by empirical studies, which gives clients, therapists, managers, and policy makers a strong argument to consider schema therapy as a treatment option.

In the dissemination and implementation of new treatments, comprehensive handbooks such as this are essential. Such books should discuss the theory underlying the treatment in a thorough yet accessible way, describe the therapeutic relationship that should be strived for, offer clear descriptions of methods and techniques, discuss the phases of therapy, address different forms of application, and offer solutions for possible problems that can be encountered with the application of the treatment. This book offers all of this. Hence, it is an excellent guide for learning schema therapy (along with video examples and training), as well as a reference for those who are more advanced practitioners. As one of the most comprehensive in the field, authored by leading experts in schema therapy, it is highly recommended.

Professor Arnoud Arntz

Preface

We were delighted to be invited by our colleagues at Cambridge University Press to write this book on schema therapy, where it could take its place alongside other established, evidence-based therapy approaches in this clinicians' series. This represented, for us, further evidence that the popularity and reach of schema therapy is growing rapidly. It also underscored the fact that the research base for schema therapy has become more widely recognised amongst our therapist peers (see Chapter 2 for an overview of the evidence). Since the schema therapy model was developed by its originator, Jeffrey Young, during the 1980s and 1990s, a new generation of schema therapists has emerged to further develop the model for application in novel treatment contexts, and to drive its empirical evaluation. This new generation of schema therapists, many of whom were trained directly by Jeffrey Young and colleagues through his New York Schema Therapy Institute, returned to their home countries and seeded much of the interest that we see today globally in the schema therapy approach.

There are, of course, already many other schema therapy books and descriptions of the model. This led us to consider what contribution our book could make to the dissemination of the schema therapy model more broadly. For our team, the answer was clear. The schema therapy model has undergone significant development since its early days, a process which is ongoing. We aimed to provide a contemporary overview of modern schema therapy as it is being practised today, almost three decades after Jeffrey Young's seminal text [1]. Further, we wanted to give more attention and depth to issues not extensively addressed elsewhere in the literature (e.g., the phasing of schema therapy, increasing therapist attunement, ending therapy/termination issues, schema therapy in online settings, and schema therapy supervision). We also wanted to showcase how the model is increasingly being extended into novel populations and treatment settings (e.g., complex trauma, eating disorders, chronic depression, anxiety disorders, violent forensic offenders, and via group delivery). The book is written in four sections. In Part I of the book, we provide an in-depth overview of the schema therapy model referencing its theoretical background (Chapter 1) and growing evidence base (Chapter 2). Part II represents the core of the book, a set of ten chapters (Chapters 3–12) demonstrating the model of schema therapy in practice. In Part III – Application and Adaptations for Mental Health Presentations (Chapters 13–15) – we provide an overview of the application of schema therapy to a range of mental health disorders outside of its traditional scope of personality disorders. Finally, in Part IV of the book – Application of Schema Therapy in Different Populations and Settings (Chapters 16–21) – we demonstrate how schema therapy may be applied in a diverse range of clinical contexts.

References

1. Young J. *Cognitive therapy for personality disorders: A schema focused approach.* Professional Resource Press; 1999.

A Note from the Series Editor

I remember when I first met Sarah Marsh, Editor at Cambridge University Press – it seems like a lifetime ago now. We met at a café in central Edinburgh in June 2017 to discuss an idea that she had to create a series of books focussed on evidenced based Psychological Therapies. The idea was simple – the books would be attractive to a trainee and simultaneously to an expert clinician. We wanted to enable readers to conceptualise a psychological difficulty using different theoretical models of understanding, but not become overwhelmed by the volume of information. We saw the need for a series of books that could be easily read and yet would examine complex concepts in a manage- able way.

So, when Sarah asked me if I would become the Series Editor, I couldn't say no. What we could never have predicted back then, when making early plans for the series, was that we would soon face a global pandemic. There were days when we didn't even know whether we could leave our house or if our children could go to school – the world effectively stopped. Yet through all the chaos, uncertainty and fear, I saw the determin- ation and successes of those around me shine through. I was in awe of the resilience of my own son, Patrick, who lived his adolescence in 'lock-down'. I watch him now and the young man he has become – he walks tall with a quiet confidence. I am so proud as he and his friends laugh together and now enjoy what most of us had previously taken for granted: their freedom at university. In a similar way, I watched the many authors of these books, most of whom are busy and tired clinicians, continue to dedicate their precious time to this venture – an incredible achievement through a most challenging time. They each welcomed me into their academic, clinical and theoretical worlds, from all over the globe. They have all been an honour to work with. I would personally like to thank every contributor and author of this series for their hard work, determination and humour even in the darkest of days. Despite all of the unknowns and the chaos, they kept going and achieved something wonderful.

I would like to thank Sarah, and Kim Ingram at Cambridge, for giving me the opportunity to be Series Editor. I have loved every minute of it; it has been a longer journey than we anticipated but an amazing one and for that I am incredibly grateful. Sarah and Kim are my friends now – we have literally lived through a global pandemic together. It has been my absolute pleasure to work together and in collaboration with Cambridge University Press.

Patricia Graham, Series Editor
Consultant Clinical Psychologist, NHS Lanarkshire, UK

Acknowledgements

We would like to acknowledge the many people that have supported us or contributed in some way to the ideas contained in this book. First, to the many clients we have had the pleasure of working with using schema therapy: we have learned so much from you and your struggles, and sincerely hope we have helped to make a difference in your lives.

To Dr Jeffrey Young, who imagined this new and powerful approach to therapeutically working with clients who at the time were often deemed 'untreatable': we live in something of a golden age of psychotherapy these days, where we now have strong evidence that even the most troubled people can and should be helped. You have contributed a great deal to that reality. Similarly, Wendy Behary, you were also there from the start and have given so much to support us and the schema therapy community globally.

Next, we would like to acknowledge all our Dutch colleagues, led by Professor Arnoud Artnz, who have achieved so much in pushing a research agenda to better understand the effects and processes of schema therapy practice. This includes Professor David Bernstein, for sharing his knowledge and wisdom related to the emerging forensic schema therapy model described in Chapter 16. Dr Lars Madsen, also, for sharing his ideas and experiences in providing schema therapy in forensic settings and providing feedback on drafts of Chapter 16. Similarly, we would like to acknowledge Andrea Papitsch-Clark for her feedback on some early drafts and ideas for this book. Big thanks also to Clodagh Coyle for her editorial work on all chapters, and to Maria Brockman for the drawings and artwork she provided for the book.

Thanks to the whole ISST (International Society for Schema Therapy) community for being a forum for creativity and support in schema therapy practice.

Last, but not least, we all wish to thank our families for their love, support, and patience. Without you, writing projects like this would not be possible, and they would not mean so much.

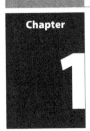

From Core Emotional Needs to Schemas, Coping Styles, and Schema Modes
The Conceptual Model of Schema Therapy

Introduction
In this chapter we provide a brief overview of the history of the development of schema therapy, and an overview of its model of the development of psychopathology and psychological health. This chapter will introduce the primary theoretical constructs of schema therapy – core emotional needs, early maladaptive schemas (EMS), coping styles, and schema modes – and explain how need deprivation gives rise to EMS, how coping styles interact with EMS to produce schema modes, and how these concepts produce psychopathology.

The Basic Schema Therapy Model
The Heart of Schema Therapy: Core Emotional Needs
It may be said that schema therapy could have very easily been named *needs therapy*, so central is the concept of *core emotional needs* to its practice. Although schema therapy began as an attempt by leading cognitive therapists to modify entrenched 'core beliefs' [1], schema therapy has evolved over the past three decades into a therapy whose central precept is the satisfaction of core emotional needs.

A core impetus for the development of schema therapy was Jeff Young and colleagues' observation in working with traditional cognitive therapy that, despite impressive outcomes in many clients, a substantial proportion (up to 50%) did not benefit significantly or enduringly [2]. Most of these cases appeared to have symptoms with clear links to childhood experiences and associated negative or traumatic memories. At the time, based on clinical observation, this group of therapists suspected that these 'schema patterns' reflected long-term 'characterological' issues with clear developmental antecedents.

Informed by the burgeoning developmental literature on psychological needs [4, 5, 6], and clinical observation, Young and colleagues described five core emotional needs that emerge in the developmental period. Understanding the extent to which these needs were met or unmet is pivotal to understanding chronic mental health problems [2]:

1. Secure attachments to others (includes safety, stability, nurturance, and acceptance).
2. Autonomy, competence, and sense of identity.
3. Freedom to express valid needs and emotions.
4. Spontaneity and play.
5. Realistic limits and self-control.

The heart of Young and colleagues' treatment model is that need satisfaction during childhood leads to the development of healthy schemas and related functional affective and behavioural patterns, while early need frustration leads directly to the development of EMS and related negative patterns of behaviour and maladaptive coping. The emphasis on early childhood development and the explicit causal role of unmet core emotional needs in producing EMS distinguished schema therapy from the prevailing theories of cognitive therapy at the time. Especially relevant types of early life experience were thought to be one or more of the following: (a) toxic frustration of needs; (b) exposure to overt trauma or victimisation; (c) a lack of boundaries or limits ('too much of a good thing'); and (d) selective internalisation or identification with significant others [2].

The Influence of Attachment Theory in Schema Therapy

Since their beginnings in the 1960s, theories of attachment [3] were quick to influence the hearts and minds of therapists in the field. The parallels between the experiences of clients' early patterns of attachment and their present-day problems appeared obvious. However, practical applications of this powerful new theory were lacking. Young was quick to recognise the importance of the theory for his emerging schema therapy model, integrating its emphasis on secure attachment as a core emotional need. Young acknowledged that the most important need for the developing child was the need for safe, stable, nurturing, and validating attachments. For Young, attachment to others was not a preference but a core emotional need, required for healthy development and well-being. To the degree that this need was thwarted during development, EMS would ensue. As noted earlier, children have a range of needs but, according to Young, attachment needs are of primary importance, laying the groundwork for other needs to be satisfied. The need for attachment and its relationship to a set of schemas in the Disconnection and Rejection domain is a primary focus for schema therapy interventions, especially *limited reparenting* interventions (see Chapter 6: Intervention Strategies for Schema Healing 1: Limited Reparenting for more detail). The original set of eighteen EMS – organised by their original domains and described in core belief terms – is described in Table 1.1.

Young's Schema Concept

Expanding upon earlier conceptions of schemas from authors such as Piaget [7], Young and colleagues [2] conceptualised schemas as a normal and central human phenomenon: an organising principle that enables humans to interpret and make sense of their experiences and the world. As children navigate and interpret the world, they will generally develop functional scripts, or schemas, which are representations of the world that are activated according to situational demands. Many schemas are mundane, representing what to expect (expectancies) or the kind of rules likely to be operating in one's environment, based on past experiences. In the broad field of cognitive psychology, schemas can be positive or negative, adaptive or maladaptive, and can be formed during childhood or later in life. Young's EMS refer to a core set of *problematic* schemas that tend to develop during childhood or adolescence, and which are centrally implicated in the development of various forms of psychopathology. For Young and colleagues [2], EMS can be defined as:

- a broad, pervasive theme or pattern
- comprised of memories, emotions, cognitions, and bodily sensations

Table 1.1 Schema domains and corresponding early maladaptive schemas*

Disconnection and Rejection Domain

1. *Abandonment/Instability* **(AB)**: Expectation that significant others will not be available to provide support, connection, strength, or protection.
2. *Mistrust/Abuse* **(MA)**: Expectation that others will hurt, abuse, humiliate, lie, cheat, steal, or manipulate.
3. *Emotional Deprivation* **(ED)**: Expectation that one will not receive adequate emotional support or be understood by others. Three major subtypes of deprivation include:

    (a) *Deprivation of Nurturance*: The absence of attention, affection, warmth, and companionship – 'No one cares . . .'
    (b) *Deprivation of Empathy*: The absence of understanding and attunement – 'No one really gets me . . .'
    (c) *Deprivation of Protection*: The absence of direction, strength, and guidance – 'I am all alone (in facing the world)'.

4. *Defectiveness/Shame* **(DS)**: Belief that one is defective, unlovable, bad, unwanted, inferior, inadequate, and/or shameful.
5. *Social Isolation/Alienation* **(SI)**: Belief that one is socially isolated, different from others, and does not belong to any group or community.

Impaired Autonomy and Performance Domain

6. *Dependence/Incompetence* **(DI)**: Belief that one is helpless and unable to cope with everyday responsibilities without significant help from others, leading to lack of autonomy and self-reliance.
7. *Vulnerability to Harm or Illness* **(VH)**: Expectation that a catastrophe is imminent, and one will be unable to prevent it.
8. *Enmeshment/Underdeveloped Self* **(EM)**: Tendency to be overly emotionally involved with one or more significant others, resulting in impaired social development, inner direction, and individuation.
9. *Failure* **(FA)**: Belief that one has failed or will fail in areas of achievement and that one is incompetent, stupid, inept, untalented, etc.

Impaired Limits Domain

10. *Entitlement/Grandiosity* **(ET)**: Belief that one is superior to others, should receive special treatment, and should not be required to follow the same rules as others.
11. *Insufficient Self-Control/Self-Discipline* **(IS)**: Inability to appropriately restrain impulses and emotions; difficulty tolerating frustration and boredom to accomplish goals.

Other-Directedness Domain

12. *Subjugation* **(SB)**: Surrender of control to others and suppression of one's own emotions and needs to avoid anger, retaliation, or abandonment.
13. *Self-Sacrifice* **(SS)**: Hypersensitivity to emotional pain and suffering in others, and a tendency to take on responsibility for their needs and feelings at one's own expense.
14. *Approval-Seeking/Recognition-Seeking* **(AS)**: Excessive emphasis on gaining approval, recognition, or attention from others, resulting in an underdeveloped authentic sense of self. Often involves overemphasis on status, achievement, and/or money.

Table 1.1 (cont.)

Overvigilance and Inhibition Domain

15. *Negativity/Pessimism* **(NP)**: Exaggerated expectation that things will go wrong, or of making mistakes, leading to excessive worry. Focusing on the negative aspects of life and minimising positives.
16. *Emotional Inhibition* **(EI)**: Inhibiting spontaneous actions, feelings (especially anger), or communication to prevent being disapproved of, ridiculed, or losing control.
17. *Unrelenting Standards/Hypercriticalness* **(US)**: Belief that whatever one does is not good enough, that one must strive to meet very high standards of performance, usually to prevent criticism; and/ or excessive emphasis on status, power at expense of health and happiness.
18. *Punitiveness* **(PU)**: Belief that people (self and others) should be severely punished for making mistakes or not meeting one's internalised expectations or standards.

* *Adapted from Young, Klosko, & Weishaar (2003)*

- regarding oneself and one's relationships with others
- developed during childhood or adolescence
- elaborated throughout one's lifetime, and
- dysfunctional to a significant degree.

EMS represent patterns of self-defeating affect and cognition that begin early in development and are repeated and elaborated throughout one's lifetime. They are triggered by current situations or circumstances relevant to the schema theme.

Key to this definition is the emphasis not only on cognitive content (e.g., core beliefs, negative automatic thoughts), but the interplay between all four components of EMS activation: (1) cognitive content; (2) memory/imagery – negative memories and imagery become more salient when the schema is triggered; (3) emotions; and (4) bodily sensations. Young and colleagues' definition highlights the significance of imagery-based, affective, and somatic processes in any approach to understanding and healing schemas. Young [2] argues that EMS are usually adaptive and accurate representations of the general tone of the family and childhood environment during the developmental period but may come to bias subsequent experience outside of that family context. EMS that were relatively accurate and perhaps adaptive during childhood can be maladaptive later in adult life. It is worth noting that in Young and colleagues' view of EMS, maladaptive coping behaviours are not themselves part of the EMS but are ways of coping with the EMS. These coping behaviours are said to be 'schema-driven' rather than representing a direct component of the schema per se.

Three Broad Maladaptive Coping Styles

Young argued that EMS are perpetuated through three broad styles of coping. Each represents a different type of adaptation to the EMS and functions to provide some sense of subjective relief from the emotions involved in the activation of the EMS. The coping behaviour usually blocks access to information that would otherwise disconfirm EMS-driven expectancies and maintains a longer-term disconnection from the satisfaction of core emotional needs. This is how coping styles reinforce and maintain schemas (*schema perpetuation*). The three main coping styles are:

Schema Avoidance (Flight): Schema avoidance refers to coping by avoiding or escaping full activation of the EMS. Common examples include overt avoidance or escape from people, places, activities, or situations that could potentially trigger EMS, and actions that dull aversive emotional arousal, such as drug use or other compulsive behaviour, self-harm, and emotional detachment.

Schema Overcompensation (Fight): Schema overcompensation refers to a person responding to the threat of schema activation by 'fighting back' in some way against the core message of the EMS. This means thinking, acting, and feeling as though the opposite of the EMS is true. Recent authors have relabelled this coping style as *schema inversion* [6]. For example, someone with a Defectiveness/Shame EMS might overcompensate by displaying arrogance and acting as if they are better than others (i.e., the opposite of feeling less worthy).

Schema Surrender (Freeze): Schema surrendering involves resignation to the EMS – accepting its core message and acting as though it was true [8]. For example, someone with an Abandonment/Instability EMS might surrender by seeking out or committing to relationships that are not secure or stable (i.e., believing that no partner will ever provide them consistent, committed emotional and physical availability). Such clients may believe they 'should not expect any better'. Alternatively, they might surrender in a potentially healthy relationship by constantly seeking reassurance or checking up on their partner because they 'believe the schema' that tells them that 'their partner will leave them sooner or later', even in the absence of objective evidence.

The Schema Mode Model

Thus far we have described the first iteration of schema therapy, which has come to be known as the *basic schema therapy model*. Treatment with the basic schema therapy model emphasises focusing on changing EMS. However, in applying schema therapy to the most complex cases, involving personality disorders and serious and chronic mental health problems, Young recognised the need to modify and expand the model to account for the issue of multiplicity of self that is a common characteristic of these clients, especially those with borderline personality disorder (BPD) [2]. BPD clients often presented with what appeared to be various – often dissociated – 'parts' which had the quality of rapidly shifting mood states. BPD challenged the conceptualisation and treatment guided by the basic model. In response, Young and colleagues [2] offered a reformulated model – what has become known as the *schema mode model* – with schema modes as the central organising construct. This 'mode model' has become the dominant form of schema therapy and is the version of schema therapy that has garnered almost all of the available empirical support for schema therapy in clinical trials (see Chapter 2: Research Support for Schema Therapy).

Schema modes are defined by Young and colleagues [2] as 'those schemas or schema operations – adaptive or maladaptive – that are currently active for an individual' (p. 37). Modes are the state-like manifestation of the interaction between the person's currently activated EMS and their coping response at any given time. Personality is conceptualised as a group of distinct 'parts' with potentially separate affective, cognitive, behavioural, and motivational qualities. Young [2] initially presented four classes of modes: child modes, parent (critic) modes, coping modes, and the Healthy Adult mode. Research and theoretical development has since expanded the mode model [9, 10, 11, 12] to better account for a broader range of psychopathology. An up-to-date mode listing is given in Table 1.2. Our

Table 1.2 Schema modes

Child Modes

1. ***Vulnerable Child* (VCM)**: The Vulnerable Child mode is the 'storehouse' of EMS, whereby the person feels the emotions associated with EMS activation and unmet emotional needs but without the perspective of a Healthy Adult (e.g., a stable sense of self that transcends temporary emotional states, confidence in ability to cope). Typical emotions include feeling lonely, lost, frightened, frantic, sad, anxious, hurt, ashamed, and guilty. The core emotional 'flavour' of a Vulnerable Child mode varies according to the specific underlying EMS: for example, someone with an Emotional Deprivation EMS likely has a Lonely Child mode; someone with an Abandonment/Instability schema probably has an Abandoned Child mode; Dependence/Incompetence EMS manifests as a Dependent Child mode, and Mistrust/Abuse EMS as an Abused Child mode.

Vulnerable (Lonely) Child Mode

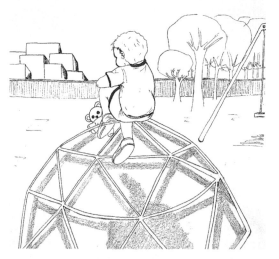

Illustration 1.1 'Vulnerable (Lonely) Child mode'

2. ***Angry Child* (ACM)**: Angry Child mode involves experiencing strong feelings of anger, rage, frustration, impatience, or indignation because core emotional or physical needs of the vulnerable child have not adequately been met. Anger is alternately suppressed and then expressed in inappropriate ways, such as through uncontrolled venting, without consideration of the consequences for themselves and others. The person may also act in a manner which is entitled or spoiled, expecting others to meet their needs immediately and perfectly, without consideration of others' needs or feelings.

Table 1.2 (cont.)

ANGRY CHILD MODE

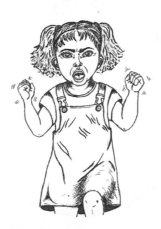

Illustration 1.2 'Angry Child mode'

3. *Enraged Child* **(ECM)**: Enraged Child mode involves experiencing extreme feelings of anger and fury, leading to destructive acts towards other people and/or objects. Others are seen as aggressors and anger is aimed at annihilating them either directly or indirectly. The person may scream, yell, and act in an uncontrolled way towards another. The tone is of a child who is enraged and has lost control.

4. *Impulsive Child* **(ICM)**: Impulsive Child mode responds to urges, impulses, cravings, and wants in the moment in an impulsive, uncontrolled way, without consideration of the medium- and longer-term impact on themselves or others. The person struggles to resist powerful desires and defer gratification. They may appear self-centred.

5. *Undisciplined Child* **(UCM)**: Undisciplined Child mode struggles to take responsibility and complete routine tasks. The person has difficulty tolerating the boredom or discomfort required to achieve longer-term goals.

6. *Happy Child* **(HCM)**: The person in Happy Child mode is contented, spontaneous, hopeful, calm, and embodied, due to having their core needs met. The person feels valued, cared for, understood, capable, effectual, energetic, motivated, playful, confident, protected, and safe. The person is flexible and able to adapt to the requirements of situations without compromising their own needs. They are emotionally and joyfully connected to others and to nature.

Coping Modes

Surrender Coping Modes (Resignation)

7. *Compliant Surrenderer* **(CSM)**: In Compliant Surrenderer mode the person is compliant, passive, submissive, pleasing, excessively agreeable, and allows others to take control in order to avoid conflict or criticism and/or to gain acceptance or nurturance. The person neglects their own needs so that they can prioritise the needs of others. They maintain a 'downtrodden' position through selecting relationships and/or behaving in a 'one-down' position.

Table 1.2 (cont.)

8. *Helpless Surrenderer* **(HSM)**: In Helpless Surrenderer mode the person feels helpless, impotent, dependent, ineffectual, passive, or stuck. They idealise others, perceiving them to be strong, competent, and potential rescuers, able to solve their difficulties. They may 'talk about' struggles and needs, but authentic connection to vulnerability is missing. The person in Helpless Surrenderer mode may have internalised the message that, to be worthy and deserving of care, they must demonstrate their needs through observable displays such as of helplessness, physical vulnerability, or frailty. The Helpless Surrenderer mode may be linked to 'learned helplessness' from childhood experiences that resulted in them feeling overpowered, helpless, overwhelmed, paralysed by fear of rejection, abandoned, or humiliated.

9. *Self-Pity Victim* **(SPVM)**: In Self-Pity Victim mode, the person sees themself as a victim. They perceive the world as unfair and feel that they have been uniquely singled out and persecuted. Others are perceived to hold power whilst they themselves are powerless. Therefore, they refuse to take responsibility for change.

Avoidance Coping Modes

10. *Detached Protector* **(DPM)**: The person in Detached Protector mode escapes from emotional suffering associated with schema activation through numbing, detachment, spacing-out, sleeping (excessive), dissociation, or somatisation. They may experience feelings of emptiness and boredom or depersonalisation. They may continue to cope with daily life in an apparently 'normal' or 'autopilot' way, whilst remaining emotionally distant from others.

11. *Detached Self-Soother* **(DSS)**: In Detached Self-Soother mode, the person escapes from overwhelming emotions through solitary activities designed to self-soothe, self-stimulate, or divert attention away from emotions. Coping behaviours frequently have an addictive or compulsive quality. Self-stimulation can include substance misuse, promiscuous sex, gambling, workaholism, extreme sports, online gaming, binge eating, alcoholism, online shopping, watching television (excessively), or fantasising.

12. *Avoidant Protector* **(AvPM)**: The person in Avoidant Protector mode attempts to prevent the risk of activating EMS through avoiding any overt situation (people, place, conversation, activity) which could potentially trigger vulnerable feelings.

13. *Angry Protector* **(APM)**: The Angry Protector mode protects the self via a wall of angry hostility, due to expecting that others will threaten, humiliate, or shame them if their underlying vulnerability is exposed. The anger is passive, but strategic, aimed at ensuring that others have no opportunity to hurt, reject, or exert power over them.

Overcompensation (Inversion) Modes

14. *Approval/Recognition Seeker* **(ASM)**: In the Approval/Recognition Seeker mode the person tries to impress others through ostentatious, flamboyant, or theatrical behaviours to overcome underlying loneliness or feeling 'unseen'.

15. *Self-Aggrandiser* **(SAM)**: The person in the Self-Aggrandiser mode seeks greater status, admiration, power, and control through behaving in a grandiose, entitled, abusive, or competitive manner. They devalue and diminish others in order to establish a 'one-up' position in relationships. The person in Self-Aggrandiser mode only values others insofar as they contribute to their status or glorify them in some way. The person believes themselves to be superior to others and expects to be treated as such. The person behaves in a self-absorbed way without consideration or empathy for others, and elevates their status through boasting, self-promotion, or humble-bragging.

Table 1.2 (cont.)

16. *Overcontroller modes*: A person in one of the Overcontroller modes seeks to gain a sense of control through rumination, overanalysing, ritualised behaviour, overplanning, or obsessionality. The person may have a strong focus on productivity and time efficiency to attain a sense of achievement or worth and overcome an underlying sense of helplessness, impotence, or failure. People in Overcontroller modes attempt to reduce uncertainty, unpredictability, and vulnerability to potential harm through excessive attention to detail and adhering to rules in a rigid manner. There are several subtypes:

   a. *Perfectionistic Overcontroller* (**POCM**): focuses on getting things 'right' and avoiding mistakes to minimise the possibility of criticism, disappointment, and failure.

   b. *Suspicious Overcontroller* (**SOCM**): hypervigilant, wary, and suspicious of others' motives. The person may be controlling towards others to protect against a perceived threat and persecutory behaviour.

   c. *Overanalysing Overcontroller* (**OACM**): characterised by the predominance of verbal-linguistic processing of past- and/or future-oriented material (e.g., rumination, worry, or obsessive thinking), at the expense of attending to the contextual and emotional qualities of present-moment experience.

   d. **Scolding Overcontroller* (**SOCM**): attempts to control others through blaming, criticising, scolding, and/or presiding over them in an overbearing manner.

   e. **Flagellating Overcontroller* (**FOCM**): overcompensates for fear of attack or punishment by punishing and blaming oneself, with the aim of restoring the illusion of control. Self-punishment or deprivation may also function as an attempt at self-improvement, to appease, to reduce the risk of being humiliated or punished (either by others or their own internal Critic), to increase predictability and perceived control over suffering and pain, or to atone for unresolved guilt or shame.

   f. **Invincible/Hyperautonomous Overcontroller* (**IOCM**): feels invincible, indestructible, and powerful. The person seeks to be completely invulnerable and eliminate or be 'on top' of emotional needs by behaving in a manner which is self-sufficient and denies the need for emotional connection to others.

17. *Bully and Attack* (**BAM**): In Bully and Attack mode, the person intimidates or attacks others strategically through threat or abusive acts (physical, sexual, emotional). The person attacks first to pre-empt attacks from others.

18. *Conning and Manipulative* (**CMM**): In Conning and Manipulative mode, the person manipulates, cheats, deceives, or victimises others to achieve their own objectives, including exploitation or escaping consequences of their own actions.

19. *Predator* (**PM**): The person in Predator mode plans and manoeuvres in a cold, calculating, and callous manner to eliminate others who represent a potential threat, enemy, competitor, or obstruction.

Maladaptive Inner Critic (Parent) Modes

20. *Punitive Critic* (**PuCrM**): The Punitive Critic mode stores and replays internalised messages from childhood and adolescence that are harshly critical and punishing. This mode conveys the belief that vulnerability, needs, and emotions are signs of weakness and must be punished or eliminated. The person in the Punitive Critic mode may experience repeated re-enactment of previous experiences of self-blame, criticism, punishment, or deprivation.

21. *Demanding Critic* (**DeCrM**): The Demanding Critic mode consists of the internalised voice that pushes, pressures, and prioritises achievement and high standards over health, well-being, and happiness. The person in Demanding Critic mode experiences thoughts containing black-and-white messages about the 'correct' way to behave through achieving the highest

Table 1.2 (cont.)

standards; being perfect, time efficient, and humble; devoting oneself to the needs of others; and retaining full control over the self and expression of emotions or needs.

22. *Guilt-Inducing Critic* **(GICr)**: The person in the Guilt-Inducing Critic mode experiences thoughts containing messages – received directly or implied, throughout their life – that others' needs are more important or urgent, and that the person is somehow a burden and undeserving of care. The person may also have internalised the message that the expression of their needs and emotions is selfish, potentially harmful or a threat to others and must be suppressed at all costs.

23. *Healthy Adult (HAM)*: In the Healthy Adult mode, the person recognises, protects, and nurtures the inner Vulnerable Child and their needs, and demonstrates compassion for self and others. This mode demonstrates flexibility, seeking to balance prioritising the needs of self and others, and can manage adult responsibilities (sustaining a job, self-care, managing finances, caring for others). The Healthy Adult strives for a flexible balance between pleasant adult activities (intellectual/cultural/physical) and maintaining commitments. This mode experiences the body and mind as integrated aspects of the self, can give and receive nurturance and care, and gains meaning from authentic self-expression and connection with others and the world. This mode, when activated, can step back with awareness from one's automatic schema-based reactions and choose adaptive reactions with respect to one's longer-term needs.

**Proposed additional modes based on recent theoretical developments [8, 11, 12, 13]

approach to schema therapy assessment and case conceptualisation using the mode model is described in Chapter 3: Schema Therapy Assessment, and Chapter 4: Case Conceptualisation and Mode Mapping in Schema Therapy, respectively.

Schema Therapy Treatment Model

The schema therapy model was initially formulated as an alternative conceptualisation to the diagnostic categorisation approach (e.g., DSM5, ICD-11) to personality disorders. Young and colleagues argued that EMS lie at the heart of personality disturbance, and that the dysregulated behaviour captured by diagnostic labels such as 'borderline' and 'antisocial' are primarily *responses* to core EMS. Schema therapy has been demonstrated to successfully treat personality disorders and their traits by targeting EMS and their related coping styles or modes. Over the past twenty years, the schema therapy model has increasingly been applied to a broader range of psychological disorders, including chronic and treatment-resistant cases of those formerly known as DSM Axis I disorders. See Chapter 2: Research Support for Schema Therapy for an overview.

Mechanisms of Change (The Four Aims of Schema Therapy)

The schema therapy model suggests four related, but distinct mechanisms of change that become the central levers for schema therapy intervention:

1. **(Re)Connect to Core Emotional Needs.** Schema therapists aim to help clients experience increased satisfaction of their core emotional needs. Most clients referred for schema therapy have either disconnected from attending to their core emotional needs or have experienced chronic thwarting of need satisfaction during childhood and

adolescence. Schema therapists aim to 'kick start' or resume the client's emotional development by addressing those needs that were not adequately fulfilled in childhood and that are most connected to their set of current problems.

2. **Support Schema Healing.** Young and colleagues [2] argued that the ultimate goal of schema therapy is schema healing. Schema healing involves weakening all aspects of EMS: the intrusiveness and intensity of negative memories or images, the schema's emotional charge (including any bodily sensations), and maladaptive cognitions.

3. **Reverse Maladaptive Coping Responses.** Because maladaptive coping responses can maintain EMS and threaten long-term emotional need satisfaction, these behaviour patterns must be identified and replaced with more adaptive behavioural repertoires.

4. **Build the Healthy Adult Mode.** While schema healing and reversing maladaptive coping responses addresses deficits in personality functioning, schema therapy also aims to build positive capacities of personality functioning by 'building the Healthy Adult mode' [14, 15]. The client needs a strong Healthy Adult mode in order to take care of their emotional functioning when therapy finishes. Throughout therapy, schema therapists balance developing the Healthy Adult alongside schema healing tasks.

Four Broad Intervention Methods

1. **Therapy Relationship Strategies (Limited Reparenting)**: The foundation upon which change occurs in schema therapy is a strong *limited reparenting relationship*. In using limited reparenting strategies, the therapist aims to go beyond a 'standard' level of therapist care and warmth and makes attempts to directly meet the needs of clients, within the appropriate bounds of a therapy relationship. These strategies include providing not only care, attunement, and warmth, but also empathic confrontation and limit setting. These are discussed at length in Chapter 6: Intervention Strategies for Schema Healing 1: Limited Reparenting.

2. **Cognitive Techniques**: To the extent that clients are fused with EMS-driven beliefs, they will struggle to make significant change. Schema therapists initially help clients to challenge their negative and distorted schema-based view of themselves and the world, on a rational level. This will not necessarily lead to lasting emotional or behavioural change, but is often a necessary preparatory step to enable such change. An in-depth overview of cognitive strategies as they are applied in schema therapy is the focus of Chapter 7: Intervention Strategies for Schema Healing 2: Cognitive Strategies.

3. **Experiential Techniques**: Jeff Young and colleagues [2] and others [16] have argued that EMS are encoded on an emotional and implicational level and that, as such, strategies that are purely cognitive or 'cold' or logic-based are rarely enough to provide lasting change. The schema therapist provides opportunities for *corrective emotional experiences* that directly heal EMS on the emotional and implicational levels. We describe these 'experiential' strategies in depth in Chapter 8: Intervention Strategies for Schema Healing 3: Experiential Techniques.

4. **Behavioural Pattern-Breaking Techniques**: Perhaps the most important and, in some cases, time consuming aspects of schema change involves changing clients' maladaptive patterns of coping behaviour. Often significant work in the preceding techniques is required before large-scale changes can be made. Nonetheless, without changing maladaptive patterns of behaviour and learning more adaptive means to get needs met in

daily life, clients' schemas are unlikely to fully heal and remain vulnerable to relapse. Behavioural Pattern-Breaking strategies are the focus of Chapter 9: Intervention Strategies for Schema Healing 4: Behavioural Pattern-Breaking Techniques.

Six Flexible Developmental Treatment Phases

We have found it useful to think of schema therapy as a set of phases of change. Young originally conceived of two phases: (1) an assessment and education phase, and (2) a change phase. Other authors have proposed further stages that include periods where there is a distinct focus in the therapy on rapport building, safety and bonding, and the development of mode awareness [17]. Here we describe a set of phases the therapist might focus on as the therapy (and client) progresses. Generally speaking, the phases can be seen as sets of developmental tasks, in which each phase supports the growth and healing capacity of the client and is somewhat necessary for the next step. This is not meant to be a rigid set of steps. In practice, the focus of therapy might move back and forth between the steps depending on the client and the particular issues or challenges they are facing at that time.

1. *Assessment and Education Phase.* In this phase, the therapist conducts their schema and mode assessment (see Chapter 3: Schema Therapy Assessment) and starts the process of educating the client about their prominent modes and/or schemas and making links to their life patterns and current presenting issues. This culminates in attempts to convey the overall case conceptualisation and derive informed consent to start treatment in the change phase (i.e., focusing on steps 2–6). See Chapter 4: Case Conceptualisation and Mode Mapping in Schema Therapy for an overview of case conceptualisation and education using 'schema mode maps'.

2. *Safety and Bonding.* As the assessment unfolds and the client starts to view their experience in schema therapy terms, the schema therapist also works on bonding with the client and developing a strong limited reparenting relationship. In doing so, the therapist also looks for opportunities to help the client feel safe enough to be in therapy, addressing any therapy issues that come up early and, where possible, helping the client find the safety and stability in their life to make room for therapy and commit to change.

3. *Schema/Mode Awareness.* One of the initial goals of schema therapy is to help the client develop schema and mode awareness. Before clients can adequately benefit from phases 4–6, they must be able to understand their problems and understand the link between their life patterns and the underlying schemas and modes that underpin them.

4. *Schema/Mode Management.* As therapy progresses and the client develops an initial understanding of their problems, the schema therapist starts to help the client manage schema activation in their daily life. This often occurs through the use of behavioural pattern-breaking techniques and schema/mode flashcards.

5. *Schema/Mode Healing.* As clients attempt to change, they will invariably encounter having their schemas or modes triggered. The schema therapist uses sessions to work on healing schemas, particularly those which have been triggered during the previous week, usually with a focus on limited reparenting and experiential treatment strategies.

6. *Autonomy Phase.* Towards the end of treatment there is more of a focus on empowering the client to meet their own needs and activate their Healthy Adult mode to self-manage and overcome obstacles and challenges. In this stage, the therapist pushes more assertively for concrete behavioural change and prepares the client for eventual

termination of therapy (see Chapter 12: Preparing for Termination and the End Phase of Schema Therapy for more detail).

Recent Developments in the Model

The strong research focus within schema therapy means that the model is continuously undergoing development and refinement. Recently, some new and potentially important developments to the schema therapy model have been proposed by Arntz and colleagues [8]. Two additional core emotional needs have been proposed, building on the original five core needs: (1) The *need for Self-Coherence,* and (2) the *need for Fairness.* These two additional needs are, in turn, directly linked to three new EMS: (1) *Lack of a Coherent Identity* (2) *Lack of a Meaningful World,* and (3) *Unfairness.* Further, we have proposed an additional need for *Connectedness to Nature,* and an associated EMS, *Lack of Nature Connectedness* [18]. Whilst research is currently underway to verify the validity of these newly proposed needs and EMS, we have included descriptions of these in Chapter 3.

Arntz and colleagues [8] further propose that dysfunctional modes may be better understood as a combination of an activated EMS and coping. They propose that the term 'Surrender' be replaced with 'Resignation'. Resignation refers to the process whereby the person behaves as if the EMS were completely true, and the person 'acquiesces' to the assumptions and rules associated with the active EMS. This refinement of theory more explicitly states that Child and Critic modes reflect resignation to EMS. It is within these modes that the strongest EMS-associated affect is experienced and dominates the person's state of mind. Furthermore, all coping modes can be considered forms of either Avoidance or Inversion (formerly Compensation), in which the emotional suffering associated with specific EMS is either avoided or inverted. The two healthy functional modes described by Young, the Happy Child, and the Healthy Adult mode, remain within their current form.

Recent research [19, 20, 21, 22] also proposes new taxonomies of EMS which include EMS clusters rather than domains. In addition, new domains related to 'positive adaptive schemas' (PAS) have also been proposed and the reader is referred to the literature in this field [23]. The impact of this empirical work on EMS and PAS clusters on schema therapy practice has yet to be fully realised but will no doubt be of influence over time.

Concluding Remarks

Schema therapy aims to heal critical deficits in a client's developmental trajectory. The model guiding schema therapy can be daunting for therapists new to the approach, but it is enormously rich and can account for a comprehensive diversity of clinical presentations. We recommend that students of the approach take time to revise and familiarise themselves with concepts of core emotional needs, EMS, coping styles, and schema modes, as the quality of individual case formulation and treatment planning will depend on how attuned the therapist is to the presence of each of these in their clients. Self-help books by Young and Klosko [23], and Jacob, van Genderen and Seebauer [24] may be particularly helpful for therapists new to schema therapy and looking for elaborations of descriptions of schemas and modes. In the next chapter, we discuss in detail how to conduct clinical assessments of this critical theoretical information.

References

1. Lockwood G, Perris P. A new look at core emotional needs. In van Vreekswijk M, Broersen J, Nadort M, eds. *The Wiley-Blackwell handbook of schema therapy*. Wiley-Blackwell; 2012, pp. 41–66.

2. Young J, Klosko J, Weishaar M. *Schema therapy: A practitioner's guide*. Guilford Press; 2003.

3. Bowlby J. The Bowlby-Ainsworth attachment theory. *Behavioral and Brain Sciences*. 1979;2(4):637–8.

4. Maslow A. *Motivation and personality*. Harper & Row; 1970.

5. Baumeister RF, Leary MR. The need to belong: Desire for interpersonal attachments as a fundamental human motivation. *Psychological Bulletin*. 1995;117(3):497.

6. Deci EL, Ryan RM. The 'what' and 'why' of goal pursuits: Human needs and the self-determination of behavior. *Psychological Inquiry*. 2000;11(4):227–68.

7. Piaget J. *Play dreams and imitation in childhood*. Norton Libr

8. Arntz A, Rijkeboer M, Chan E, et al. Towards a reformulated theory underlying schema therapy: Position paper of an international workgroup. *Cognitive Therapy and Research*. 2021; 45:1007–20. https://doi.org/10.1007/s10608-021-10209-5.

9. Bamelis LL, Renner F, Heidkamp D, Arntz A. Extended schema mode conceptualizations for specific personality disorders: An empirical study. *Journal of Personality Disorders*. 2011;25(1):41–58.

10. Bernstein DP, van den Broek E. Schema Mode Observer Rating Scale (SMORS). Unpublished Empirical Article manuscript, Department of Psychology, Maastricht University, The Netherlands. 2006.

11. Talbot D, Smith E, Tomkins A, Brockman R, Simpson S. Schema modes in eating disorders compared to a community sample. *Journal of Eating Disorders*. 2015;3(1):1–4.

12. Stavropoulos A, Haire M, Brockman R, Meade T. A schema mode model of repetitive negative thinking. *Clinical Psychologist*. 2020;24(2):99–113.

13. Edwards D. Overcoming obstacles to reparenting the inner child. Workshop presented at the Conference of the International Society of Schema Therapy, World Trade Center, New York; 2012.

14. Simpson S, Smith E. *Schema therapy for eating disorders: Theory and practice for individual and group settings*. Routledge; 2019.

15. Aalbers A, Engels T, Haslbeck J, Boorsboom D, Arntz A. The network structure of schema modes. *Clinical Psychology & Psychotherapy*. 2021;28(5):1065–78. https://doi.org/10.1002/cpp.2577.

16. Farrell J, Reiss N, Shaw I. *The schema therapy clinician's guide: A complete resource for building and delivering individual, group and integrated schema mode treatment programs*. John Wiley & Sons; 2014.

17. ISST Environmental Awareness & Action Group. Schema therapy and connection with nature. *Schema Therapy Bulletin*, issue 23, https://schematherapysociety.org/Schema-Therapy-Bulletin/.

18. Bach B, Lockwood G, Young JE. A new look at the schema therapy model: Organization and role of early maladaptive schemas. *Cognitive Behaviour Therapy*. 2018;47(4):328–49.

19. Edwards D. Using schema modes for case conceptualization in schema therapy: An applied clinical approach. *Frontiers in Psychology*; 2, 763670. https://doi.org/10.3389/fpsyg.2021.763670.

20. Karaosmanoglu, A. An investigation of the second order factor structure of the Young Schema Questionnaire – Short Form 3 (YSQ-SF3); Empirical Article manuscript (in preparation).

21. Yalcin O, Lee C, Correia H. Factor structure of the Young schema

questionnaire (long Form-3). *Australian Psychologist*. 2020 Oct 1;**55**(5):546–58.

22. Louis J, Wood A, Lockwood G, Ho M, Ferguson E. Positive clinical psychology and Schema Therapy (ST): The development of the Young Positive Schema Questionnaire (YPSQ) to complement the Young Schema Questionnaire 3 Short Form (YSQ-S3).

Psychological Assessment. 2018 Sep;**30**(9):1199.

23. Young J, Klosko J. *Reinventing your life: How to break free from negative life patterns and feel good again*. Penguin; 1994.

24. Jacob G, van Genderen H, Seebauer L. *Breaking negative thinking patterns: A schema therapy self-help and support book*. Wiley-Blackwell; 2015.

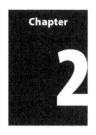

Research Support for Schema Therapy

Introduction

From its inception, Jeffrey Young has actively and consistently sought to establish schema therapy as an empirically supported therapy, having worked alongside Aaron Beck to build the evidence base for cognitive therapy. Schema therapy research was bolstered in the late 1990s and early 2000s when a group of Dutch researchers, led by Arnoud Arntz, collaborated with Young on the first of several clinical investigations into the efficacy of schema therapy for borderline personality disorder (BPD). This body of research has grown substantially over the past 20 years; we estimate there to be hundreds of empirical studies that now support various aspects of the schema therapy model and which have investigated the efficacy of schema therapy, the most important of which will be summarised in this chapter.

Research Supporting the Schema Therapy Conceptual Model

Evidence for the Existence of Universal Core Emotional Needs

When Young, Klosko, and Weishaar [1] identified the five *core emotional needs* they saw as universal (see Chapter 1), they acknowledged that the list of needs was drawn from existing theory and clinical observation but had limited empirical support at that time. Since then, multiple factor analyses have been undertaken of the various versions of the Young Schema Questionnaire (YSQ) which provide indirect support for the basic schema therapy model; if early maladaptive schemas (EMS) arise from a core set of unmet emotional needs, the EMS proposed to result from a common unmet need should correlate more highly together than EMS from different domains (related to different unmet needs). For example, the EMS thought to arise from disrupted and deprived attachments within the Disconnection and Rejection domain – Abandonment, Emotional Deprivation, Social Isolation, Mistrust/Abuse, and Defectiveness/Shame – should correlate more closely with each other than those thought to arise from deprivation of limit setting: Entitlement/Grandiosity and Insufficient Self-Control/Self-Discipline. Principal component and factor analyses from across countries over the last 15 years have found differing optimal component structures but more consistently supported a four-factor structure, which has become regarded as more theoretically coherent than the original five-domain grouping [2]. Thus, the currently favoured taxonomy of the need deficits arising from inadequate parenting consists of Disconnection and Rejection; Impaired Autonomy and Performance, Excessive Responsibility and Standards, and Impaired Limits. However, research into the precise number of EMS and their factor structure remains ongoing, with recent research supporting an alternative 4-factor structure [3], and some authors arguing for a fifth *Emotional Dysregulation* domain [4]. The number of EMS and factors obtained from the YSQ appear to be influenced by whether the short or long form is used, which language version is used, whether the sample is predominantly clinical or non-clinical [4], and whether items are presented in random order or grouped according to their presumed EMS [5]. In summary, correlation patterns between EMS provide one line of support for the idea within the schema therapy model that a certain type of need frustration will have predictable effects. The results of factor analyses are relatively consistent with Young's model – especially for the EMS associated with disconnection and rejection – but nevertheless vary sufficiently between studies that, together with proposals to investigate new EMS [3], further studies will be needed to solidify our understanding of unmet need–EMS relations.

Although much of the schema therapy literature has focused on elucidating need deficits and the resulting damage – which was understandable given the primary aim of understanding severe psychopathology – complete evidence for the existence of needs requires demonstrating that need *fulfilment* also produces psychological well-being. In the past 10 years, measures of early adaptive schemas – positive counterparts to EMS – have been developed [6]. Recently, Louis, Davidson, Lockwood and Wood's [7] confirmatory factor analysis of the Young Positive Schema Questionnaire (YPSQ) across cultures supported a four-factor structure mirroring that of the YSQ, consisting of domains of Connection and Acceptance, Healthy Autonomy and Performance, Realistic Standards and Reciprocity, and Reasonable Limits.

Most of the research that is recognisably focused on the schema therapy model has employed retrospective self-report designs with adult participants. Longitudinal research studying children would provide stronger evidence for the role of thwarted core emotional needs on the development of EMS. Recently, an international schema therapy workgroup [3] endorsed Carol Dweck's [8] taxonomy of needs, providing explicit recognition that the broader developmental psychology literature provides relevant evidence for the existence of core psychological needs as understood in schema therapy.

Dweck [8] organised her taxonomy of needs to both bridge disparate theoretical research programmes and to reflect the sequence in which different needs emerge during early childhood development. This extends the precision and specificity with which needs have been discussed in the schema therapy literature to date. Dweck [8] argued that there were three basic needs which are present at birth or very early in infancy: needs for acceptance, optimal predictability, and competence. Dweck also outlined four 'compound' needs produced from combinations of basic needs after greater cognitive development has occurred: the need for trust (which emerges from needs for acceptance and predictability), the need for control (which develops from needs for competence and predictability), the need for self-esteem or status (which grows from needs for acceptance and competence), and the need for self-coherence (a stable and integrated sense of self, which emerges from monitoring whether all other needs are being met). Much of the evidence Dweck [8] cites to support the existence of these basic needs consists of observations that the stimuli infants are most attentive to, and the learning infants most readily achieve, is consistent with humans having innate propensities to form attachments, learn causal relations and operate on the environment.

The clearest correspondence between Dweck's and Young's catalogue of needs is that of Dweck's need for acceptance, which overlaps largely with Young and colleagues' [1] need for secure attachment, which is met when caregivers provide acceptance, predictability, and trustworthiness [3]. Labelled as 'acceptance', Dweck saw this need as overlapping with what others had labelled 'relatedness' [9], 'belongingness' [10], 'attachment' [11]; [12], 'warmth and comfort' [13], 'affection' [14], 'affiliation' [15], and 'love' [16]. Elsewhere, Young's needs straddle developmental periods according to Dweck's system. Young's autonomy, competence, and sense of identity entails both the basic need for competence – to build basic skills for acting on or in the world – and the more developed sense of personal agency and autonomy in the needs for control and for experiencing self-worth and social standing from Dweck's model. Young's freedom to express needs, opinions, and emotions is seen to overlap with basic needs for competence and acceptance as well as the more developed sense of self-esteem/status in Dweck's system. Young's need for spontaneity and play was seen by the schema therapy workgroup as a specific means of meeting Dweck's basic need for competence. Young's needs for realistic limits and self-control were seen to be captured by Dweck's needs for competence, optimal predictability (to understand the orderly way that events connect in the world), and control. To reiterate, schema therapy experts view Young et al.'s core emotional needs as fully encapsulated by the list of needs which have been subject to research in the broader psychological literature, which we will now review.

Although Young and colleagues [1] did not define how 'needs' might differ from other psychological constructs, Baumeister and Leary [10] provided a widely accepted definition, wherein needs:

> a) produce effects readily under all but adverse conditions; b) have affective consequences; c) direct cognitive processing; d) lead to ill effects (such as on health or adjustment) when thwarted; e) elicit goal-oriented behaviour designed to satisfy it; f) [are] universal in the sense of applying to all people; g) [are] not be derivative of other motives; h) affect a broad variety of behaviours; and i) have implications that go beyond immediate psychological functioning. (p. 498)

The challenge for needs research is that needs cannot be directly demonstrated; they must be inferred from the consequences that result from different conditions and behaviours which aim to meet the hypothesised needs.

The need for acceptance or secure attachments is supported by attachment theory research. Ainsworth and colleagues' [11] strange situation studies provided a means to assess the different attachment consequences of how well caregivers have been meeting their infants' needs. During these studies, an infant's mother temporarily left the infant in a new room full of toys, with an unfamiliar adult, before returning. The period of separation from their mother was usually a stressful experience. Infants who were 'securely attached' to their mothers sought comfort from them upon their return, and after a couple of minutes of close bodily contact were soothed and ready to resume exploration of the toys. Mothers were then observed in their homes. Mothers of securely attached infants appeared more sensitive and responsive to their infants' communications; they were quicker to pick them up when they cried; they handled their babies tenderly and carefully and for longer periods than parents of children who were not securely attached; they were quicker to feed their infants when showing signs of hunger and kept feeding until their infant appeared satiated. This style of parenting has come to be called *sensitive parenting*. In contrast to infants whose mothers provide less warm comforting physical contact, who are less facially expressive, and who do not time their care provision according to the infant's signals, securely attached infants thrive, becoming more exploratory, more cooperative, and show more positive affect and less frustration. Caregiver sensitivity has shown small to medium effects on attachment by preschool, measured prospectively or concurrently [17].

Mapping the need for reasonable limits to the broader psychological literature is increasingly challenging. Although there is widespread agreement that authoritative parenting is associated with superior well-being in children and adolescents compared to authoritarian parenting [18], the components of effective limit setting within authoritative parenting have often been inconsistently or inaccurately conceptualised [19]. Permissive parenting, which is characterised by low limit-setting [20], is generally associated with poorer outcomes for children than authoritative parenting, including higher substance abuse; school misconduct and lower school engagement [21]; greater affiliation with delinquent peers and associated externalising symptoms in adolescence [22]; and academic entitlement, poorer well-being, and increased depressive symptoms among college students [23]. On the other hand, a three-year longitudinal study found that permissive parenting was not associated with poor adjustment in fifth graders, although the authors expressed concerns about the quality of the permissiveness measure [24].

Nevertheless, the evidence seems reasonably consistent that limit setting, when done in a way that does not compromise the fulfilment of other core emotional needs (e.g., acceptance), is associated with increased childhood well-being. Gray and Steinberg [25] found that the extent of parental supervision and limit setting had a medium–large effect on fewer behaviour problems in adolescents (e.g., stealing, carrying a weapon) and was more related to number of behaviour problems than autonomy-granting or acceptance. In the self-determination theory literature, limit setting is part of parents providing structure: teaching children how their actions affect outcomes (which in Dweck's terminology would be an example of how a parent might contribute to meeting the child's need for optimal predictability) through clear consistent rules; guidelines and expectations; and clear, consistent consequences contingent on actions [26]. Children of parents who provided more structure for unsupervised time felt more competent and in control of outcomes in their lives [27]. Seventh and eighth grade children whose parents provided more structure perceived themselves to have more control over their academic success or failure, were more competent at school, were more engaged, and achieved better grades according to school records [26]. Simultaneously meeting children's needs for autonomy while meeting their need for realistic limits appears especially important. When parents attempted to set limits on who their adolescent children associated with in a controlling way, their children were more likely to associate with deviant peers than when the parents communicated their prohibition in an autonomy-supporting manner [28].

Although needs as a topic of psychological research has come in and out of vogue over time, substantial support has amassed for the existence of several psychological needs, especially belongingness/secure attachment [29, 30], competence, and autonomy [19]. Both maladaptive and adaptive schemas appear to cluster according to themes of whether or not early experiences provided connection, autonomy, and reasonable limits. Research continues to explore and refine how many psychological needs must be adequately met to ensure healthy psychological development, but as a plank of schema theory model development there appears to be adequate support for the existence of basic psychological needs [31].

Evidence that Schemas Result from Unmet Needs

A key hypothesis of the schema therapy model is that EMS occur when basic needs are inadequately met during childhood. Accordingly, Pilkington, Bishop, and Younan [32] conducted multiple meta-analyses of available studies ($k = 33$) investigating the association between EMS and two types of childhood adversity: toxic frustration of needs and traumatisation or victimisation. All but one study measured childhood adversity via adults' retrospective self-reports and approximately one-third of studies employed clinical samples. Consistent with Young and Klosko's [33] hypothesis that the Emotional Deprivation EMS often has its origins in insufficient maternal nurturance, the strongest correlation between a form of childhood adversity and an EMS was between maternal emotional neglect (which in these studies was indicated by low endorsement of questionnaire items measuring amount of parental warmth, interest, and attention) and Emotional Deprivation ($r = 0.51$, $k = 9$).

Emotional abuse – being ridiculed, insulted, shamed, and 'destructively' criticised – might be expected to correlate most strongly with Defectiveness/Shame and Mistrust/Abuse [33]. However, Pilkington et al. [32] found emotional abuse was most strongly associated with Emotional Deprivation ($r = 0.44$ [0.35, 0.51]), and also had moderate correlations of similar strength ($\sim0.3 - 0.35$) with Mistrust/Abuse, Social Isolation/Alienation, Defectiveness/Shame, Failure, Vulnerability to Harm and Subjugation. It was also perhaps surprising that the correlations between other types of abuse and the Mistrust/Abuse EMS were not higher, with $r = 0.25$ (0.14, 0.35) for physical abuse and $r = 0.25$ (0.13, 0.38) for sexual abuse. Also, somewhat surprisingly, the EMS most associated with sexual and physical abuse was Social Isolation/Alienation. Overall, approximately half of the adversity–EMS correlations aggregated across studies were significant. Only Entitlement/Grandiosity did not appear associated with toxic frustration of needs or traumatisation, which is consistent with Young and Klosko's [33] hypothesis that Entitlement/Grandiosity results from being over-indulged or receiving insufficient limit setting and coaching in frustration tolerance and impulse control. Establishing empirical support for unmet need–EMS links is a formidable exercise and retrospective reports are not the ideal methodology to test these hypotheses. The heterogeneity of effect sizes in the meta-analyses was also found to be large, suggesting several unaccounted-for moderators. This body of studies is supportive of a central tenet of schema therapy theory: that the thwarting of basic needs in childhood (childhood adversity) increases the strength of most EMS, although the pattern of relationships between specific needs and specific EMS is not always consistent with predictions.

The schema therapy model would predict that the effects of unmet needs in childhood on later psychopathology should be mediated by maladaptive schemas or schema modes. Mertens, Yilmaz, and Lobbestael [34] found partial support for this idea. In their study, of the different types of adversity measured, only emotional abuse had effects on personality disorder that were mediated by schema modes. The effect of emotional abuse on BPD symptom severity was mediated by child modes and coping modes. The effect of emotional abuse on antisocial personality disorder (ASPD) severity was mediated by parent modes, and the effect of emotional abuse on avoidant and dependent personality disorders (AvPD and DPD) severity was mediated by healthy modes (Healthy Adult and Happy Child). The authors interpreted these relationships as follows: In BPD, emotional abuse leads to the development of vulnerable and angry modes and the need to develop maladaptive coping strategies; In AvPD and DPD, the stronger the healthy modes, the less intense are Cluster C symptoms in response to emotional abuse; and in ASPD, the more overdeveloped the Demanding Critic, the less ASPD develops from emotional abuse. These may be reasonable explanations, but they await prospective testing. It should be noted that the study was underpowered to detect more complex relationships and so the 14 modes of the schema mode inventory (SMI) needed to be collapsed into only four categories. In an earlier study of incarcerated females looking at EMS, associations between childhood adversity and BPD symptoms were no longer significant when controlling for Disconnection and Rejection and Impaired Limits EMS, consistent with the idea that EMS mediate the relationship between childhood adversity and BPD symptoms [35]. Elsewhere, The Punitive Critic and Angry Child modes were found to mediate the effect of low parental care on early age of onset and longer duration of non-suicidal self-injury in psychiatric outclients [36]. More theoretically predictable relationships were obtained in a sample of depressed adolescents [37]. The association between emotional maltreatment and anxious arousal was mediated by the Vulnerability to Harm EMS, a threat-related schema, whereas the effect of emotional maltreatment on anhedonic depression was mediated by Self-Sacrifice and Social Isolation/Alienation EMS. The association between physical abuse and anxious arousal was also mediated by Vulnerability to Harm, but the effect of physical abuse on anhedonic depression was mediated by Emotional Deprivation. In summary, there is ample evidence that various forms of childhood adversity reflecting inadequate need fulfilment are associated with various symptoms of psychopathology, and a portion of this relationship can consistently be accounted for by one or more EMS or maladaptive modes, although the specific EMS or modes involved can vary considerably between studies.

Specific Schema and Mode Profiles and Their Relationship to Psychopathology

Several studies have been carried out with the primary aim of establishing the schema and mode profile of BPD. These have generally yielded consistent results. Bach and Farrell [38] compared large samples of clients with BPD, personality disorders other than BPD, and healthy non-clients and found that BPD clients showed higher scores on measures of Mistrust/Abuse and Defectiveness/Shame EMS, and Angry Child and Impulsive Child modes, and lower Happy Child mode scores than non-BPD personality disordered participants. BPD clients also showed higher Insufficient Self-Control/Self-Discipline EMS and Vulnerable Child and Enraged Child mode scores than non-clients. Bach and Lobbestael [39] examined unique associations between self-reported schemas and modes and specific BPD symptoms identified by diagnostic interview within a sample of mixed personality disorder outpatients. Although most specific BPD symptoms had unique associations with one or more specific modes, 43% variance in the total BPD criteria count was accounted for by Abandonment and Mistrust/Abuse EMS alone when just considering EMS as predictors. When just considering modes, 46% variance in total BPD symptom count was accounted for by Angry Child and Impulsive Child modes. Similar results were obtained in a study of 220 Iranians with Cluster B personality disorders from psychiatrists' and psychologists' clinics: Vulnerable Child and Impulsive Child modes were associated with BPD but not ASPD or NPD [39]. Potentially, this is because ASPD and NPD involve strong overcompensator modes which may block awareness of underlying child modes. Furthermore, clients often confuse overcompensatory modes for Healthy Adult mode, which may explain why ASPD clients reported higher Healthy Adult mode scores. An earlier study contradicted these more recent findings, with the only significant difference between BPD and ASPD being that Healthy Adult mode scores were relatively high in ASPD and low in BPD; however, this study should perhaps be given less weight as it employed a more primitive version of the SMI [40]. In summary, Mistrust/Abuse EMS, Impulsive Child modes and low Healthy Adult modes appear characteristic of BPD, although other schemas and modes may be more or less prominent for any individual.

Bamelis and colleagues [41] aimed to elucidate the distinct mode profiles of individuals with Cluster C, Paranoid, Narcissistic or Histrionic personality disorders using a newly expanded Schema Mode inventory (SMI-2). Personality disorder status was determined both by self-report and clinician interview, and the authors reported the modes which had high partial correlations with personality disorder pathology after controlling for the effect of all other personality disorders: Paranoid PD was characterised by Angry Child and Suspicious Overcontroller modes; Histrionic PD characterised by Attention and Approval Seeker mode; Narcissistic PD by Undisciplined Child, Self-Aggrandiser, and Attention and Approval Seeker modes; Avoidant PD by Lonely Child, Abandoned Child, Compliant Surrenderer, Detached Protector, and Avoidant Protector modes; DPD by Abandoned Child, Dependent Child, Compliant Surrenderer, Punitive Critic, and a weak Healthy Adult mode; and OCPD by Perfectionistic Overcontroller and Demanding Critic modes. It should be noted that the use of partial correlations has been criticised for attenuating relationships and making the patterns less interpretable [41].

Jacobs, Lenz, Wollny, and Horsch [42] demonstrated that the schema modes could be conceptualised as driven by three higher-order factors: internalisation (low Healthy Adult mode, high Vulnerable Child and Compliant Surrenderer modes); externalisation (high Bully and Attack, Impulsive Child, and Enraged Child modes), and compulsivity (high Demanding Critic and Detached Self-Soother modes). This somewhat approximates the hierarchical structure of personality disorders: internalising (BPD), externalising (BPD, NPD, HPD, ASPD, PPD) [43]. In a study of 70 forensic mental health inpatients with BPD, NPD, or ASPD, Keulen-de Vos et al. [44] found that ASPD was distinguished by the combination of low internalising modes and high externalising modes, whereas BPD was associated with high internalising modes.

In summary, distinct combinations of modes for specific forms of psychopathology have been found in various studies; however, to date there has been considerable variation between studies in the mode profile found for a specific personality disorder. Allowing the emerging consensus on the taxonomy of psychopathology [43] to guide mode model specification is likely to produce more consistent findings in the future.

Research Supporting the Efficacy of Schema Therapy

Borderline Personality Disorder

The effectiveness of schema therapy has most often been investigated in the treatment of BPD. A number of early uncontrolled trials established that participation in schema therapy was associated with improvements in BPD symptomatology [45], and stronger evidence has accumulated since. The first randomised controlled trial by Giesen-Bloo and colleagues [46] assigned 86 participants (93% female) to three years of two individual sessions per week of either schema therapy or transference-focused psychotherapy (TFP). Schema therapy followed the approach manualised by Arntz and van Genderen [47]. More people dropped out of TFP (51%) than schema therapy (26%), and those who quit schema therapy completed significantly more sessions ($Mdn = 98$) than those who quit TFP ($Mdn = 34$). This has been a feature of schema therapy outcome studies generally; drop out is low, suggesting a high level of acceptability. Intent-to-treat (ITT) analyses showed that participants in both groups made significant improvements which were evident by the end of the first year, but schema therapy achieved greater reductions in BPD symptoms, general psychopathology, and personality disorder beliefs and 'defence styles'. At four-year follow-up, more schema therapy recipients (52%) no longer met BPD diagnostic criteria than TFP recipients (27%), and a higher proportion had achieved reliable change on BPD symptom measures. Interestingly, those who had recovered within schema therapy at three-year follow-up achieved normal hypervigilance responses to negative emotional stimuli whereas those not recovered maintained high hypervigilance, suggesting that schema therapy potentially alters an important causal mechanism of BPD pathology [48]. Furthermore, schema therapy was later found to also be more cost effective, mainly due to less use of informal care supports [49].

The Giesen-Bloo efficacy study was followed by a large-scale implementation study which tested whether schema therapy could be delivered more efficiently and remain effective when delivered by mental health clinicians in routine practice. Individual 45-minute sessions were delivered twice per week for only the first year, and once per week thereafter, to 62 clients diagnosed with BPD. After 18 months, 42% had recovered according to having Borderline Personality Disorder Severity Index scores below diagnostic threshold [50].

The next major randomised controlled trial evaluated a group schema therapy protocol as described by Farrell and Shaw [51]. Participants (all female) were assigned to either [1] treatment as usual (TAU), which was primarily supportive psychotherapy or [2] Group Schema Therapy (30 weekly 90-minute group schema therapy sessions over 8 months) plus TAU. Farrell and colleagues' approach to group schema therapy was notably distinct from previous group schema therapy formats: it emphasised ensuring that all group members remained involved throughout each session and were not merely watching the therapist work with one of the members at a time; there were more group rules to enhance feelings of safety and security; more structure; written psychoeducation materials; homework assignments; and more attention to the Happy Child mode [52]. Remarkably, at post-treatment there was 100% retention in the schema therapy group and 94% no longer met diagnostic criteria for BPD. By contrast, 25% had dropped out of TAU and only 16% no longer met criteria for BPD. The schema therapy group also achieved large reductions in general psychopathology. Attempts to replicate and further understand these results are underway. A 3-year uncontrolled study has begun in Germany with 10 BPD clients with frequent psychiatric hospital admissions. Results from the first year showed that weekly group schema therapy programme members experienced a reduction in BPD symptoms, schema mode activation, and hospitalisations [52]. Finally, a 15-site, 5-country RCT involving 495 participants has just been completed comparing two years of treatment with a predominantly group schema therapy and a balanced individual plus group schema therapy with TAU [53]. Although all groups achieved large reductions in BPD symptom severity, the schema therapy groups achieved greater reduction than TAU, which was statistically significant by 18 months of treatment. Furthermore, the balanced individual/group condition produced greater reductions than the predominantly group format which was statistically significant by 6 months post-treatment and had higher retention rates.

Recent studies have aimed to explore how briefly schema therapy for BPD can be delivered whilst retaining efficacy. Dickhaut and Arntz [52] piloted a 2-year-long combined weekly 60-minute individual plus 90-minute group schema therapy session programme. This study involved two cohorts (all female) and altered the form of group therapy the second cohort received to incorporate Farrell and Shaw's [51] practises. These changes were associated with a higher immediate recovery rate at the end of 24 months in the second cohort (66.5%, n = 10, no longer met BPD criteria) compared to the first (18.7%, n = 8). Combining the cohorts at 30 months, 77% no longer met BPD criteria and achieved large reductions in BPD symptoms, as well as improvements in happiness and quality of life. Hilden and colleagues [54] randomised 42 clients (83% female) to receive either a 20-session group schema therapy programme plus TAU (consisting of psychiatric consultations plus monthly therapy sessions from a psychiatric nurse) or TAU alone. The programme shortened Farrell and Shaw's [51] protocol by reducing the cognitively focused content. At 5-month follow-up there was no difference between BPD symptoms as measured by the Borderline Symptom List (BSL-23) [54] and the means for both groups were in the 'moderate' range at both baseline and post-treatment. Hamid and colleagues [56] randomly assigned 45 BPD clients (100% male) to 12 – presumably, individual – sessions of schema therapy, Dialectical Behaviour Therapy (DBT), or no treatment. After 6 months, both DBT and schema therapy had produced equivalent reductions in emotional and behavioural dysregulation symptoms compared to no treatment, but DBT produced significantly greater reductions in disrupted communication symptoms. The results of this study are somewhat difficult to compare with previous studies as a more limited range of measures was used and the percentage who no longer met criteria for BPD was not reported. Nevertheless, the reductions in BPD symptomatology in response to a relatively brief intervention are encouraging.

In summary, there is reasonably strong support for the idea that long-term individual schema therapy for females with BPD is efficacious in reducing BPD symptomatology and comorbid psychopathology. There is encouraging evidence that group schema therapy does likewise; however, critics might argue that comparisons with bona fide psychotherapies, employing assessors blind to treatment condition, would be needed to demonstrate efficacy conclusively. With the exception of Hamid et al. [56], the efficacy of schema therapy for men with BPD has received little investigation. Future studies should also continue to explore the efficacy of shorter forms of schema therapy, and it has been recognised that there is a need to compare schema therapy against the best alternative specific therapies for BPD such as DBT, with several trials underway to address these gaps. Fassbinder et al. [57] are undertaking an extensive comparison of 18-month schema therapy and DBT interventions.

Other Personality Disorders

Several uncontrolled trials have investigated brief forms of group schema therapy for mixed personality disorder populations. An abbreviated 20-session group schema therapy protocol, Group Schema Cognitive-Behavioural Therapy (SCBT-g), was tested in a mixed outpatient sample of 63 people (73% female), in which 75% were assessed as having personality disorders [58]. SCBT-g is condensed by concentrating on the application of schema therapy methods to recent and present situations rather than past events. Results showed that half of the participants achieved clinically significant reductions in general psychopathology, and maladaptive schema and mode activation, while 34% remained unchanged and 13% showed significant worsening, with 24% dropping out. Skewes, Samson, Simpson, and van Vreeswijk [59] adapted SCBT-g to increase the experiential exercises and mode-focused content with a single outpatient group containing six people with AvPD and two with BPD. At the end of treatment, four members no longer met diagnostic threshold according to the Millon Clinical Multiaxial Inventory (MCMI-III) at post-treatment and five were subthreshold by six-month follow-up. Schaap, Chakhssi, and Westerhof [60] conducted an uncontrolled trial of twice per week group schema therapy for 12 months in an inpatient setting with 65 people (72% female), 79% of which had at least one personality disorder (47% of which was personality disorder not otherwise specified). All clients had more than 3 months of previous treatment, 92% in outpatient settings and 42% in inpatient settings. The programme was not manualised but based on an earlier version of Farrell and Shaw's [51] approach. Following group schema therapy there were significant mean reductions at post-treatment and 6-month follow-up in general psychopathology, EMS, and mode frequency/intensity. As might be expected in a severe sample, there was a 35% dropout rate; however, effect sizes were substantially larger for those who completed treatment. Finally, Schema Mindfulness-Based Cognitive Therapy (SMBCT) consists of 8 weekly 90-minute group sessions which educate clients about schema modes experientially through mindfulness exercises. Van Vreeswijk, Spinhoven, Zedlitz, and Eurelings-Bontekoe [61] randomised 58 outpatient clients (76% female) with personality disorders (43% Cluster C, 22% BPD) to either SMBCT plus TAU (medication and psychiatrist consults) or TAU plus an 8-week competitive memory therapy (COMET) intervention, which involved clients bringing unhelpful personal images to mind while stimulating positive emotions through posture, facial expressions, and self-talk. Both groups achieved symptomatic improvements with no significant differences between groups. SMBCT produced improvement or recovery from general psychopathology in 37% recipients, while 40% were unchanged and 23% showed reliable deterioration. On average, there were also small improvements in self-esteem, Disconnection and Rejection EMS, Other Directedness EMS, Overvigilance and Inhibition EMS and Critic modes, but no significant improvements in mindfulness, Impaired Limits schemas, or child modes. Personality disorders are typically challenging to treat. These findings are promising but further research is needed to ascertain whether group schema therapy is more effective than any other manualised approach for mixed personality disorders.

The largest completed randomised controlled trial of schema therapy involved 323 people (57% female) with a range of personality disorders other than BPD (and not including ASPD, schizotypal, or schizoid personality disorder) [62]. At three of the 12 sites, people were randomised to either individual schema therapy or clarification-oriented psychotherapy (COP), a non-directive insight-oriented psychotherapy designed for personality disorders; at the remaining nine sites, people were randomised to schema therapy or TAU. Schema therapy was delivered according to Arntz and Jacob's [63] protocol over 40 weekly sessions plus 10 monthly booster sessions. At 3-year follow-up, a higher proportion of those who received schema therapy no longer met criteria for their primary personality disorder diagnosis (82%), compared to TAU groups (55%). Those who received schema therapy also had significantly higher rates of recovery than COP when controlling for personality disorder type, although this difference did not hold when recovery was defined as the absence of subthreshold symptoms (79% [0.65, 0.88] ST v 59% [0.40, 0.75] COP). Although there were few differences between groups on other measures, there was a lower rate of depressive disorders and higher social functioning among schema therapy recipients at three-year follow-up. The study has been criticised for the lack of generalised improvement across measures and the use of an arguably uncommon or weak control condition [64]. Nevertheless, given the severity of these disorders and the dearth of empirical evaluations of psychotherapies for these conditions, the study represents an important step in the development of more effective approaches for working with those affected by personality disorder.

Personality Disorders in Forensic Settings

Bernstein and colleagues [65] randomly assigned 103 male offenders from 8 high-security forensic hospitals in the Netherlands to 3 years of either schema therapy or TAU. This represented a severe sample and a stringent test of the efficacy of schema therapy; 54% were admitted for physically violent offences, 26% for sexually violent offences, and 16.5% for threats or coercion. The psychiatric profile was arguably more severe than had been seen in any previous psychotherapy study: 60% met criteria for ASPD, 21% NPD, and 17% BPD. Randomisation was effective: the distribution of crime and PD was effectively identical between conditions. No external incentives for participation were provided. Schema therapy was provided twice per week until participants began obtaining leave to reintegrate into the community, at which point frequency reduced to once per week. TAU received weekly individual psychotherapy (group therapy at one site) but overall 'attention' was matched by TAU participants receiving more hours of ancillary therapy (e.g., art therapy).

Results indicated that both groups improved, with statistically significant advantages for schema therapy recipients. A higher proportion of schema therapy recipients were granted both supervised and unsupervised leave throughout each year. Self-reported PD symptoms decreased faster over time among schema therapy recipients than in TAU alone. Schema therapy participants also made greater reductions in EMS scores over the study, and faster reductions in maladaptive schema mode scores and faster increases in healthy mode scores, although TAU participants had mostly 'caught up' by the end of the study. There was a significant difference in treatment retention during the first year favouring schema therapy (93% schema therapy v 80% TAU remained in treatment), but no significant difference at 3 years (75% schema therapy, 68% TAU). Arguably, the most important findings of the study were that almost all forensic mental health clients in the study were able to achieve supervised leave within 3 years (97% schema therapy, 91% TAU) and the majority achieved unsupervised leave (67% schema therapy, 59% TAU). The differences between groups were reported as small to moderate, but nevertheless favoured schema therapy. The authors speculated that the differences between groups early in the study may have diminished because as schema therapy recipients achieved leave sooner, they may have encountered a greater range of challenges and setbacks than the TAU group. The authors acknowledged that group outcome differences could be due to schema therapy being delivered more intensively rather than to its content per se, so further studies comparing schema therapy with a bona fide therapy are required to speak more conclusively to its efficacy. Readers should also be aware that the study did not include clients who displayed psychotic symptoms; who met criteria for schizophrenia, bipolar disorder, current substance dependence, or autism spectrum disorder; who had an IQ below 80 or serious neurological impairment (which are common exclusion criteria in psychotherapy studies); or whose offending was exclusively related to paedophilia. Nevertheless, the study demonstrates that positive outcomes using the schema therapy approach are possible even with a severely violent and psychiatrically disabled sample.

Personality Disorders in the Elderly

The application of schema therapy to elderly people is especially worth highlighting, given the limited efficacy of psychotherapies in this population and the relatively lower rate of research in this area. A multiple-baseline study demonstrated the promise of individual schema therapy. Eight people aged over 69 with Cluster C personality disorders were provided 40 weekly sessions of schema therapy plus 10 booster sessions over 6 months using the Young et al. [1] manual. Results showed that improvement trends were evident during the treatment phase but not the baseline or follow-up phase. All but one participant no longer met diagnostic criteria according to the SCID-II and achieved improved quality of life scores, while five produced significantly improved YSQ scores [66]. Previously, an uncontrolled trial of the 20-session SCBT-g intervention was undertaken with 42 people aged 60–78 (74% female) whom a multidisciplinary team agreed had either a chronic mood or adjustment disorder with comorbid personality disorder traits [67]. Although 26% dropped out, those who completed therapy achieved medium effect size reductions in general psychopathology, EMS, and mode activation. A multi-centre randomised controlled trial is now underway to compare the cost-effectiveness of 20 sessions combining 2 hours of schema therapy and an additional hour of psychomotor therapy group programme to TAU for elderly adults with Cluster B or C personality disorders [68].

Anxiety and Related Disorders

To our knowledge, only two historical comparisons and no randomised controlled trials have evaluated schema therapy for anxiety disorders. Gude and Hoffart [69] compared two sequential cohorts treated for 12 weeks as inpatients for agoraphobia; one received psychodynamic TAU (n = 18, 67% female) and the other TAU plus schema-focused cognitive therapy (n = 24, 71% female). The programme consisted of five weeks of daily group CBT focusing on behavioural experiments to test fears about anxiety and EMS-driven beliefs, followed by six weeks consisting of eight group sessions and 9–10 individual sessions focusing on changing EMS. Controlling for the effects of phobic avoidance, those who received schema therapy–informed CBT showed greater reductions in interpersonal problems. Cockram, Drummond, and Lee [70] compared a historical cohort (n = 127) of male Vietnam veterans who received a 190-hour CBT-only PTSD group plus individual treatment programme with a cohort (n = 54) who received a version that substituted a focus on EMS for six of its fifteen 90-minute cognitive restructuring sessions. Those whose treatment included schema therapy components experienced greater reductions in PTSD symptoms, anxiety and depression symptoms, and YSQ scores. Finally, an open trial of schema therapy-enhanced exposure and response prevention for obsessive compulsive disorder (OCD) has been evaluated in ten inpatients (50% female) who had failed to respond to CBT [71]. The programme consisted of twice-weekly individual sessions for 12 weeks. A schema mode conceptualisation and limited reparenting-style guided preparation for and execution of exposure exercises. Schema therapy interventions – for example, chair mode dialogues – might have been used to ensure that clients undertook exposure exercises in a 'Healthy Adult mode' state of mind. As clients became able to undertake self-guided exposure, therapeutic focus shifted more to schema therapy. The group achieved large reductions in observer-rated and self-reported OCD symptoms and depressive symptoms, maintained at 6-month follow-up. Although randomised controlled trials are needed to establish its efficacy, these studies suggest that schema therapy interventions may be helpful for people with chronic anxiety-related problems, especially if they have not responded to first-line evidence-based therapies.

Eating Disorders

An uncontrolled study of an adapted form of SCBT-g for a group of eight women with mixed eating disorders (75% Eating Disorder Not Otherwise Specified) was conducted by Simpson, Morrow, van Vreeswijk, and Reid [72]. Sessions were lengthened to two hours and focused on a mode conceptualisation and mode-based treatment focus of eating behaviour and negative body image. Although two dropped out, the remaining six members achieved a 43% reduction in EMS severity post-treatment and a 59% reduction by 6-month follow-up. Four of the completers achieved clinically significant change in EMS activation, anxiety and depression symptoms, and eating disorder symptoms. A similar trial which evaluated a 25-session group schema therapy programme for eating disorders is currently nearing completion, with the protocol published by Calvert and colleagues in 2018 [73]. In a case report, Simpson and Slowey [74] described a brief mode formulation-informed therapy delivered via videoconferencing for a 39-year-old woman with Eating Disorder Not Otherwise Specified characterised by a 15-year history of yoyo dieting and daily self-induced vomiting. Following one telephone and seven video appointments over 11 weeks, she achieved a 77% improvement in eating disorder symptoms, 28 days abstinence from vomiting, and improvements in general psychopathology, distress, and self-esteem. Finally, 112 females were randomly assigned to 6 months of individual weekly sessions plus 6-monthly booster sessions of either CBT, appetite-focused CBT, or schema therapy for reducing binge eating [75]. There were no differences between groups; by post-treatment, 49% of participants had abstained from binge eating and were within one standard deviation of the mean on a measure of eating disorder symptoms. Although we would not yet recommend schema therapy as a first-line treatment for anorexia nervosa or bulimia nervosa, these studies suggest schema therapy may be used to improve binge eating and transdiagnostic eating disorder symptoms, particularly if first-line evidence-based therapies had been first tried with limited success.

Other Applications

Research continues to explore applications of schema therapy for a myriad of concerns. Mohtadijafari, Ashayeri, and Banisi [76] compared a 10 × 2-hour session group schema therapy intervention to a no-treatment control group for Iranian women with premenstrual dysphoric disorder and found improvements in quality of life and reduced distress in the schema therapy group. Nameni, Saadat, Afshar, and Askarabady [77] compared 11 sessions of a weekly 2-hour group schema therapy programme plus TAU (33 sessions of counselling) to TAU only for Iranian women seeking divorce, which was a relatively new opportunity in that country, but which brought additional challenges. The schema therapy programme was associated with improvements in resilience (hardiness) and differentiation, and the ability to balance one's own identity with maintaining relationships with others.

Caveats for Readers When Applying Schema Therapy in Their Own Work

Conducting psychotherapy treatment outcome studies is an expensive and labour-intensive task. Schema therapy researchers are especially heroic in working with severe populations, intensively, and over long timeframes. The outcomes achieved are truly encouraging and are providing clinicians with optimism and direction for providing services with clients that have traditionally been viewed as being 'treatment resistant'. Notwithstanding this progress, it has been our experience that clinicians learning new psychotherapy approaches can hold unrealistic expectations not only of themselves, but also of what can be achieved even with the best interventions in the hands of the world's best therapists, so we would like to highlight a couple of things about the schema therapy literature so the reader can manage their expectations.

Unless clinicians are working in specialised services with strict eligibility criteria, they may not choose – or be able – to practise much systematic selection over the clients they see. As described herein, most schema therapy efficacy studies – as is common practice in most psychotherapy research – have purposely excluded people with comorbid problems that include bipolar disorder, psychotic disorder, ASPD, dissociative identity disorder (DID), attention deficit hyperactivity disorder (ADHD) and substance use disorders requiring detoxification. In Farrell et al. (2009) [78], the schema therapy group had a lower proportion of people with a recent suicide plan, step, or attempt at baseline, despite randomisation. If the reader is considering applying schema therapy to a client who does have one or more of these disorders, it may not be reasonable to expect similar rates of improvement to highly controlled published studies. In Giesen-Bloo et al. [46] only 50.9% of those screened for the study were eligible and participated. In Farrell et al. [78] all participants were to remain in weekly outpatient psychotherapy for six months prior to being enrolled and be willing to remain in weekly therapy for a further eight months. Further studies of the effectiveness of schema therapy with these complex presentations (as opposed to highly controlled studies of efficacy) are needed to understand how well schema therapy performs in routine clinical practice where such comorbidity is the norm. In our experience, clinicians new to schema therapy are often excited to apply this new approach with clients in their caseload who have been least responsive to their existing repertoire of interventions. While such energy is probably useful in a lot of respects in treating such 'tough cases', therapists should be aware of the potential limitations in the evidence and adjust their expectations accordingly.

Evidence That Schema and Mode Change Mediates Psychopathology Improvements Resulting from Schema Therapy

Yakın et al. [79] examined changes in mode frequency within Bamelis and colleagues' [62] study and their relationship to outcomes. Across both psychotherapies, self-reported increased frequency in Healthy Adult mode and decreased frequency in Vulnerable Child, Impulsive Child, and Avoidant Protector modes prospectively predicted improved PD pathology. Increases in Healthy Adult mode and decreases in Self-Aggrandiser Mode frequency predicted improvements in social and occupational functioning. Schema therapy was no more effective than COP in changing Healthy Adult, Vulnerable Child, Impulsive

Child, and Avoidant Protector mode frequency. However, schema therapy was more effective than COP at reducing Self-Aggrandiser mode frequency and, in turn, in improving social and occupational functioning. Importantly, while decreased Vulnerable Child and increased Healthy Adult mode frequency prospectively predicted decreased PD pathology, decreased PD pathology did not prospectively predict decreased Vulnerable Child mode and increased Healthy Adult mode frequency. These results suggest that schema modes are a potentially important treatment target: reductions in maladaptive modes and increases in adaptive modes led to reductions in psychopathology, irrespective of whether current schema therapy methods are especially optimised to change their frequency.

Evidence Supporting the Efficacy of Specific Components of Schema Therapy

Imagery Rescripting

Outside of schema therapy, a large and growing number of studies have evaluated imagery rescripting (ImRS) as a stand-alone intervention for a range of conditions, including PTSD, depression, social anxiety, OCD, and body dysmorphic disorder. A meta-analysis of 19 such studies found a large within-group effect of ImRS on symptoms of the primary disorder at post-treatment ($g = 1.22$ [1.00, 1.43]), and larger at follow-up, typically 3 months later ($g = 1.79$ [1.54, 2.03]) [80]. Only five studies at that time had used a control condition (2 wait list, 3 attention placebos); however, within this set of studies, ImRS still produced a large between-group effect ($g = 1.00$ [0.27, 1.74]).

Since this meta-analysis, at the time of writing, at least 28 further studies have quantitatively evaluated the impact of ImRS on key outcomes; only 16 were randomised controlled trials and only 6 of these involved clinical populations. Results mirror most psychotherapy studies whereby specific interventions out-perform no-treatment or wait-list controls by large effect sizes but produce equivalent outcome changes to bona fide interventions. In recent ImRS studies, the bona fide comparisons were typically either imaginal exposure or cognitive restructuring. However, although ImRS may not produce superior changes in outcomes, there has been some evidence that ImRS produces its outcomes via different processes to comparison interventions. For example, in a comparison of a single session of ImRS or cognitive restructuring, despite there being no consistent differences on self-report measures, ImRS uniquely produced reductions in heart rate variability measures [80]. Furthermore, in a study of their efficacy to reduce nightmare frequency and distress, ImRS and imaginal exposure were equally effective, but were mediated via different mechanisms; ImRS exerted half of its effect through increasing mastery over nightmare content, whereas imaginal exposure exerted its effects via emotional tolerance [81]. Finally, Romano, Moscovitch, Huppert, Reimer, and Moscovitch [82] examined the relative impact of ImRS, imaginal exposure (IE), and supportive counselling on representations in memory of the event targeted by these interventions among people with social anxiety disorder. Memory descriptions were elicited via structured interviews 1 week, 2 weeks, and 3 months after receiving one of the three interventions. ImRS was found to only enhance recall of positive and neutral details about the event, whereas IE enhanced recall of both positive and negative details about the event, and supportive counselling had no effect on memory detail. Furthermore, at the end of each intervention session, participants were asked to revise their core belief (assessed pre-intervention); ImRS participants were more likely to 'update' this belief (i.e., generate a new more positive and/or realistic statement about themselves or others). Researchers continue to work on elucidating exactly how ImRS works [81], but the emerging evidence suggests it has distinct effects which do not merely represent a placebo effect.

A particularly relevant study was a large randomised controlled trial comparing twelve 90-minute sessions of eye movement desensitisation reprocessing therapy (EMDR) compared with ImRS delivered twice per week to 155 people with PTSD associated with childhood sexual abuse [83]. Both conditions produced equivalent large improvements in the primary outcome (PTSD symptoms) after 8 weeks ($d = 1.7$), which were sustained at 1-year follow-up, with very low drop out (7.7%). There was a non-significant trend for EMDR to have its effects a little faster, and for the superiority of ImRS at the 1-year follow-up mark, suggesting the two trauma-processing methods may work through separate mechanisms. Further analyses based on this study are currently underway to compare mechanisms of change and predictors of improvement. Based on the evidence to date, ImRS compares very well to established treatments for PTSD (e.g., prolonged exposure and EMDR).

A final study worth highlighting, given the severity of symptoms and the poverty of empirically supported interventions to treat them, is Paulik, Steel, and Arntz's [84] case series of twelve individuals with PTSD who experienced auditory hallucinations thematically related to traumatic events. Participants received a 10-session intervention involving eight sessions of ImRS in routine private practice and achieved significant mean reductions in voice distress and frequency, and trauma intrusions. Significantly, most of the sample met diagnostic criteria for a psychotic disorder (e.g., schizophrenia, schizoaffective disorder). This study provides initial evidence for the acceptability and potential effectiveness of ImRS with this population.

Evidence Regarding Therapist-led vs Client-led Rescripting

One of the decisions schema therapists may contend with in ImRS is whether to ask the client to imagine their present-day self intervening to protect and comfort their past self in a schema-relevant memory, or to imagine a third-party helper intervening to protect their past self (see Chapter 8: Intervention Strategies for Schema Healing 3: Experiential Techniques for an overview). At present, there are no studies employing clinical clients as participants, but a recent analogue study may be informative. University students were exposed to a traumatic movie clip and then randomly assigned to either (1) ImRS-A, where they were taught to imagine themselves intervening to disempower the perpetrator and save the victim in the aversive film scene; (2) ImRS-P, where they were taught to imagine a trustworthy other person intervening to disempower the perpetrator and help the victim; (3), Imagery rehearsal,where they were asked to recall the aversive film scene; and (4) no intervention control. Both ImRS conditions were less distressing than reimagining the aversive film scene, with the passive form (ImRS-P) less distressing than the active form (ImRS-A); however, only the ImRS-A condition was associated with increased positive affect [85]. It was noteworthy that there were no differences between ImRS conditions in participants' levels of self-efficacy. Overall, the findings support the common schema therapy practice of guiding clients toward imagining third-party helpers as their first ImRS step because it is the easier task, but also supports the additional value of transferring agency within ImRS exercises to the client.

Chairwork Exercises

Part of the rationale for using chairwork rather than traditional counselling dialogues is to intensify activation of schemas – thoughts and emotions – which in turn is thought to lead to greater schema change in both explicit and implicit memory systems [86]. Some support for these ideas came from early small, randomised trials with students [87] and clinical clients [88, 89] in which exploration of inner conflict via two-chair dialogues led to greater depth of feeling and perspective shifts than in empathic counselling. Emotional intensity was also a key theme of participants' experience of chairwork in a recent qualitative study of compassion-focused therapy [90]. When a single session of either a two-chair decision-making dialogue or another CBT strategy have been compared, there have been equivalent improvements on primary outcome measures (e.g., Conoley, Conoley, McConnell, and Kimzey [91]), with inconsistent additional benefits to chairwork. For example, Greenberg and Clarke [87] found the two-chair dialogue produced greater reductions in ambivalence than problem-solving therapy. Trachsel, Ferrari, and Holtforth [92] found no differences in indecisiveness but found chairwork produced higher self-reported and observer-rated emotional activation than a decision cube task. Compared with ImRS, there are relatively fewer evaluations of chairwork as a stand-alone procedure and no meta-analyses that we are aware of.

A further source of evidence for the efficacy of chairwork comes from studies evaluating emotion-focused therapy (EFT). One of the key two-chair dialogues used in EFT is between the 'Critic' and the 'Criticised Self'. Early studies identified characteristics of participants who resolved inner conflicts through chairwork as those who demonstrated a 'softening' of the Critic part, which changed from lecturing at the Criticised part, to describing its own feelings and sharing a similar depth of experience to the Criticised part, and then toward empathy, self-compassion, and discussion of mutual understanding [93]. Those who experienced resolution improved their indecisiveness and made more progress with their target complaints than those who did not [94]. In a multiple-baseline study, a five-session phase of the two-chair Critic–Criticised dialogue was associated with more change in anxiety and depression symptoms than the baseline phase [95]. In a study of people with major depressive disorder, people were randomised to receive either 16 weeks of Process-Experiential Therapy (PET, a precursor to EFT that contained significant amounts of chairwork) or CBT [96]. Both groups experienced equivalent improvements in all outcomes, except that the PET group achieved a significantly greater reduction in interpersonal problems.

For clients with trauma symptoms from childhood sexual abuse, EFT often employs a two-chair dialogue between the client and the perpetrator (in the empty chair). Clients are encouraged to voice their thoughts and feelings about the traumatic events and their consequences directly to the perpetrator. Greenberg and Malcom [97] studied those who had completed a course of EFT for childhood maltreatment and/or interpersonal problems and found that clients who had been able to express unmet needs through chair dialogues achieved larger reductions in general psychopathology and interpersonal problems than those who had not. Paivio, Harry, Chagigiorgis, Hall, and Ralston [98] compared two forms of EFT ($M = 17$ sessions); one involved the perpetrator-confrontation chair dialogue and the other involved addressing the consequences of traumatic events by simply exploring the client's feelings and meanings via empathic counselling. There were no significant differences between the groups in trauma symptom change, but there was higher attrition in the group that involved perpetrator-confrontation chairwork (20%) than empathic counselling alone (7%).

The implications of this research for schema therapy are arguably modest given that the use of chair dialogues in EFT diverges in important ways from their use in schema therapy. Nevertheless, schema therapists can be assured that the use of chairwork as a means to effect change has received at least some empirical scrutiny. There is evidence that chairwork achieves greater emotional activation, which is its intended purpose in schema therapy: to bypass avoidant coping modes. As a means of cognitive change, chairwork appears to work at least as well as more 'rational' cognitive restructuring methods. This initial research also suggests that the benefits of this component are not so profound that a schema therapist ought to feel compelled to use them, although the study by Paivio and colleagues [98] provides some caution that there are risks in pursuing emotional stimulation too aggressively. It should be noted that none of these chairwork studies has assessed for DSM personality disorder diagnoses. To date, the evidence for the safety and effectiveness of chairwork with cases of severe psychiatric disability (e.g., BPD) comes from evaluations of complete integrated courses of schema therapy, rather than stand-alone or dismantled designs.

Concluding Remarks

In this chapter, we aimed to provide an overview of the research studies to date that support schema therapy theory and treatment. The strongest evidence for the efficacy of schema therapy is for the treatment of personality disorders, especially BPD, but there is preliminary support for its use in a range of other conditions, especially if they have not responded to CBT (e.g., Eating Disorders, ImRS for PTSD). We hope that the evidence reviewed here, gives schema therapists confidence in the basic theory and treatment model, and knowledge about those presentations for which schema therapy has proven most helpful to date, while also providing some realistic boundaries and expectations for those cases that are not yet represented well by the evidence base.

References

1. Young J, Klosko J, Weishaar M. *Schema therapy: A practitioners guide*. New York: Guilford; 2003.

2. Bach B, Lockwood G, Young J. A new look at the schema therapy model: Organization and role of early maladaptive schemas. *Cognitive Behaviour Therapy*. 2017;47 (4):328–49.

3. Arntz A, Rijkeboer M, Chan E et al. *Towards a Reformulated Theory Underlying Schema Therapy: Position Paper of an International Workgroup*. Cognitive Therapy and Research. 2021.

4. Yalcin O, Lee C, Correia H. Factor structure of the Young Schema Questionnaire (Long Form-3). *Australian Psychologist*. 2020;55 (5):546–58.

5. Marais I, Moir VK, Lee, CW. The effects of item placement in the Young Schema Questionnaire. *Journal of Applied Measurement*, 2017;18(4):370–82.

6. Lockwood G, Perris P. A new look at core emotional needs. In van Vreekswijk M, Broersen J, Nadort M, eds. *The Wiley-Blackwell handbook of schema therapy*. Wiley-Blackwell, pp. 41–66.

7. Louis J, Davidson A, Lockwood G, Wood A. Positive perceptions of parenting and their links to theorized core emotional needs. *Journal of Child and Family Studies*. 2020;29 (12):3342–56.

8. Dweck C. From needs to goals and representations: Foundations for a unified theory of motivation, personality, and

development. *Psychological Review.* 2017;**124**(6):689–719.

9. Deci E, Ryan R. The 'what' and 'why' of goal pursuits: Human needs and the self-determination of behavior. *Psychological Inquiry.* 2000;**11**(4):227–68.

10. Baumeister R, Leary M. The need to belong: Desire for interpersonal attachments as a fundamental human motivation. *Psychological Bulletin.* 1995;**117**(3):497–529.

11. Ainsworth M. Attachment as related to mother-infant interaction. In Rosenblatt J, ed. *Advances in the Study of Behaviour.* Academic Press; 1979. pp. 1–51.

12. Bowlby J. *Attachment and Loss: Attachment (Vol 1).* Basic Books; 1969.

13. Harlow H. The nature of love. *American Psychologist.* 1958;**13**(12):673–85.

14. Murray, H. A. *Explorations in personality: A clinical and experimental study of fifty men of college age.* Oxford University Press; 1938

15. McClelland DC. *Human motivation.* Cambridge; 1987

16. Maslow A. A theory of human motivation. *Psychological Review.* 1943;**50**(4):370–96.

17. O'Neill M, Pillai Riddell R, Bureau J et al. Longitudinal and concurrent relationships between caregiver–child behaviours in the vaccination context and preschool attachment. *Pain.* 2020;**162**(3):823–34.

18. Calders F, Bijttebier P, Bosmans G et al. Investigating the interplay between parenting dimensions and styles, and the association with adolescent outcomes. *European Child & Adolescent Psychiatry.* 2019;**29**(3):327–42.

19. Ryan, R. M., & Deci, E. L. *Self-determination theory: Basic psychological needs in motivation, development, and wellness.* The Guilford Press; 2017.

20. Baumrind D. Rearing competent children. In Damon W, ed. *Child development today and tomorrow.* Jossey-Bass/Wiley; 1988. pp. 349–78.

21. Lamborn S, Mounts N, Steinberg L, Dornbusch S. *Patterns of competence and*

adjustment among adolescents from authoritative, authoritarian, indulgent, and neglectful families. *Child Development.* 1991;**62**(5):1049.

22. Hinnant J, Erath S, Tu K, El-Sheikh M. Permissive parenting, deviant peer affiliations, and delinquent behavior in adolescence: The moderating role of sympathetic nervous system reactivity. *Journal of Abnormal Child Psychology.* 2015;**44**(6):1071–81.

23. Barton A, Hirsch J. Permissive parenting and mental health in college students: Mediating effects of academic entitlement. *Journal of American College Health.* 2015;**64**(1):1–8.

24. Shumow L, Vandell D, Posner J. Harsh, firm, and permissive parenting in low-income families. *Journal of Family Issues.* 1998;**19**(5):483–507.

25. Gray M, Steinberg L. Unpacking authoritative parenting: Reassessing a multidimensional construct. *Journal of Marriage and the Family.* 1999;**61**(3):574.

26. Farkas M, Grolnick W. Examining the components and concomitants of parental structure in the academic domain. *Motivation and Emotion.* 2010;**34** (3):266–79.

27. Grolnick W, Raftery-Helmer J, Marbell K et al. Parental provision of structure: Implementation and correlates in three domains. *Merrill-Palmer Quarterly.* 2014;**60**(3):355.

28. Soenens B, Vansteenkiste M, Niemic C. Should parental prohibition of adolescents' peer relationships be prohibited? *Personal Relationships.* 2009;**16**(4):507–30.

29. Feeney B, Collins N. The importance of relational support for attachment and exploration needs. *Current Opinion in Psychology.* 2019;**25**:182–6.

30. Silvia P, Kwapil T. Aberrant asociality: How individual differences in social anhedonia illuminate the need to belong. *Journal of Personality.* 2011;**79** (6):1315–32.

31. Stanley P, Schutte N, Phillips W. A meta-analytic investigation of the

relationship between basic psychological need satisfaction and affect. *Journal of Positive School Psychology.* 2021;**5**(1):1–16.

32. Pilkington P, Bishop A, Younan R. Adverse childhood experiences and early maladaptive schemas in adulthood: A systematic review and meta-analysis. *Clinical Psychology & Psychotherapy.* 2020;**28**(3):569–84.

33. Young JE, Klosko JS. Reinventing your life: The breakthrough program to end negative behavior and feel great again. *Plume*; 1994.

34. Mertens Y, Yılmaz M, Lobbestael J. Schema modes mediate the effect of emotional abuse in childhood on the differential expression of personality disorders. *Child Abuse & Neglect.* 2020;**104**:104445.

35. Specht M, Chapman A, Cellucci T. Schemas and borderline personality disorder symptoms in incarcerated women. *Journal of Behavior Therapy and Experimental Psychiatry.* 2009;**40**(2):256–64.

36. Saldias A, Power K, Gillanders D, Campbell C, Blake R. The mediatory role of maladaptive schema modes between parental care and non-suicidal self-injury. *Cognitive Behaviour Therapy.* 2013;**42**(3):244–57.

37. Lumley M, Harkness K. Specificity in the relations among childhood adversity, early maladaptive schemas, and symptom profiles in adolescent depression. *Cognitive Therapy and Research.* 2007;**31**(5):639–57.

38. Bach B, Farrell J. Schemas and modes in borderline personality disorder: The mistrustful, shameful, angry, impulsive, and unhappy child. *Psychiatry Research.* 2018;**259**:323–9.

39. Bach B, Lobbestael J. Elucidating DSM-5 and ICD-11 diagnostic features of borderline personality disorder using schemas and modes. *Psychopathology.* 2018;**51**(6):400–7.

40. Dadashzadeh H, Hekmati I, Gholizade H, Abdi R. Schema modes in cluster B personality disorders. *Archives of Psychiatry and Psychotherapy.* 2016;**18**(2):22–8.

41. Bamelis L, Renner F, Heidkamp D, Arntz A. Extended schema mode conceptualizations for specific personality disorders: An empirical study. *Journal of Personality Disorders.* 2011;**25**(1):41–58.

42. Jacobs I, Lenz L, Wollny A, Horsch A. The higher-order structure of schema modes. *Journal of Personality Disorders.* 2020;**34**(3):348–76.

43. Kotov R, Krueger R, Watson D et al. The hierarchical taxonomy of psychopathology (HiTOP): A dimensional alternative to traditional nosologies. *Journal of Abnormal Psychology.* 2017;**126**(4):454–77.

44. Keulen-de Vos M, Bernstein D, Clark L, et al. Validation of the schema mode concept in personality disordered offenders. *Legal and Criminological Psychology.* 2017;**22**(2):420–41.

45. Sempértegui G, Karreman A, Arntz A, Bekker M. Schema therapy for borderline personality disorder: A comprehensive review of its empirical foundations, effectiveness and implementation possibilities. *Clinical Psychology Review.* 2013;**33**(3):426–47.

46. Giesen-Bloo J, van Dyck R, Spinhoven P et al. Outpatient psychotherapy for borderline personality disorder: Randomizedtrial of schema-focused therapy vs transference-focused psychotherapy. *Archives of General Psychiatry.* 2006;**63**(6):649.

47. Arntz A, van Genderen H. *Schema therapy for borderline personality disorder.* Wiley. 2009.

48. Sieswerda S, Arntz A, Kindt M. Successful psychotherapy reduces hypervigilance in borderline personality disorder. *Behavioural and Cognitive Psychotherapy.* 2007;**35**(4):387–402.

49. van Asselt A, Dirksen C, Arntz A, Severens J. The cost of borderline personality disorder: Societal cost of illness in BPD-clients. *European Psychiatry.* 2007;**22**(6):354–61.

50. Nadort M, Arntz A, Smit J et al. Implementation of outpatient schema therapy for borderline personality disorder with versus without crisis support by the therapist outside office hours: A randomized trial. *Behaviour Research and Therapy*. 2009;47(11):961–73.

51. Farrell JM, Shaw JM. *Group schema therapy for borderline personality disorder a step-by-step treatment manual with patient workbook*. Wiley-Blackwell. 2012

52. Dickhaut V, Arntz A. Combined group and individual schema therapy for borderline personality disorder: A pilot study. *Journal of Behavior Therapy and Experimental Psychiatry*. 2014;45(2):242–51.

53. Arntz A, Jacob GA, Lee CW et al. Effectiveness of predominantly group schema therapy and combined individual and group schema therapy for borderline personality disorder: A randomized clinical trial. *JAMA Psychiatry*. 2022;79 (4):287–99.

54. Hilden H, Rosenström T, Karila I et al. Effectiveness of brief schema group therapy for borderline personality disorder symptoms: a randomized pilot study. *Nordic Journal of Psychiatry*. 2020;75 (3):176–85.

55. Bohus M, Kleindienst N, Limberger M et al. The short version of the borderline symptom list (BSL-23): Development and initial data on psychometric properties. *Psychopathology*. 2008;42(1):32–9.

56. Hamid N, Molajegh R, Bashlideh K, Shehniyailagh M. The comparison of effectiveness of dialectical behavioral therapy (DBT) and schema therapy (ST) in reducing the severity of clinical symptoms (disruptive communication, emotional deregulation and behavioral deregulation) of borderline personality disorder in Iran. *Pakistan Journal of Medical and Health Sciences*. 2020;14:1354–62.

57. Fassbinder E, Assmann N, Schaich A et al. PRO*BPD: Effectiveness of outpatient treatment programs for borderline personality disorder: A comparison of Schema therapy and dialectical behavior therapy: Study protocol for a randomized trial. *BMC Psychiatry*. 2018;18(1).

58. van Vreeswijk M, Spinhoven P, Eurelings-Bontekoe E, Broersen J. Changes in symptom severity, schemas and modes in heterogeneous psychiatric patient groups following short-term schema cognitive-behavioural group therapy: A naturalistic pre-treatment and post-treatment design in an outpatient clinic. *Clinical Psychology & Psychotherapy*. 2012;21(1):29–38.

59. Skewes S, Samson R, Simpson S, van Vreeswijk M. Short-term group schema therapy for mixed personality disorders: A pilot study. *Frontiers in Psychology*. 2015;5(1592):1–9.

60. Schaap G, Chakhssi F, Westerhof G. Inpatient schema therapy for nonresponsive clients with personality pathology: Changes in symptomatic distress, schemas, schema modes, coping styles, experienced parenting styles, and mental well-being. *Psychotherapy*. 2016;53 (4):402–12.

61. van Vreeswijk M, Spinhoven P, Zedlitz A, Eurelings-Bontekoe E. Mixed results of a pilot RCT of time-limited schema mindfulness-based cognitive therapy and competitive memory therapy plus treatment as usual for personality disorders. *Personality Disorders: Theory, Research, and Treatment*. 2020;11 (3):170–80.

62. Bamelis L, Evers S, Spinhoven P, Arntz A. Results of a multicenter randomized controlled trial of the clinical effectiveness of schema therapy for personality disorders. *American Journal of Psychiatry*. 2014;171(3):305–22.

63. Arntz A, Jacob G. *Schema therapy in practice: An introductory guide to the schema mode approach*. Wiley-Blackwell; 2013

64. Hopwood C, Thomas K. Schema therapy is an effective treatment for avoidant, dependent and obsessive-compulsive personality disorders. *Evidence Based Mental Health*. 2014;17(3):90–1.

65. Bernstein D, Keulen-de Vos M, Clercx M et al. Schema therapy for violent PD offenders: A randomized clinical trial. *Psychological Medicine*. 2021:1–15.

66. Videler A, van Alphen S, van Royen R et al. Schema therapy for personality disorders in older adults: A multiple-baseline study. *Aging & Mental Health.* 2017;**22** (6):738–47.

67. Videler A, Rossi G, Schoevaars M, van der Feltz-Cornelis C, van Alphen S. Effects of schema group therapy in older outpatients: a proof of concept study. *International Psychogeriatrics.* 2014;**26**(10):1709–17.

68. van Dijk S, Veenstra M, Bouman R et al. Group schema-focused therapy enriched with psychomotor therapy versus treatment as usual for older adults with cluster B and/or C personality disorders: a randomized trial. *BMC Psychiatry.* 2019;**19**(1):26.

69. Gude T, Hoffart A. Change in interpersonal problems after cognitive agoraphobia and schema-focused therapy versus psychodynamic treatment as usual of inpatients with agoraphobia and Cluster C personality disorders. *Scandinavian Journal of Psychology.* 2008;**49**(2):195–9.

70. Cockram D, Drummond P, Lee C. Role and treatment of early maladaptive schemas in vietnam veterans with PTSD. *Clinical Psychology & Psychotherapy.* 2010;**17** (3):165–82.

71. Thiel N, Jacob G, Tuschen-Caffier B et al. Schema therapy augmented exposure and response prevention in clients with obsessive-compulsive disorder: Feasibility and efficacy of a pilot study. *Journal of Behavior Therapy and Experimental Psychiatry.* 2016;**52**:59–67.

72. Simpson S, Morrow E, van Vreeswijk M, Reid C. Group schema therapy for eating disorders: A pilot study. *Frontiers in Psychology.* 2010;**1**(182):1–10.

73. Calvert F, Smith E, Brockman R, Simpson S. Group schema therapy for eating disorders: study protocol. *Journal of Eating Disorders.* 2018;**6**(1):1–7.

74. Simpson S, Slowey L. Video therapy for atypical eating disorder and obesity: A case study. *Clinical Practice & Epidemiology in Mental Health.* 2011;**7**(1):38–43.

75. McIntosh V, Jordan J, Carter J et al. Psychotherapy for transdiagnostic binge eating: A randomized controlled trial of cognitive-behavioural therapy, appetite-focused cognitive-behavioural therapy, and schema therapy. *Psychiatry Research.* 2016;**240**:412–20.

76. Mohtadijafari S, Ashayeri H, Banisi P. The effectiveness of schema therapy techniques in mental health and quality of life of women with premenstrual dysphoric isorder. *Iranian Journal of Psychiatry and Clinical Psychology.* 2019;**25**(3):278–91.

77. Nameni E, Saadat S H, Keshavarz-Afshar H, Askarabady F. Effectiveness of group counseling based on schema therapy on quality of marital relationships, differentiation and hardiness in women seeking divorce in families of war veterans. *Journal of Military Medicine.* 2019; **21** (1):91–9.

78. Farrell J, Shaw I, Webber M. A schema-focused approach to group psychotherapy for outpatients with borderline personality disorder: A randomized controlled trial. *Journal of Behavior Therapy and Experimental Psychiatry.* 2009;**40**(2):317–28.

79. Yakın D, Grasman R, Arntz A. Schema modes as a common mechanism of change in personality pathology and functioning: Results from a randomized controlled trial. *Behaviour Research and Therapy.* 2020;**126**:103553.

80. Hyett M, Bank S, Lipp O et al. Attenuated psychophysiological reactivity following single-session group imagery rescripting versus verbal restructuring in social anxiety disorder: Results from a randomized controlled trial. *Psychotherapy and Psychosomatics.* 2018;**87**(6):340–9.

81. Kunze A, Lancee J, Morina N, Kindt M, Arntz A. Mediators of change in imagery rescripting and imaginal exposure for nightmares: Evidence from a randomized wait-list controlled trial. *Behavior Therapy.* 2019;**50**(5):978–93.

82. Romano M, Moscovitch D, Huppert J, Reimer S, Moscovitch M. The effects of imagery rescripting on memory outcomes in social anxiety disorder. *Journal of Anxiety Disorders.* 2020;**69**:102169.

83. Boterhoven de Haan K, Lee C et al. Imagery rescripting and eye movement desensitisation and reprocessing as treatment for adults with post-traumatic stress disorder from childhood trauma: randomised clinical trial. *The British Journal of Psychiatry.* 2020;**217**(5):609–15.

84. Paulik G, Steel C, Arntz A. Imagery rescripting for the treatment of trauma in voice hearers: A case series. *Behavioural and Cognitive Psychotherapy.* 2019;**47**(6):709–25.

85. Siegesleitner M, Strohm M, Wittekind C, Ehring T, Kunze A. Improving imagery rescripting treatments: Comparing an active versus passive approach. *Journal of Behavior Therapy and Experimental Psychiatry.* 2020;**69**:101578.

86. Rafaeli E, Young J, Bernstein D. *Schema therapy: Distinctive features.* Routledge. 2011

87. Greenberg L, Clarke K. Differential effects of the two-chair experiment and empathic reflections at a conflict marker. *Journal of Counselling Psychology.* 1979;**26**(1):1–8.

88. Greenberg L, Dompierre L. Specific effects of Gestalt two-chair dialogue on intrapsychic conflict in counselling. *Journal of Counselling Psychology.* 1981;**28**(4):288–94.

89. Greenberg L, Higgins H. Effects of two-chair dialogue and focusing on conflict resolution. *Journal of Counseling Psychology.* 1980;**27**(3):221–24.

90. Bell T, Montague J, Elander J, Gilbert P. 'A definite feel-it moment': Embodiment, externalisation and emotion during chair-work in compassion-focused therapy. *Counselling and Psychotherapy Research.* 2019;**20**(1):143–53.

91. Conoley C, Conoley J, McConnell J, Kimzey C. The effect of the ABCs of rational emotive therapy and the empty-chair technique of gestalt therapy on anger reduction. *Psychotherapy: Theory, Research & Practice.* 1983;**20**(1):112–17.

92. Trachsel M, Ferrari L, Holtforth MG. Resolving partnership ambivalence: A randomized controlled trial of very brief cognitive and experiential interventions with follow-up. *Canadian Journal of Counselling and Psychotherapy.* 2012; **46**(3):239–58.

93. Greenberg L. The intensive analysis of recurring events from the practice of Gestalt therapy. *Psychotherapy: Theory, Research & Practice.* 1980;**17**(2):143–52.

94. Greenberg L, Webster M. Resolving decisional conflict by Gestalt two-chair dialogue: Relating process to outcome. *Journal of Counseling Psychology.* 1982;**29**(5):468–77.

95. Stiegler J, Molde H, Schanche E. Does an emotion-focused two-chair dialogue add to the therapeutic effect of the empathic attunement to affect? *Clinical Psychology & Psychotherapy.* 2017;**25**(1):e86–e95.

96. Watson J, Gordon L, Stermac L, Kalogerakos F, Steckley P. Comparing the effectiveness of process-experiential with cognitive-behavioral psychotherapy in the treatment of depression. *Journal of Consulting and Clinical Psychology.* 2003;**71**(4):773–81.

97. Greenberg L, Malcolm W. Resolving unfinished business: Relating process to outcome. *Journal of Consulting and Clinical Psychology.* 2002;**70**(2):406–16.

98. Paivio S, Jarry J, Chagigiorgis H, Hall I, Ralston M. Efficacy of two versions of emotion-focused therapy for resolving child abuse trauma. *Psychotherapy Research.* 2010;**20**(3):353–66.

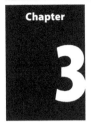

Schema Therapy Assessment

Introduction

In this chapter we provide a detailed description of how to conduct assessments to produce good-quality schema therapy case conceptualisations (see Chapter 4) which, in turn, direct effective treatment provision. A clear understanding of the client's experiences throughout their life allows the therapist to fine-tune their limited reparenting (see Chapter 6) to specifically address needs which were not met in childhood and deeply attune to the client. This profound level of understanding enables the therapist to work collaboratively with clients to set highly personalised therapy goals that help them learn how to meet their emotional needs in healthy ways.

Traditionally, for complex cases, 5–8 sessions are dedicated to the schema therapy assessment phase, not only because more information is gathered than in typical psychotherapy assessments but also because doing so facilitates a safe and constructive therapeutic bond. Assessment is also a process of hypothesis testing; as information is gathered, the schema therapist will start to form hypotheses about the central modes, schemas, and unmet needs contributing to the client's problems, which will eventually produce a collaborative case conceptualisation. Psychoeducation is interwoven throughout the assessment phase via a collaborative and curious stance that helps the client 'make sense' of their problems and builds the therapeutic alliance. Rather than depending heavily on any one method, the schema therapist relies on a triangulation of multiple methods, which are listed here and are outlined throughout the rest of this chapter.

1. Clinical interview
2. Identification of key problem areas and related therapy goals
3. Functional assessment of key problem areas
4. Self-monitoring forms
5. Downward arrowing techniques
6. Mode assessment
7. Questionnaire/psychometric data
8. Diagnostic imagery
9. Process assessment/transference data

Part I: Schema Therapy Assessment: Focus and Considerations

A central goal of any schema therapy assessment is to gain a clear understanding of the client's presenting problems, and to begin to conceptualise how underlying EMS and modes cause and perpetuate such problems. In schema therapy, many of the presenting problems or 'key problem areas' may be conceptualised as behavioural and/or cognitive manifestations of coping modes, designed to escape the emotional pain associated with unmet needs in childhood. Common problems associated with coping modes might include substance use disorders (e.g., Self-Soother mode), eating disorders (e.g., Overcontroller mode), or a range of interpersonal problems related to being excessively compliant or reliant on others (e.g., Compliant Surrenderer mode), being too aloof from or avoidant of others (e.g., Detached Protector mode), or being highly antagonistic (e.g., Bully and Attack mode). A detailed assessment will reveal that these coping mechanisms usually make sense in the context in which they developed. In the short term, they tend to provide relief, and thereby function primarily as 'solutions' to underlying emotional pain. This conflict between the relief provided by coping mechanisms and the secondary distress that they cause often results in ambivalence about change: on the one hand the person wants to get rid of the self-harm, binge eating, or drug use, but on the other hand they find it difficult to relinquish the benefits and sense of safety they provide. In contrast to presenting issues related to coping modes, when clients describe their difficulties in terms of overwhelming emotions and difficulties with regulating distress, these might be conceptualised as manifestations of child modes. Many clients come to therapy with the perception that their Vulnerable Child mode is the 'problem', and that this part of themselves needs to be eliminated, 'fixed', or controlled. Such clients may present with issues such as chronic anxiety, overwhelm, or anger dysregulation. Other problems – like 'low self-esteem', self-injury, and other forms of self-defeating behaviour – might reflect the dominance of maladaptive parent or critic modes. It is equally important to pay attention to the strength of the client's Healthy Adult mode. Generally, the strength of maladaptive modes is likely to indicate relative weaknesses or 'blind spots' in a client's Healthy Adult mode. For example, a client with a strong Punitive Critic mode is likely to have poor Healthy Adult mode functioning in the domain of self-compassion (a positive schema which is the antithesis of the Punitiveness EMS).

Mode Assessment: Identification of Modes for the Case Conceptualisation

Identifying which modes account for most of the client's problematic experiences is arguably the most important objective of schema therapy assessment. The therapist looks to answer two key questions: (1) Which mode/s dominate/s the client's presentation in session? (2) Which modes are implicated in the client's problems? Modes can be identified 'in the moment' through three main sources of information: the *content* of speech (what the person says), non-verbal communication (e.g., the *tone* of their voice, facial expressions, postures, and gestures), and *countertransference* (feelings and behavioural urges that the client's responses elicit within the therapist). Examples of ways in which the modes can manifest are presented in Table 3.1.

Identifying Key Problem Areas

Identifying specific and clear 'Key Problem Areas' is critical for at least three reasons. First, they provide initial clues as to which EMS and/or modes are likely problematic for the client. Second, a clear problem list focuses the treatment, avoiding a common technical flaw of repeatedly 'putting out spot fires' without reducing the frequency of crises over the long

Table 3.1 Assessment questions linked to each schema

Early Maladaptive Schemas	Unmet Needs	Interpersonal Problems (e.g., Signs in Relationships)	Typical Relevant Modes	Assessment Queries
Emotional Deprivation	Insufficient: Warmth, nurturance, affectionate touch, guidance, empathy, validation, attunement, being cherished.	Resignation (Surrender): Detachment, lack of overt expression of needs, attraction to partners who cannot commit; Feels bored/ smothered when with loving partners. Avoidance: Keeps others at an arm's length, avoids intimacy/commitment, uses compulsive coping (e.g., bingeing, alcohol, substances, promiscuous sex, gaming) to block emptiness and self-soothe when alone. Inversion (Overcompensation): Co-dependency, emotionally (&/or practically) demanding toward friends and partners.	Resignation Coping Modes: Vulnerable (Lonely, Unlovable) Child; (Overt or Suppressed) Angry Child; Impulsive Child; Inner Critic ('You're undeserving') Avoidant Coping Modes: Detached Protector; Detached Self-Soother; *Funny Protector, Compliant Surrenderer; *Helpless Surrenderer (function = 'See me') Inversion Coping Modes: Perfectionistic Overcontroller; *Clown; Attention/Approval Seeker	How close were you to your parents as you were growing up? Were your parents present emotionally? How did they show their love (e.g., warmth, affection, connecting, vs. through gifts, working hard to pay for a good school, food/cooking)? How much time was spent *being with* your parents (e.g., playing, conversing, having fun), without the pressure to perform or achieve? To what extent can you talk to your parents about the things that really upset or bother you? If you were upset about something that happened to you as a child, who would you have gone to? Why/ why not? If you had gone to mum/dad/grandma, how do you think they would have responded? What did you fear would happen (to you or to them) if you had shared your feelings and needs more? Who provided guidance about managing difficult emotions, making decisions in your family? Who (if anyone) would you have spoken with if you were upset about an incident at school? Do you feel as though others in your family really 'get' who you are and understand you? Did you feel loved and cherished? If yes, how did you know? What indicated to you that you were cherished? Were your parents able to overtly show warmth, such as through affectionate touch, hugs, telling you they loved you?

Table 3.1 (cont.)

Early Maladaptive Schemas	Unmet Needs	Interpersonal Problems (e.g., Signs in Relationships)	Typical Relevant Modes	Assessment Queries
				Did anyone play with you as a child, and spend time laughing and having fun or being silly together?
				Did you feel really understood as your own person (rather than what that you were expected to be)?
				When you talk about emotions, to what extent are others able to listen to you and really understand your struggles?
				To what extent were your parents able to meet your needs? Did you have any role in taking care of your parents' needs?
Defectiveness/ Shame	Insufficient: Unconditional love, acceptance, inadequate protection from criticism, put-downs, abuse.	Resignation: Tolerates friends who are critical, rejecting. Puts others on a pedestal whilst blaming & demeaning self. Avoidance: Keeps others at an emotional distance; Doesn't allow others to see vulnerability or to get close. Inversion: Puts others on a pedestal to elevate own status; Critical and demeaning toward others to elevate own status; Acts hyper-'nice' and caring to prevent potential rejection.	Resignation Coping Modes: Vulnerable (Inferior/Ashamed) Child; Angry Child; Impulsive Child; Inner Critic (Punitive; Demanding): 'You're bad, worthless, unlovable' Avoidant Coping Modes: Detached Protector; *Avoidant Protector; Detached Self-Soother; *Helpless Surrenderer Inversion Coping Modes: Self-Aggrandiser; Overcontroller (*Flagellating/ Scolding/Perfectionistic); Attention/Approval Seeker; *Clown	Did you feel criticised or judged by anyone in your family as a child? Did you feel accepted for who you are, or was there an expectation that you should be a certain way in order to be lovable? Did you ever feel rejected by your parents? Did anyone make you feel ashamed for your needs or feelings? Did you experience punishment (emotional/physical) that made you feel ashamed or defective? Did anyone hurt you or touch you in an unwanted or sexual way as a child? As an adult, do you ever think of yourself as unlovable, or defective in any way? Do you compare yourself negatively with others, and think of yourself as less worthy or lovable? Are you hypersensitive to criticism (or have others noticed this about you)?

Schema	Early experiences	Coping styles	Coping modes	Questions
Abandonment/ Instability	Insufficient: Consistent emotional availability of caregivers; support & guidance to help deal with loss; emotional stability. Too much: Emotional unavailability/ inconsistency; loss.	Resignation: Chooses & tolerates partners who are unable to commit. Avoidance: Avoids close relationships and commitment. Uses compulsive coping (e.g., bingeing, alcohol, substances) to self-soothe when alone. Inversion: Clings to partners, friends. Becomes angry and attacking of partner for any separations.	Resignation Coping Modes: Vulnerable (Abandoned) Child; Angry Child; Impulsive Child Avoidance Coping Modes: Detached Protector; *Reassurance Seeker; *Funny Protector; *Slacker/Oblomov; Detached Self-Soother; Compliant Surrenderer; *Helpless Surrenderer Inversion Coping Modes: Bully and Attack; *Clown; *Conning & Manipulation; *Hyperautonomous Overcontroller	Were your parents consistently available to provide support and care? Did grandparents or previous generations experience any abandonment that affected your parents? Were either of your parents emotionally unavailable for any reason (e.g., working away, mood swings, alcohol or drug use)? Were there any periods of time that you were separated from your parents/caregivers as a child? Did anyone important to you leave or die during your childhood? If so, how much emotional support did you have from your parents (or others) following this event? As an adult, do you struggle with feeling abandoned, desperate, or alone when you are apart from others who are close to you? Or do you close yourself off by leaving others before they leave you? Do you expect others to leave you?
Mistrust/Abuse	Insufficient: Protection, safety, stability, reliability of caregivers Too much: Abuse, deception, lies, duplicity.	Resignation: Attracted to partners/friends who turn out to be abusive; Tolerates abuse; Copes in ways which provoke rage/outbursts from others. Avoidance: Keeps others at a distance; Avoids trusting others with secrets and vulnerabilities. Inversion: Mistreats, abuses, manipulates others. Writes others off as soon as they are not of use.	Resignation Coping Modes: Vulnerable (Abused) Child; Angry Child; Impulsive Child; Inner Critic (Punitive): 'You're dirty, damaged, bad' Avoidant Coping Modes: Detached Protector (Dissociation); *Avoidant Protector; Detached Self-Soother; *Slacker/Oblomov Inversion Coping Modes: Overcontroller (*Flagellating, Paranoid); Bully and Attack;	Did anyone hurt, abuse, cheat on you, or lie to you as a child? Did anyone hurt you or touch you inappropriately as a child? Did either of your parents lie to you, use you for their own benefit, or try to manipulate you? Were you humiliated by parents or other family members? Did anyone in your family act to protect you when/if you were mistreated? Was anyone in the family duplicitous, or underhand in the way they managed situations? As an adult, do you find yourself trusting the wrong people? Do you notice higher chemistry with people who end up being untrustworthy?

Table 3.1 (cont.)

Early Maladaptive Schemas	Unmet Needs	Interpersonal Problems (e.g., Signs in Relationships)	Typical Relevant Modes	Assessment Queries
			*Idealiser; *Clown; Conning & Manipulation	Does it feel like you can trust people 100% or not at all? Do you end your relationships abruptly due to feeling let down or hurt by others?
Social Isolation	Insufficient: Opportunities to gain a sense of *belonging* and community with both family and peers.	Resignation: Stays on the periphery of groups, doesn't join in with group activities, joins 'outcast' groups, exaggerates differences (e.g., through dress, attire, hair, makeup). Avoidance: Stays away from social gatherings, groups. Inversion: Works hard to fit in, through 'acting the part'.	Resignation Coping Modes: Vulnerable (Alienated/ Misunderstood) Child; Angry Child; Impulsive Child; Inner Critic: 'You don't belong, you don't fit in' Avoidant Coping Modes: Detached Protector; *Avoidant Protector; Detached Self-Soother; *Funny Protector; Compliant Surrenderer Inversion Coping Modes: Attention-Seeker; Self-Aggrandiser; *Superior Loner; *Clown	Did you feel that you belonged in your family? In what ways was your family the same as other families? Did you ever feel that your family was different from other families in any way? Were you ever part of a peer group or community where you felt you belonged? Did you ever feel excluded from your peers? Did you feel part of a peer group when you were at school? Did you ever feel different to others, like you didn't fit in? As a child/adolescent (and now as an adult) have you ever been part of a community (e.g., church, sports club, interest group)? As an adult, when you are with a group, do you join in, or stay on the periphery watching others?
Dependence/ Incompetence	Insufficient: Practical support, help, guidance (under- or overprotectiveness).	Resignation: Seeks partners & friends who appear dominant/confident. Relies on others to take on day-to-day responsibilities; Constantly seeks advice and reassurance Avoidance: Avoids making decisions, taking responsibility for own life	Resignation Coping Modes: Vulnerable (Dependent) Child; Angry Child; Impulsive Child; Inner Critic: 'You're too incompetent, you can't cope' Avoidant Coping Modes: Detached Protector; Detached Self-Soother; *Funny Protector;	Were you over-protected by either of your parents? Did they prefer to do things for you rather than letting you have a go and learn by your own mistakes? Did you feel like you had to grow up and take responsibility too quickly? Did you feel like you had to take care of yourself and had no one to depend on for periods of your life? As an adult, do you find it difficult to take care of yourself in practical ways? Do you lean on others to

Schema	Unmet Need	Coping Behaviours	Coping Modes	Questions
		choices. Sticks to comfort zone whilst avoiding new challenges. Inversion: Hyper-self-reliant and autonomous; doesn't ask for help; takes on 'helper' role for others.	Compliant Surrenderer *Helpless Surrenderer Inversion Coping Modes: Overcontroller (Perfectionistic/ *Invincible/ *Hyperautonomous); *Clown	take responsibility for day-to-day issues (e.g., financial matters, fixing things)? Do you find yourself looking for answers or direction from others? Do you notice that you are easily drawn into the next gimmick?
Vulnerability to Harm or Illness	Insufficient: Safety and protection from harm/illness. Reassurance and support to build trust in body, thoughts, emotions and own resources.	Resignation: Seeks reassurance & speaks obsessively about fears around illness, deaths and other catastrophes; Obsessionally checks own and family members for signs and symptoms of illness. Reassurance-seeking; Cossets family members due to fears of harm. Avoidance: Sticks to same routine and doesn't venture anywhere new (including family holidays) due to fear of harm/illness. Inversion: Takes risks and ignores safety regulations. Behaves as though invincible.	Resignation Coping Modes: Vulnerable (Anxious) Child; Angry Child; Impulsive Child Avoidant Coping Modes: Detached Protector; Detached Self-Soother; *Funny Protector; *Reassurance Seeker/*Helpless Surrenderer Inversion Coping Modes: *Invincible Overcontroller; *Clown	As a child, did you or anyone in your family experience any harm or illness that felt frightening? Did grandparents or previous generations experience any serious illness or harm that affected your parents? Did any family members worry or talk a lot about illness or death? Do you recall worrying excessively about illness and death as a child? As an adult, do you find yourself seeking reassurance from others? Do you notice yourself avoiding going to certain places, or venturing far due to a fear of illness or death? Do you worry about the impact or meaning of your thoughts? Do you try to control or suppress thoughts that frighten you? Do you ever worry that you are losing control or going mad?
Enmeshment (undeveloped self)	Insufficient: Encouragement and praise to support development of	Resignation: Excessively close contact with parents/partner; Lack of privacy, tells them everything; Lives	Resignation Coping modes: Vulnerable (Invisible; non-individualised) Child; Angry Child/Sulking/Rebellious Child	As a child, did you feel that stating your own views, or wanting/believing something different from one or both parents would lead to them acting hurt or disappointed?

Table 3.1 (cont.)

Early Maladaptive Schemas	Unmet Needs	Interpersonal Problems (e.g., Signs in Relationships)	Typical Relevant Modes	Assessment Queries
	autonomy. Attunement and recognition of individual preferences, character traits. Encouragement to develop express own views and values.	through children and/or partner. Avoidance: Avoids closeness, intimacy. Avoids stating own opinions, preferences. Inversion: Rebels against expectations and asserts individuality through behaving in opposite way to parents.	Inner Critic (Guilt-Inducing): 'You're hurting me by separating from me and making life choices that don't involve me' Avoidant Coping Modes: Detached Protector; *Funny Protector; Detached Self-Soother; Compliant Surrenderer Inversion Coping Modes: *Clown; *Hyperautonomous Overcontroller	Were there any barriers in your family to you becoming separate or independent? As an adult, do you find it difficult to state your opinions without fearing that you will hurt one or both of your parents? Has it been difficult to make your own life choices without feeling that you are letting one or both of them down? Do you find it difficult to know what you feel or want from your life?
Failure (to achieve)	Insufficient: Encouragement, praise, support, guidance, opportunities for mastery.	Resignation: Makes minimal effort; Looks up to others on the assumption that they are more intelligent, capable. Avoidance: Procrastinates, avoids work tasks. Inversion: Relentless striving, prioritises work over health, and relationships with partner, family, friends.	Resignation Coping Modes: Vulnerable (Anxious; Failed) Child; Angry Child; Impulsive Child; Undisciplined Child; Inner Critic (Punitive, Demanding): 'You're a failure, stupid, inept' Avoidant Coping Modes: Detached Protector, Detached Self-Soother; *Reassurance Seeker; *Funny Protector Inversion Coping Modes: Perfectionistic Overcontroller; *Clown; Self-Aggrandiser (The Winner)	Were either of your parents critical of your abilities or achievements? Did you experience excessive criticism from teachers or significant others? As a child/adolescent, did you ever receive praise or encouragement for your work/study? Did you struggle with learning at school for any reason? How was it dealt with by parents/teachers? Was there any area of your life where you felt a sense of mastery and competence? As an adult, do you ever feel that you are not reaching your true potential (at work/study)? Do you compare yourself negatively with others, and think of yourself as less capable?

Schema			Coping Modes	Questions
Entitlement-grandiosity	Insufficient: Healthy consistent limits; support with developing compassion/empathy for others; opportunity to learn how to function in relationships on an equal footing with others. Too much: Spoiled, over-indulged. Focus on material expression of love, at expense of emotional presence/attunement.	Resignation: Boasts about achievements; competes with others, one-up-manship; Bullying, demanding, controlling toward others. Takes advantage of others in relationships. Avoidance: Avoids being with others who are of higher status – except to gain status via association. Inversion: Focuses excessively on others' needs.	Resignation Coping Modes: *Grandiose Child; *Spoiled Child; Angry/Enraged Child; Impulsive Child; Inner Critic (usually Demanding): 'You should strive to be better than others; anything less than perfect is unacceptable' Avoidant Coping Modes: Detached Self-Soother; Detached Protector; *Avoidant Protector Inversion Coping Modes: *Over-humble mode	Did your parents ever give you the impression that the rules and conventions that others have to follow don't apply to you? Did they give you the impression that you were special in some way? How did your parents show love? Was there an emphasis on material gifts? How important is/was success, wealth, and status to your parents? Did you experience any pressure from your parents to get into a particular school/university, or to aim for a particular job or position? Did your parents have trouble setting limits or consistent boundaries? Did they make you follow the rules, even if you resisted? As an adult, do you have trouble following the rules that others follow? Do you feel like you deserve better than others, or should be treated differently? Do you ever justify doing what you want by reassuring yourself, e.g. 'Others won't mind if I ....?
Insufficient self-control (or self-discipline)	Insufficient: Lack of consistent boundaries and parental presence. Child was not made to complete boring or routine tasks and to take on normal responsibilities (e.g., homework and household chores).	Resignation: Doesn't stick with tasks until completed, gives up easily. Avoidance: Avoids responsibility and allows others to do the boring or routine tasks. Avoids employment or turns up late and does not complete required tasks. Expects others to do boring/routine tasks and doesn't do their share.	Resignation Coping Modes: Undisciplined Child Angry/Enraged/*Sulking Child Avoidant Coping Modes: *Avoidant Protector; Detached Protector; Detached Self-Soother Inversion Coping Modes: Perfectionistic Overcontroller	As a child, did anyone ensure that you completed homework and took on other appropriate responsibilities within your family? Were consequences set in a healthy consistent way to ensure that you followed the family rules/boundaries? Were steps taken to ensure that you and your siblings were not disrespectful or hurtful toward others? As an adult, do you find it difficult to complete routine or boring tasks? Do others notice that you tend to pass responsibility on to them? Do you often feel like you can say or do whatever you want, without thinking about the consequences or

Table 3.1 (cont.)

Early Maladaptive Schemas	Unmet Needs	Interpersonal Problems (e.g., Signs in Relationships)	Typical Relevant Modes	Assessment Queries
		Inversion: Tightly controlled or self-disciplined; Overly responsible; Demands high standards from self and others.		effects on others? Do you often lose control of your emotions?
Subjugation	Insufficient: Freedom to make decisions based on own feelings and needs, and to follow own intuition. Too much: Control, anger, coercion in response to non-compliance and expression of needs/feelings.	Resignation: Goes along with others' views and decisions, doesn't stand up for own opinions or needs. Allows others to be in control without asserting own needs. Avoidance: Avoids situations that may result in conflict. Hides information from others to avoid conflict, anger. Inversion: Controlling and domineering toward others.	Resignation Coping Modes: Vulnerable (Intimidated) Child; Angry Child; Rebellious Child; Inner Critic (Guilt-Inducing): 'you're selfish, you cause trouble' Avoidant Coping Modes: Compliant Surrenderer; Detached Protector; Detached Self-Soother; *Funny Protector Inversion Coping Modes: Bully & Attack; Overcontroller (*hyperautonomous; *scolding); Self-Aggrandiser; *Clown	As a child, were either of your parents overcontrolling and/or overprotective? Were you made to feel guilty if you said what you felt or needed? Did either of your parents become angry or act as if you had hurt them if your needs or feelings clashed with theirs? Did you feel smothered and/or unable to express your own views in your relationship with either/both parents, for fear of repercussions? As an adult, do you struggle to say 'no' and set limits on others, due to fears that others will get angry at you? Do you often feel controlled/coerced into doing things that you would not choose to do of your own volition? Are you fearful of standing up for yourself due to expectations that others will get angry at you? As an adult, do you find it difficult to know what you want or need?
Self-Sacrifice	Insufficient: Encouragement and support to prioritise own needs	Resignation: Tuned in to others' needs and feelings; Takes care of others; Shuts off from own feelings and	Resignation Coping Modes: Vulnerable (Parentified) Child; *Aggrieved Child; Angry Child;	As a child (and adult), did (do) you have a high sensitivity to the feelings, and emotional suffering of others?

Schema	Insufficient / Too much	Description	Inner Critic / Coping Modes	Assessment questions
	and self-care; Lack of role model or guidance in balancing own needs with others'. Too much: Exposure to others' troubles, pain and suffering.	needs. May be disdainful toward own needs. Avoidance: Avoids situations and relationships which involve being the recipient of care and nurturance; May avoid situations that involve giving, to avoid impending burnout. Inversion: Withholding and resentful when others express their needs.	Inner Critic (Guilt-Inducing/Absent/Over-Anxious): you're selfish, your needs are not important' Avoidant Coping Modes: Detached Protector; *Funny Protector; Detached Self-Soother Inversion Coping Modes: Overcontroller (*hyperautonomous); Self-Aggrandiser; *Clown	Did you tend to feel responsible for managing one or both of your parents' emotions and needs? As a child, did you ever worry that your feelings and needs were a burden on others? Did you ever feel that by stating your feelings and needs you would overwhelm your parents? Do you feel guilty if you do something for yourself, or find yourself feeling happy, whilst others are suffering? As an adult, do others typically seek you out for support and guidance? Do you struggle to say 'no' and set limits on others, due to feelings of responsibility and guilt?
Approval/Recognition-seeking	Insufficient: Unconditional love, approval, recognition, attention, praise. Too much: Approval conditional on success, status.	Resignation: Seeks recognition or approval from others through trying to impress (through knowledge, skills, status, success, appearances). Avoidance: Avoids interacting with those from whom approval is desired. Inversion: Reacts by being 'invisible', not standing out; Rebels against perceived expectations of others to elicit disapproval.	Resignation Coping Modes: Vulnerable (Invisible) Child; Attention-seeking Child; Angry/Sulking Child; Impulsive Child Avoidant Coping Modes: Detached Protector; Detached Self-Soother Inversion Coping Modes: Self-Aggrandiser; Overcontroller (*hyperautonomous)	As a child, did you find it difficult to get the approval and attention you needed? Were there any circumstances in your family that made it difficult to get the recognition you needed from your parents (e.g., a sibling with emotional problems or learning difficulties; a parent with mental health problems)? Did you feel that in order to get the love and attention you needed, you had to perform well or be 'good'? What type of behaviours did your parents reward or value when you were a child? Do you feel like you turned out to be the person they wanted you to be? Can you explain more about that? What were the qualities that they were impressed by? How did you know? How did they let you know about that? Did you ever feel that you had to eliminate aspects of yourself to be acceptable to others? Did you learn to use achievement, status, or success as a way of seeking approval and recognition from others?

Table 3.1 (cont.)

Early Maladaptive Schemas	Unmet Needs	Interpersonal Problems (e.g., Signs in Relationships)	Typical Relevant Modes	Assessment Queries
				As an adult, do you ever feel that by seeking approval and recognition from others, you can end up neglecting yourself and giving yourself 'time to just 'be' and have fun?
Negativity/ Pessimism	Insufficient: Balance of positive and negative life events; Support with managing difficult events and regulating emotions in healthy ways. Too much: Discussions focused on negative outcomes, disappointments, and not getting hopes up.	Resignation Coping Modes: Worries & ruminates about potential negative outcomes whilst dismissing positives; Discussions with others are focused on complaining about problems, worrying about circumstances going wrong; Obsessionally prepares for every possible scenario in attempt to avoid negative outcomes. Avoidance: Avoids situations perceived to be 'risky'; Stays within narrow comfort zone; Uses avoidant self-soothing (e.g., alcohol, drugs, bingeing, promiscuous sex, gambling) to block depression. Inversion: Sees the positive in every situation; denies negative feelings or fears; Overly buoyant and positive whilst ignoring negative emotions and	Resignation Coping Modes: Vulnerable (Disappointed; downhearted) Child; Angry Child Avoidant Coping Modes: Detached Protector; *Funny Protector; Detached Self-Soother Inversion Coping Modes: *Pollyanna; *Clown	As a child, was there an excessive focus on negativity, pessimism, and things going wrong in your family? Was there less focus on talking about the positive side of life? How much play, joy, and spontaneity did your family engage in when you were a child? Were either of your parents depressed/highly anxious/ a worrier? Did either of your parents talk about their worries and anxieties, predicting all of the possible problems that could emerge? *As an adult*, do you focus a lot on things that could go wrong? Do you spend a lot of energy planning and avoiding situations that might not be guaranteed of a 100% positive outcome?

minimising difficult life circumstances; Takes on 'expert' role to compensate for underlying insecurities.

Schema	Parenting origins	Coping styles	Coping Modes	Questions
Emotional Inhibition	Insufficient: Expression of vulnerability, emotions, and needs. Too much: Disapproval/judgement for expressing emotions, especially anger.	Resignation: Stays detached, calm, emotionally unexpressive in relationships. Controls and suppresses expression of emotions, including joy, spontaneity. Avoidance: Steers clear of relationships and situations that may result in overt expression of emotions. Inversion: Tries to fit in, and act in a vivacious or outgoing way, but feels stiff and fabricated.	Resignation Coping Modes: Vulnerable (Inhibited) Child; Vulnerable (Frightened) Child; Angry Child; Inner Critic (Demanding); Avoidant Coping Modes: Detached Protector; Detached Self-Soother; *Avoidant Protector; *Funny Protector Inversion Coping Modes: *Clown; Attention-Approval Seeker; *Overcontroller (Invincible)	As a child, did your parents express and talk openly about their feelings? Did your parents/caregivers encourage you to express your feelings? How was anger expressed by members of your family? How do members of your family express happiness, joy? As an adult, do others see you as emotionally uptight? Is it difficult for you to show emotions to others? Do you feel self-conscious expressing affection?
Unrelenting Standards (hypercriticalness)	Insufficient: Unconditional acceptance; balance of fun, spontaneity, play alongside work/study. Too much: Family culture of pressure to achieve; emphasis on work; role modelling of prioritisation of work/striving over health & happiness.	Resignation: Strives for perfection; prioritises work over health & happiness; prepares in excessive, over-inclusive manner in attempt to reach excessive standards. Avoidance: Procrastination/avoidance to prevent being scrutinised by peers; avoids mistakes. Inversion: Relinquishes standards; haphazard, slap-dash, careless approach.	Resignation Coping Modes: Vulnerable (Disappointing/Short-Falling) Child; *Over-Diligent Child; Angry/*Sulking/*Rebellious Child; Impulsive Child; Inner Critic (Demanding); Avoidant Coping Modes: Detached Protector; Detached Self-Soother Inversion Coping Modes: *Slacker/Oblomov, *Helpless Surrenderer	As a child, what messages did you receive from your parents about work-life balance? How much balance did your parents demonstrate in their own lives? Were they able to take time for fun, enjoyment, spontaneity, and play? What was your attitude toward people who didn't uphold these high standards (in terms of study/ success (e.g. academic, sports, appearance, etc.))? How much pressure did you feel under to perform well and get good grades at school? Were you expected to strive in order to be accepted into a particular school/university as you grew up? As an adult, do you strive to be the best? Do you find it hard to forgive yourself for making mistakes?

Table 3.1 (cont.)

Early Maladaptive Schemas	Unmet Needs	Interpersonal Problems (e.g., Signs in Relationships)	Typical Relevant Modes	Assessment Queries
				Do you ever notice an urge to avoid work presentations due to fears about being scrutinised by your peers?
Punitiveness	Insufficient: Love, warmth, affection, nurturance. Too much: Punishment, harshness, criticism, judgement.	Resignation Coping Modes: Critical, punitive, harsh toward self & others. Avoidance: Keeps others at a distance due to fear of being punished. Inversion: Lacks assertiveness, forgives everything.	Resignation Coping Modes: Vulnerable (Bad) Child; Angry or *Sulking Child; Impulsive Child; Inner Critic (Punitive) Avoidant Coping Modes: Detached Protector; Detached Self-Soother Inversion Coping Modes: *Overforgiving merciful mode	As a child, were you punished harshly (e.g., shouted at, hit) for making mistakes? Were you humiliated or made to feel bad about yourself when you got something wrong? As an adult, if you make a mistake, do you believe that you deserve to be punished? Do you feel compelled to punish others when they get things wrong? Do you worry that others will punish you?
*Lack of Connectedness to Nature	Insufficient: Opportunity to connect to nature in a meaningful way, insufficient opportunity to develop connectedness with place (natural environment).	Resignation Coping Modes: Operates in disconnected and disembodied way, materialism; has no active relationship with Nature. Avoidance: Actively avoids spending time in nature; or spends time in nature in disengaged manner. Inversion: Consumerism; domination and exploitation of nature; use of nature purely as resource to be manipulated, and profited from.	Resignation Coping Modes: Vulnerable (Empty) Child Avoidant Coping Modes Detached Protector, *Avoidant Protector; Detached Self-Soother Inversion Coping Modes: Self-Aggrandiser; Predator	As a child, what were your favourite places where you felt most alive and free? How much time did you spend in nature in childhood? What aspects of the natural environment do you recall most clearly? As you focus on those places in your mind's eye, are there any images or sensations that you notice? What does it feel like in your body to recall those memories? Did you and/or anyone in your family have a special connection with animals or other aspects of nature? What kinds of things did your family members do that might indicate they cared about nature and the environment? Do you ever find yourself affected or anxious about current environmental crises?

			Coping Modes	Questions
*Unfairness	Insufficient: Culture of fairness, equality, opportunity to explain point of view. Too much: Treated unfairly, blamed when things go wrong; Treated differently from siblings; victimised, bullied.	Resignation: Interprets others' behaviours as signs of victimisation and unfair treatment; interprets negative events as evidence that they are being unfairly victimised; Expects others to take care of them or makes things right. Avoidance: Avoids relationships, closeness based on equality and trust. Inversion: Dominating, controlling, manipulating, attacking others to give feeling of power and dominance to prevent being used/treated badly by others. Alternatively, naively idealises others as fair and equal, and does not take adequate steps to protect oneself.	Resignation Coping Modes: Vulnerable (Victimised) Child; Angry Child; Impulsive Child. Avoidant Coping Modes: Detached Protector; Detached Self-Soother; *Helpless Surrenderer; *Victim/Self-Pity. Inversion Coping Modes: Bully & Attack, Predator; *Invincible/Idealising Overcontroller; *Conning Manipulator	As a child, were you treated differently from other children – by your parents, school, peers? Were you treated differently from your siblings in any way? E.g., were you made to feel less important, or to do an unfair share of the chores around the house? As an adult, do you ever feel like you are a victim and that the world is unfair? Do you feel like you have to prepare yourself for the worst? Do you feel that there is no point in getting your hopes up? Alternatively, do you always assume the best of everyone and not take precautions even when others would do so?
*Lack of a Coherent Identity	Intersection of needs across all schemas. Insufficient: Identity grounded in interpersonal connectedness, self-relevant roles; opportunities to feel psychologically rooted and intact.	Resignation: Feels unable to express own views, opinions, lacks a sense of coherent self. Intimacy is superficial and lacks emotional depth. Avoidance: Derealisation, dissociation, depersonalisation, pseudoseizures, facilitates avoidance of sense of 'falling apart' or fragmentation of self.	Resignation Coping Modes: Vulnerable (Confused) Child; Angry Child. Avoidant Coping Modes: Detached Protector (dissociative); Detached Self-Soother. Inversion Coping Modes: Overcontroller; *Invincible-Pretender	As a child, did you feel like it was difficult to rely on others to be there for you? Did it feel as though you couldn't be certain that your caregivers would be there for you? Did you feel cherished by your family? Did your family celebrate special events in your life – such as your birthdays, graduation, etc.? Did you feel really 'known' or understood at a deep level by family and friends? Was there a lot of disruption or change in your childhood as you grew up? Did you feel part of a wider community that meant something to you as you grew up?

Table 3.1 (cont.)

Early Maladaptive Schemas	Unmet Needs	Interpersonal Problems (e.g., Signs in Relationships)	Typical Relevant Modes	Assessment Queries
		Use of drugs, alcohol, gaming, promiscuous sex. Inversion: Clings to false certainty and predictability such as through co-dependency, and/or overcontrolling behaviours (e.g., obsessional rituals, eating-disordered rituals); Objectifies self and others in attempt to find tangible identity; Pretends to have a strong sense of identity and sure-footedness.		Was it hard for you to make sense of what was happening in your relationships and the ways that other people behaved? Did you worry or feel anxious about your capacity to cope with all of the changes happening in your life? Did you ever worry that things were out of your control (e.g. life circumstances, relationships, your feelings, your body)? As an adult, do you cling to certain relationships or coping habits as a way of trying to feel safe and in control? Do you worry that things will go wrong if you don't keep tight control over everything? Do you worry about whether you are capable of coping when unexpected or unpredicted events crop up in your life? Do you ever feel like you don't know who you are, as if your identity is missing, or as though you only exist as separate bits (or body parts)?
*Lack of a meaningful world	Intersection of needs across all schemas. Insufficient: Opportunities to develop meaningful social connections, meaningful goals and pursuits.	Resignation: Experiences life as empty, meaningless. Sense of disconnection from others and the world. Avoidance: Derealisation, dissociation, depersonalisation, pseudoseizures, facilitates	Resignation Coping Modes: Vulnerable (Disconnected) Child; Angry Child; Avoidant Coping Modes: Detached Protector (dissociative); Detached Self-Soother; *Helpless Surrenderer	As a child, what were the values that were important to your family? Which was more important in your family: success and status, or other things? What meant most to your parents as you were growing up? How much interest did your family show in the experiences and suffering of fellow others in the world who are suffering (e.g., other people, animals, nature)?

avoidance of sense of emptiness, meaninglessness of life; Use of drugs, alcohol.

Inversion:
Clings to pseudo-control and meaning, such as by focusing on tangible materialistic life goals (e.g., accumulation of possessions, wealth, appearance, weight) and overcontrolling behaviours (e.g., obsessional rituals, eating-disordered rituals); Objectifies self and others in attempt to find tangible meaning and purpose; Pretends to have a strong sense of control and meaning.

Inversion Coping Modes:
*Pollyanna/*Pretender

Was your family part of a church or any other spiritual group? Did this resonate for you? Were you able to feel a sense of belonging of fulfilment in this community?
How much time/energy was spent on supporting charities or other people outside of the family?
How much opportunity did you have to connect with nature? How much time did you spend with your parents in the outdoors in natural or wild environments?

* Proposed additional schemas/modes and associated unmet needs are based on recent theoretical developments by Arntz et al. [13] Aalbers et al. [33], Simpson and Smith [34], and Edwards [35, 36].

Table 3.2 Common key problems in schema treatment as related to typical mode patterns

Reported Problem Area	Potential Mode
Chronic or acute anxiety or panic	Vulnerable Child mode
Chronic or acute depression	Vulnerable Child mode, Punitive (Parent) Critic mode, Detached Protector mode
Low self-esteem	Punitive (Parent) Critic mode
Anger dysregulation	Angry Child mode
Aggression	Angry Child mode, Bully and Attack mode
Relationship problem – assertiveness	Compliant Surrenderer mode
Relationship problem – control	Overcontroller mode, Self-Aggrandiser mode
Relationship problem – lack of intimacy	Detached Protector mode, Avoidant Protector mode
Worry and rumination	Overcontroller mode (Over-analyser type)
Perfectionism	Perfectionistic Overcontroller mode
Hopelessness	Helpless Surrender mode; Avoidant Protector mode
Stress/pressure/burnout	Perfectionistic Overcontroller mode, Demanding (Parent) Critic mode
Withdrawal, avoidance of relationships and activities	Avoidant Protector mode
Shut down, loss of motivation and interest, lack of connection to positive affect	Detached Protector mode
Binge drinking (or other compulsive or addictive behaviour)	Detached Self-Soother, Impulsive Child mode

term. Third, a clear problem list informs the goals of treatment, by which the effectiveness of therapy will be judged. Whether therapy has been effective can only be determined by referring to its goals and objectives. Table 3.2 outlines key problem areas that commonly present in chronic and complex clients seeking schema therapy, and the schemas and mode categories they might commonly reflect. Most clients will manifest a combination of modes, depending on their individual case conceptualisation.

Diagnosis in Schema Therapy Treatment

The challenges of assessment vary across client groups. For some presenting problems, the client will be insufficiently forthcoming with information to understand what maintains the problem. In these cases, making a formal psychiatric diagnosis (e.g., DSM-5 or ICD-10) can help the clinician access information about areas that are likely to be over- or under-reported by clients with that diagnosis. For example, clients with borderline personality disorder will often provide a detailed description of their emotional struggles but need more guidance with identifying coping behaviours that perpetuate their unmet needs. In contrast, clients with narcissistic personality disorder will require a concerted effort from the therapist to delineate what the presenting issues are, and what the client's worst fears are, should their difficulties remain unchanged. In addictions and eating disorders the focus should be on identifying the underlying suffering and unmet emotional needs that drive the urge for compulsive avoidance. Furthermore, because efficacy studies usually select clients who fit specific diagnostic categories, identifying a client who also fits these categories gives the therapist more confidence that a specific therapeutic approach or treatment format is likely to be successful. On the other hand, many clients have experienced significant stigma related to either receiving particular diagnoses or the process of being 'diagnosed'. We attest that while forming a diagnostic impression can inform the schema therapist, its ultimate usefulness will depend on the client and their experiences of diagnosis. Schema therapy can be described as a transdiagnostic model that works with common processes (e.g., self-criticism, emotional detachment, avoidance) rather than diagnostic categories per se; therefore, schema therapy can be applied with clients who are not seeking a mental health diagnosis but who can identify significant problem areas as a focus for treatment. Box 3.1 provides an overview of the initial schema-focused assessment session.

Box 3.1 Summary of Initial Assessment Session(s)

Aims

- Establish a therapeutic connection or bond
- Explore unmet needs linked to childhood or adolescent experiences
- Assess strength of schemas and modes through observation of non-verbals, language (content), countertransference, and questionnaires
- Explore the client's capacity to describe their internal world, including emotions, thoughts, and interoceptive experience
- Look for patterns within the manifestation of symptoms over time
- Develop hypotheses regarding the client's dominant modes and dynamics between modes
- Assess strength of the client's Healthy Adult self. How much compassion do they show themselves? To what degree are they able to take responsibility for their decisions and day-to-day lives, to regulate their emotions?
- Assess suitability for treatment

Therapeutic Stance

- Warmth, presence, and attunement
- Compassionate stance based on tuning in to the client, how much compassion do they show themselves? To what degree are they able to take responsibility for their problems? How is the level of eye contact?

Essential Topics to Cover

- Presenting issues (history and current manifestation)
- Begin exploration of developmental, family, and educational history throughout childhood and adolescence as it relates to current difficulties, paying particular attention to attachment disruptions. Explore relationships with caregivers within and since childhood
- Why they want treatment now: reasons (and fears) that led them to seek help at this time
- Previous therapy/treatment experiences
- Risk assessment (acute comorbid disorder or risk which requires immediate hospitalisation?)
- Enquire about personal goals for therapy: What does the client want to work on? How will you know when this has been achieved? Try to link goals to specific behavioural changes

- Ask for feedback: check in at the end of the session regarding the client's emotional reactions to you (therapist) and the session
- Clarify your (therapist's) understanding of the client's difficulties so far and ask for feedback in terms of whether this resonates with the client's experience
- Clarify what the client can expect over the assessment period, and how long this is likely to take (i.e., how many sessions)
- Identify factors which may limit efficacy or require some degree of adjustment to the treatment, such as IQ, acute psychosis, or neurodiversity (including ADHD, ASD)
- Allow venting about previous therapy experiences
- Hand out questionnaires and assign relevant reading as take-home tasks
- Begin the process of conceptualisation, the most relevant treatment format: short-term; longer-term; group/individual?

Conceptualising Modes Based on Process Information and Countertransference
- Identify client modes via patterns of speech, content, tone, and countertransference reactions
- Hypothesise about which modes are manifested by the way in which the client tells their story

- ### Assessing Suitability for Treatment

- Assess client ability for treatment: regular sessions, and management of risk through self-harm and suicide risk

Structuring the Initial Assessment Session

First Assessment Session Aims. The first session may take up to 90 minutes, with the goal of beginning to develop a therapeutic bond and simultaneously gaining a preliminary understanding of the client's difficulties. We invite the client to describe in their own words, and from their perspective, the main problems and their reasons for seeking help. As the client tells their story, the therapist's goal is to deepen their understanding of the issues and to identify 'what happened' (or didn't happen) during the client's early years that contributed to the development of their current difficulties. The therapist explores which needs may not have been met during the client's life. Throughout, the therapist assesses the extent to which the client can describe their inner experience, including emotions, thoughts, and interoceptive sensations. At this early stage, the therapist does not give corrective advice or suggestions, as the client may experience this as invalidating. This is especially true for clients whose childhood was characterised by invalidation or well-meaning but 'empty' validation consisting of platitudes, general reassurance, and advice. Instead, the therapist focuses on attuning to the client's experience and being as emotionally present and attentive as possible. The presence and strength of schemas and modes is assessed through the triangulation of multiple sources of information, including self-monitoring tools, observation of non-verbal behaviour, language (content), countertransference, questionnaire data, and imagery exercises. This information will eventually be collated into a schema therapy case conceptualisation or *mode map* depicting hypotheses about the client's dominant modes and the dynamics between modes.

First Session Therapeutic Stance: Emotional Presence and Co-Regulation. As the client tells their story, the schema therapist tries to be as emotionally present and validating as possible. Emotional presence requires the therapist to be in a centred state, aware of their own experience, so that they can 'be with' the client without becoming flooded by their own – or the client's – emotional reactions. Dan Siegel uses the acronym COAL to describe the ingredients of emotional presence: Curiosity, Openness, Acceptance, and Love [1]. The therapist remains a safe recipient of whatever the client needs to express. The therapist remains 'with' the client as they experience whatever they experience, including what will often feel like overwhelming emotions. Instead of providing advice at this early stage, schema therapists want the client to have an experience of being attuned to and getting their needs met from the very first session. To attune to the client, the therapist needs to be willing to experience feeling vulnerable so that their emotions resonate with the client's experience. In schema therapy, attunement is not simply listening and summarising/paraphrasing to show we understand – it is listening deeply and showing that we really *care* about the client's internal reactions and experience; we aim for the client to have the experience of *feeling felt and seen*. As much as possible, the therapist needs to slow the interview down: for example, 'I really want to understand this . . . can we slow this down a bit, can you tell me what that experience was like for you?' The therapist conveys warmth, empathy, and care through eye gaze and tone of voice. The therapist aims to partially recreate the relationship of mother–infant bonding: a contained, 'stable base' providing emotional co-regulation for the client as they become aware of and describe difficult psychological experiences (see Chapter 6: Intervention Strategies for Schema Healing 1: Limited Reparenting). The therapeutic relationship provides enough emotional security to enable the client to go out into the world and continue their emotional development whilst learning to express themselves and connect authentically with others. Emotional regulation and stability are provided and internalised through the process of the client exploring and expressing their emotions in the presence of a therapist who remains attentive, calm, and caring, rather than through the therapist teaching regulation skills. Just as a child learns to regulate their own emotions through the soothing, attuned presence of a parent, our clients can learn to regulate themselves via this same process (limited reparenting).

Linking Past and Present. The therapist tentatively suggests links between current difficulties and early experiences, checking whether their hypotheses resonate with the client. Box 3.2 illustrates this process.

Exploring the Client's Coping Repertoire. When enquiring about presenting symptoms, behavioural urges, and coping strategies, our goal is to identify how these have evolved since childhood, and how they are linked to underlying schemas and schema modes. Schema- and mode-driven behavioural patterns and symptoms often manifest in different ways over the lifespan, so the therapist should not assume that current coping strategies exhaust the client's repertoire and enquire about ways of coping at other times in the client's life. Box 3.3 illustrates a query to assess coping strategies.

We might also enquire about how other family members and friends perceive the client's problems and what advice they have received from them. Further, we would investigate what (if any) professional treatment they have received in the past, and to what degree this was helpful.

Recognising and Making Sense of Body Experience. As the therapist explores the client's experience, it is also important to understand their experience of physical sensations in the body – their interoceptive felt sense linked to schemas and modes. Clinically significant

---

Box 3.2 Clinical Example of Linking Past and Present During Assessment

Miriam described feeling anxious every time her partner was late or was unable to take her calls at work. As a young child, her mother frequently raised the subject of leaving, telling Miriam that she didn't want to be a parent, that she had never wanted Miriam, and that she was a burden to her. When Miriam was telling her therapist about the panic that had led to an argument with her partner the previous week, the therapist hypothesised:

Therapist: As you are speaking about your history of romantic relationships, a part of me wonders if this might be linked to your experience as a child, when your mum would come and go, leaving you feeling alone and scared? And so, when your partner is late home from work, in your mind's eye you teleport back to being that little girl, whose mother has threatened to leave you again. I might be making too much of a leap, but as you were describing the intensity of that sense of panic that you were experiencing, that possible association jumped out at me ... would that make sense to you?

Box 3.3 Clinical Example of Enquiring About Coping Strategies Across the Lifespan

Therapist: So, it seems that gambling is one way you have learned to cope ... when and how did this pattern emerge in your life? How old were you when this started? What about earlier in your life, were there any patterns of using distraction as a way of avoiding difficult emotions as a young child?

Box 3.4 Clinical Example of Identifying and Labelling Emotions During Assessment

Client: 'Well ... I notice my heart is racing, and my chest is tense, like I can't catch my breath. My throat is tight. My vision is blurry.'
   Therapist: Could you try closing your eyes, focusing on those sensations, and just notice the first image or word that comes up? I wonder if that feeling might be anxiety ... does that resonate for you? Or could it be scared, or worried? Or is there another word that might fit even better? Or alternatively, some people find it easier to use colours ... if those sensations had a colour, what would it be?

---

sensations might include smells, tastes, muscle tension, 'heaviness', fatigue, temperature changes, nausea, or agitation. We might ask 'When you are describing this event to me now, what are you noticing in your body?' Answers may reveal body-experiences linked to schema modes. For clients who have little or no experience of labelling their emotions, this begins to develop their emotional literacy; the therapist helps the client make sense of their sensations by suggesting emotion labels that are likely to fit with their experience. In the words of Dan Siegel [2], 'name it to tame it' refers to the notion that putting the felt sense of emotions into words increases one's understanding of emotions and reduces their overwhelming impact. Box 3.4 illustrates how the clinician might assist clients to label their emotions.

Assess Strength of the Client's Healthy Adult Self. From the first session we begin to assess the strength of the client's Healthy Adult self. Healthy Adult abilities include the capacity to show compassion for their own vulnerability and suffering, and to exercise self-care. Many clients will have high-functioning coping modes that mask the fact that their Healthy Adult mode is actually very underdeveloped – what Dialectical Behaviour Therapists call 'apparent competence' [3]. Detached Protector, Overcontroller, Self-Aggrandiser, and Compliant Surrenderer can all appear to fulfil the functions of Healthy Adult, but underneath there is very little self-compassion. A litmus test for the compassionate strength of the Healthy Adult is the 'Child in the Street' exercise [4], wherein the client is asked to imagine themselves approaching a child who they find crying in the street. As they approach the child, they notice their responses, emotions, and urges. Then they are guided to notice that the child is their own inner Vulnerable Child. Clients are asked to notice whether their responses stay the same or change once they realise the child is them.

Discuss Previous Therapy Relationships. Giving the client an opportunity to talk and/or complain about previous therapists is also an important option in the assessment phase that can provide some insight into the client's EMS triggers (e.g., hypersensitivity to feeling misunderstood, invalidated). This can help the therapist to anticipate potential therapeutic ruptures associated with client schema activation. For example, clients with BPD may have developed a pattern of elevating therapists to 'rescuer' status early in the relationship, and then felt abandoned when they have not been available due to therapist illness or extended leave. Miriam described several previous therapists who had terminated the therapy before she was 'ready'. She had pleaded with them to continue to work with her and was angry when therapy ended. She also described feeling anxious when therapists were away on holidays and had tried to recruit several therapists to support her all at once. This was a clear indication that her Abandonment EMS was being activated within the therapeutic setting and signalled to the schema therapist to focus on the impact of this schema on treatment from the outset.

Questionnaires. Questionnaires may be given out at the end of the first session. However, for those with a strong overcompensatory coping style, it can be worthwhile to either wait before administering the questionnaires or give the questionnaires again after 8–10 weeks of therapy, once the client is displaying some of the vulnerability and suffering that lies underneath the coping modes. A list of suggested questionnaires is included in the section on *Schema Therapy Questionnaires*.

Logistical Issues. In the first session, important aspects of the therapeutic relationship are clarified, including therapy times (length of sessions), conditions of payment (where required), and cancellation policy, and a contract for informed consent is signed. The client is invited to ask any questions they might have about the therapeutic contract. Clarification of the proposed length, phases, and format of therapy are gradually introduced towards the end of the assessment period, once the therapist has developed a clear case conceptualisation and treatment plan.

Conceptualising Modes Based on Process Information and Countertransference. Depending on which of the client's modes are active or 'front stage' in the assessment sessions, the therapist will need to adjust the content of the interview accordingly. For example, a client with an avoidant (e.g., Detached Protector mode) or overcompensatory (Self-Aggrandiser, Overcontroller) style of relating to others might discuss a history of abuse or neglect in a detached manner, whereby their emotional reaction has become disconnected from their narrative. They may dismiss the importance of early attachments or losses or describe their childhood as 'fine' or 'great'. The person may even idealise their childhood or minimise the impact of early unmet needs without being able to convey a balance of positive and negative experiences. The therapist might also notice their own 'countertransference' reaction of detachment or disinterest towards the client, in contrast to their usual attitude of interest and empathy. A client in Overcontroller mode might describe their experiences in an overly detailed way, focusing on the facts of the events but neglecting their emotional impact. The countertransference response in the therapist might be boredom, frustration, or a sense of powerlessness. A client in Compliant Surrenderer mode may also minimise the impact of childhood events whilst focusing more on others' needs and the negative impact that they have had on others by not fulfilling their expectations or aspirations. In Compliant Surrenderer mode, the client may be more tuned in to the therapist's needs, telling the therapist what they think that they want to hear. The countertransference response might initially include a positive feeling linked to a sense that 'we are on the same page', followed by feeling stuck when the therapist notices the client 'paying lip service' to the process but not authentically connecting to their Vulnerable Child self. The therapist needs to remain tuned in to the within-session presentation and behaviour of the client and to be guided by constantly questioning 'what mode could this be?' In all of these examples, the coping modes are 'front stage', dominating the client's conscious perspective on the world, whereas their child modes are likely to be 'back stage', meaning information relating to their emotional experience is less available. This informs the therapist the extent to which strategies for bypassing coping modes are needed to reach the hidden child modes.

Assessing the Client's Suitability for Schema Therapy. An important component of schema therapy assessment is evaluating the client's suitability to begin therapeutic work. Many clients experience regular crises as a central part of their mental health difficulties. This does not preclude them from accessing therapy; in fact, a significant period of therapeutic work will be dedicated to emotional bonding and stabilisation. However, if instability is so significant that the client is unable to attend sessions regularly, they may require preparatory practical support or stabilisation prior to starting schema therapy. Clients with acute comorbid disorders – such as severe depression, substance misuse, acute psychosis, and eating disorders – may require a hospital admission to bring about sufficient stability to enable them to begin a course of outpatient schema therapy. Risk posed by acute suicidality should also be assessed, with particular attention to coping resources. In schema therapy, analysing situations which provoke thoughts of suicide or self-harm is especially valuable in elucidating unmet emotional needs and associated schema modes. For example, many clients with longstanding difficulties report chronic suicidal ideation, which may represent a compulsive re-enactment of internalised messages of defectiveness and punitiveness. Alternatively, suicide or self-harm may serve one or more coping function (e.g., escape from distress). The schema therapist should explore and formulate links between schemas, modes, and suicidality, and associated risk. Which modes might be driving the risk? Which modes want the client to self-harm? This is valuable information for the risk assessment and will determine the degree to which additional mental health support services may need to be involved, and whether hospital admission and stabilisation are required before onset of therapy (e.g., in the case of severe depression and/or suicidal-ity). Other therapeutic approaches (e.g., dialectical behaviour therapy, acceptance and commitment therapy) may also be integrated during the initial phase of therapy to enhance coping and reduce risk [5] in preparation for implementing schema therapy.

Wrapping up the First Session. At the end of the first session, it can be useful to ask about the client's experience of the session and whether there were any aspects that made them feel uncomfortable. For example, a client with a history of rejection or abandonment may be highly rejection-sensitive and require more than usual reassurance about the therapist's availability to provide consistent care. Another client with a strong Mistrust/Abuse schema may be more likely to view warmth and empathy with suspicion and may react with disdain or cynicism. This 'checking in' allows the therapist to respond to any queries or anxieties that the client may have at the end of the session, to demonstrate curiosity about the client's internal experience in the here and now, and to further strengthen the therapeutic rapport through validation and attunement.

Comprehensive Schema Therapy Assessment (Sessions 2–8)

As the assessment proceeds beyond the initial 1–3 sessions, both therapist and client will be better able to gauge whether and how they will work together in the longer term. Should they continue to work together, assessment continues until sufficient information has been garnered from interviews, questionnaires, and the therapy relationship (process information and therapist countertransference reactions), to develop a preliminary case conceptualisation and mode map. This section describes all the areas the clinician should include over the course of the assessment phase to enable them to put together, and eventually present, a case conceptualisation to the client (see Chapter 4: Case Conceptualisation and Mode Mapping in Schema Therapy).

Assessment of Temperament. The therapist should enquire about the client's temperament (both as an infant and now) to help understand the mismatch between innate predisposition and parenting style that resulted in unmet needs during childhood and, in turn, to the formation of EMS. Temperament appears to influence both choice of coping style [6, 7], and emotional sensitivity and intensity [8]. Recent evidence suggests that at least 25% of the population may have a *highly sensitive* temperament, which, in turn, increases reactivity to the type of parenting received [8, 9]. These clients appear to thrive with highly nurturing parenting but are more susceptible to developing difficulties when faced with inadequate or adverse childhood circumstances.

The reader is directed to the extensive research on the role of temperament in personality development, including the work of Rothbart and colleagues [10] and Cloninger and colleagues [11]. The following dimensions were provided by Young, Klosko, and Weishaar [7] as a guide for assessing client temperament:

- Extraversion–Introversion
- Labile–Non-Reactive
- Dysthymic–Optimistic
- Anxious–Calm
- Obsessive/Perfectionistic–Distractable
- Passive–Aggressive
- Irritable–Cheerful
- Shy–Sociable

Assessment of Life History. A comprehensive life history assessment explores the inter-action between the client's temperament and unmet childhood emotional needs that have contributed to the development of EMS and schema modes. We suggest that eight main areas of *unmet needs* should be explored:

- *Secure Attachment and Connection to Others* – Children need the protection of a safe and reliable adult upon whom they can depend. Children need opportunities to connect and share their emotions, experiences, and thoughts with others. Children require attuned co-regulation during their early development to be able to modulate their emotions [12].
- *Freedom of Self-Expression* – Children need the freedom to express their emotions and views without the threat of being punished or restrained.
- *Play and Spontaneity* – Children need opportunities to play, have fun, and be spontaneous to enable them to develop a sense of connection and capacity for joy.
- *Autonomy* – Children need a secure, safe environment from which they can venture out to experience the world, discover their capacity to cope, and develop self-reliance and self-efficacy.
- *Realistic Limits* – Children need support to develop an understanding of societal rules to enable them to live in harmony alongside others, and guidance to learn how to deal with frustration.
- *Self-Coherence and Meaningful World* [13] – The healthy person knows who they are; they have an inner sense that a part of them is consistent and stable across moods and situations, and that feels secure and 'together'. The healthy person knows what they value and lives a meaningful life consistent with their values. They recognise their existence both as a separate and 'whole' individual as well as a being who is inextricably interconnected with all living beings. They have a sense of purpose that includes but extends beyond the individual. They experience a sense of self-determination and capacity to live a life that brings them joy, harmony, and purpose. Children need support to develop a sense of self and identity whereby they can feel positive about themselves and develop self-appreciation.
- *Physical Safety and Security* – Children need protection from physical harm, uncertainty, and pain. Children need to feel secure that they – and their significant others – are safe from physical harm or injury, illness, abuse, and financial collapse.
- *Connection to Nature* – People thrive when they feel connected with nature and all living creatures [14]. The ability to experience interconnectedness with all aspects of the universe, Earth, and nature is an essential source of well-being and nourishment [15, 16].

The extent to which the aforementioned needs have been met in the client's life will determine which EMS and modes are likely to have developed. Childhood physical, sexual, and emotional abuse are important areas of enquiry in a schema therapy assessment [17]. In the case of assessing emotional, physical, and sexual abuse, the therapist is looking at *experiences that happened but shouldn't have* within the person's childhood. However, many more clients have been affected by emotional neglect. In this case, the therapist is looking for ingredients that the client should have had as part of a healthy upbringing but missed out on: the *absence of childhood need satisfaction*. A significant proportion of the population are growing up 'under the radar', without adequate experiences of parental or family capacity for emotional availability, attunement, warmth, overt affection, nurturance, empathy, guidance, and feeling cherished. In these cases, the history-taking must be more nuanced, with greater use of hypothetical questions. Intergenerational sociograms or genograms [18] can be used to draw out interpersonal patterns and EMS that have been transmitted through successive generations. This may also include societal problems and traumas associated with discrimination and historical atrocities based on race and sexuality. Cultural factors and intergenerational patterns should be explored alongside intra-familial patterns, including family attitudes towards physical touch, emotional expression, gender roles, body objectification, and so on. Asking about unmet needs within the parents' and grandparents' childhoods can also be a helpful starting point, before moving on to explore ways in which the client's parents' parenting style was the same or different from their grandparents' parenting style. For example: 'What do you know about your mum's childhood? What were the good bits and the difficult bits that you know about? Is that something you could ask her more about? I wonder if she parented you in a similar way to the parenting she received, or whether she tried to do things differently? If there were improvements, what were they? What were the parts of parenting that might have been a struggle for her because of her own childhood?' For further assessment questions linked to specific schemas, see Table 3.1.

Generally, when clients can describe their childhood in a coherent, balanced way which includes both positive and negative aspects of their experience, and they are able to describe repeated instances in which a particular need was met – without the need to idealise or minimise the impact of their experiences – the therapist can assume that this need was adequately met.

In the Appendix to this chapter, you will find more detailed suggestions for questions that we have found useful to help the therapist explore the relevance of each of these needs. They are not exhaustive and should not be used as a 'checklist' per se, but offer a guide as to lines of questioning that are often useful to explore the client's childhood background through an attachment and 'needs' lens.

Schema Questionnaires. Schema therapists vary greatly in how they administer and utilise questionnaires. On most occasions, these will be handed to clients to fill out as homework between sessions. However, when working with clients with high levels of trauma or dissociation, or who are very easily overwhelmed, it can be helpful to cover the questionnaires more slowly during a session to try to keep within the 'window of tolerance' (the zone of arousal which is optimal for receiving, processing, and integrating information) [19] while completing them.

- **Young Schema Questionnaire (YSQ-L3 (Young & Brown, 2003) [20]; YSQ-S3 (Young, 2005) [21], YSQ-R [22]** measures 18 EMS, with a 6-point Likert scale that ranges from a score of 1 (*Completely untrue of me*) to a score of 6 (*Describes me perfectly*). To guide clinical use, Young has recommended looking at items with high rating (i.e., 5 or 6) and interpreting as clinically meaningful any EMS for which 3 high-rating items have been endorsed on the long version (YSQ-L3) or 2 items have been endorsed on the short version (YSQ-S3). The YSQ-S3 was validated using community as well as clinical samples [23]. Internal consistency and Cronbach's alpha reliability was >0.70 for 17 of the EMS, except for Entitlement. A validation study by Bach, Simonsen, Christoffersen, and Kriston [24] found all 18 EMS had a Cronbach's alpha value of >0.70. The subscales of the YSQ-S3 were also found to be meaningfully linked with personality disorders. Clients with strong overcompensatory modes may generate artificially low scores on core EMS in the Disconnection and Rejection domain. In this case, consider using other measures, such as the Young Parenting Inventory [25] or Young Parenting Inventory-Revised [26]. Recently, Yalcin, Marais, Lee, and Correia used item response theory analyses to create a new short version, the YSQ-R, containing only items with the best psychometric characteristics. This analysis also led to a reconceptualisation of the Emotional Inhibition schema as better representing two separate factors of Emotional Constriction and Fear of Losing Control (of emotions) and the Punitiveness schema as having separate factors: Punitiveness (Self-Directed) and Punitiveness (Other-Directed). The YSQ-R and scorer are available from the journal article's website [22].

- **Young Parenting Inventory-revised (YPI-R2; Louis, Wood & Lockwood, 2018)** [25] assesses perceived negative parenting. The YPI-R2 is a 36-item questionnaire measuring parenting styles, namely: Competitiveness and Status seeking; Degradation and Rejection; Emotional Inhibition and Deprivation; Overprotection and Overindulgence; Punitiveness; Controlling. Subscale scores are calculated as mean scores, with higher scores indicating stronger perceived negative parenting. The YPI-R has been shown to be a reliable and valid measure of perceived parenting [26].
- **The Schema Mode Inventory (SMI V1.1; Young et al., 2007)** [27] is a self-report measure consisting of 124 items designed to assess 14 schema modes, which includes 5 dysfunctional coping modes, namely Compliant Surrenderer, Detached Self-Soother, Detached Protector, Bully and Attack, and Self-Aggrandiser. A 6-point Likert scale ranging from 1 (*never or almost never*) to 6 (*all of the time*) is used to rate each item. The overall score for the individual schema mode is calculated by the sum score of each scale, which is then divided by the number of items on that scale. The higher the calculated schema mode score, the more pervasive the mode.
- **Positive Schema Questionnaire (PSQ; Louis, Wood, & Lockwood, 2018)** [28] is a self-report measure consisting of 56 items rated on a 6-point Likert scale ranging from 1 (*never or almost never*) to 6 (*all of the time*). This questionnaire was designed to assess early adaptive schemas linked to 14 themes – Emotional Fulfilment; Success; Empathic Consideration; Basic Health and Safety/Optimism; Emotional Openness and Spontaneity; Self-Compassion; Healthy Boundaries/Developed Self; Social Belonging; Healthy Self-Control/Self-Discipline; Realistic Expectations; Self-Directedness; Healthy Self-Interest /Self-Care; Stable Attachment; Healthy Self-Reliance/Competence. This scale has been found to have good factorial validity, cross-cultural stability, and excellent reliability [27].
- **Life Events Checklist (LEC-5; Weathers et al., 2013)** [29] – When it comes to clients divulging trauma in the assessment phase, we have found that for some clients it can be a case of 'don't ask, don't tell'. For these clients, if you do not ask directly about trauma, it may be many sessions down the line until the client divulges this. We have found the Life Events Checklist for DSM-5 (LEC-5) to be a useful self-report screen for potential traumatic events across a respondent's lifetime. The LEC-5 assesses exposure to 16 events known to commonly predict subsequent PTSD or distress and includes an additional open question designed to pick up events not covered explicitly by the checklist. There is no formal scoring protocol or interpretation per se. In a schema therapy assessment, the checklist will pick up potentially traumatic incidents to be followed up. It is particularly important to ascertain the impact of any of these events both on the client's current functioning, and on their childhood development, if any of these events occurred during childhood.

Questionnaire scores can be explored collaboratively in the form of bar graphs, which will enable the therapist to focus on which EMS or modes are relatively high and which are unexpectedly low. Alternatively, questionnaires can be used more qualitatively, by exploring each of the client's main schemas in turn, in terms of relevant childhood and adolescent experiences (and unmet needs) as well as current patterns that have evolved from these. The

YSQ can be used to explore schema themes and unmet needs that are linked to these. As the therapist provides feedback regarding the questionnaire scores, the client can be asked for examples from different aspects of their lives. The therapist may choose to focus on the schemas with the highest questionnaire scores, or it may be more fruitful to focus on the schemas for which scores are relatively high in the case of an individual whose scores are suppressed across all EMS. For clients who only report secondary/compensatory schemas, the therapist may choose to explore the aspects of life that the client avoids, to shed more light on the underlying core schemas. For example, a client may endorse a high Unrelenting Standards and Self-Sacrifice schema on the YSQ, but core schemas appear unsubstantial. However, the therapist notes that the client has attended therapy due to marital dissatisfaction, alongside a longstanding pattern of consistently forming relationships with emotionally unavailable partners, so explores the possibility of an underlying Emotional Deprivation schema that is hidden by powerful coping modes. If the client's responses have been obscured by a highly avoidant or overcompensatory coping mode, then it can be useful to revisit these later in therapy, once coping modes have been bypassed and the client is able to complete questionnaires from a more authentic perspective. Coping modes may also arise as the therapist provides feedback on questionnaire results, in terms of how the person describes events and associated unmet needs. For example, someone with a strong Detached Protector mode may say something like, 'that's all in the past, I'm over that now, I've dealt with it and don't see the point of dwelling on that stuff'. All responses provide data that can help the therapist make sense of the client's presentation and feed into the mode conceptualisation. The therapist can also enquire about how the client found the process of filling out the questionnaires as a means of exploring the role of schemas and modes. An exploration of both schemas and modes can enrich the case conceptualisation by fine tuning the understanding of how schemas and modes operate under different circumstances, and the 'flavours' of the modes, based on underlying schemas, unmet needs, typical triggers, and emotional felt sense. Examples of different 'core emotional flavours' of the Vulnerable Child mode are described in Table 3.3.

Imagery in Assessment. Diagnostic imagery is a powerful technique for identifying links between presenting issues, coping behaviours, early experiences of unmet childhood needs, and the origins of EMS. Many chronic and complex clients are unable to report the details of schema-related experiences (e.g., specific triggers, feelings, bodily sensations, meaning aspects) during traditional interviewing. In these cases, imagery – which has a strong connection to emotional memory [30] – can be used to activate the schema within the session to make its contents more accessible. Imaginal assessment helps the therapist and client develop a deeper, experiential understanding of the schema. There are two main types of imagery for assessment:

1) *Imagery of a recent event* – The therapist asks the client to recall a recent episode of the problem being triggered but, rather than simply discussing it, asks the client to close their eyes and relive the recent episode, relaying the experience as though they were there. Although the primary purpose of the exercise is to help identify problem-schema-coping relationships, this kind of imagery task is also a good indicator of the client's capacity to manage affect. If the client has some difficulty regulating affect during this kind of recent imagery, it is unlikely they would be ready to process imagery focused on the past, especially childhood images which tend to be more overwhelming.

2) *Imagery of a historical event via 'Affect Bridge'* – If clients can handle recent images, an imagery affect bridge can be used to establish an experiential link between recent schema

Table 3.3 Assessment and identification of schema modes

Modes	Verbal Content	Non-verbal Gestures, Behaviours and Tone	Typical Body Experience and Urges	Countertransference Reactions	Mode 'Agenda'	Therapist Pitfalls
Child Modes						
Vulnerable Child	Describes & expresses emotions in authentic manner.	Tone of voice and posture indicates vulnerability, sadness, anxiety, loneliness, overwhelm. May be child-like, terrified of abandonment, tearful.	Increased activity in the upper chest area, changes in breathing and heart rate. Decreased limb activity.	Compassion, empathy, connection. Therapist can 'feel' the client's feelings in the room. (May trigger therapist's emotional inhibition schema, leading to detachment.)	To communicate needs, emotions.	Therapist stays too cognitive and does not stay emotionally present. Limited reparenting is too general and not attuned to client's unmet needs.
Angry Child	Acting out anger in child-like way to show others how much hurt they have caused. Blames therapist or others. 'I hate you! It's not fair!'	Facial expression either overtly or passively angry. Overt: Slams doors, shouts, throws things. Covert: Silently punishes others (e.g. through missing appointments, acting in sullen manner).	Sensations of approach/ aggression in head, upper limbs, and torso.	Anxiety, defensiveness (may trigger therapist's Subjugation, Emotional Inhibition &/or Mistrust/ Abuse, and Punitiveness schemas).	To show others the hurt they have caused, by acting out or punishing them.	Therapist becomes defensive and makes excuses. Therapist becomes angry at client and fights back. Therapist detaches and loses connection with client. Therapist allows client to vent endlessly without setting limits.

Undisciplined Child	'I can't do it, it's too hard, too uncomfortable!'	Cancels or does not attend sessions at short notice. Pays 'lip service' to homework – then avoids tasks which may cause distress or discomfort. Does not complete homework, does not pay for sessions on time.	Mild discomfort in the legs and stomach.	Frustration, anger, punitiveness, urge to control (may trigger therapist's Failure or Unrelenting Standards, or Punitiveness Schema).	To escape discomfort, to avoid sense of failure.	Therapist colludes with client's avoidance of discomfort, steering away from difficult topics. Therapist takes all-or-nothing (rather than a graduated approach) to setting therapy session and homework tasks.
Impulsive Child	'I want it now!'	Seeks immediate gratification, impatient, easily frustrated or irritated.	Excitement, urge to respond to take risks/what they want. Anger in chest and extremities if thwarted.	Anxiety (regarding risk-issues).	To bypass obstacles to freedom. To take what I want/need before my freedom is taken from me.	Therapist avoids raising issue of boundary transgressions. Therapist does not recognise unmet needs associated with impulsive acting out.
Inner Critic (Internalised) Modes						
Punitive mode	'I'm a bad person; There is something wrong with me; I am defective, flawed, unlovable'.	Self-punishment, self-harm.	Increased sensations in the head, chest (shame), digestive system, and around the throat region (disgust). Urge to hide, freeze, avoid.	Intimidated.	To punish self and sabotage recovery (due to belief that they don't deserve happiness).	Therapist is not sufficiently assertive in setting limits on this mode.

Table 3.3 (cont.)

Modes	Verbal Content	Non-verbal Gestures, Behaviours and Tone	Typical Body Experience and Urges	Countertransference Reactions	Mode 'Agenda'	Therapist Pitfalls
Demanding mode	'I should try harder; Where is the extra 10%?'	Produces 'perfect' homework, tries to get everything 'right', striving for flawless recovery.		Pressure to meet client's high expectations.	To push client to reach high standards instead of taking care of self.	Therapist colludes with this mode by setting unrealistically high standards for self and client.
Guilt-Inducing mode	'I'm undeserving, a burden.'	Dismisses/ minimises own needs, and pushes for recovery only to reduce impact of client's problems on others.		Anger (on behalf of client).	To make client feel guilty for placing emphasis on own recovery and future happiness.	Therapist is not sufficiently assertive in setting limits on this mode.
Coping Modes						
Detached Protector/Self-Soother	Describes problems in detached way. When asked about how they feel, they commonly answer 'I don't know'.	Zoned out, numb, yawning, 'downloading' information in detached or cynical, or Pollyanna (excessively upbeat or positive) manner.	Deactivation of sensations, depersonalisation, body rigidity creating separation from others.	Fatigue, sleepiness, zoning out, boredom 'walking through mud', frustration. (May trigger therapist's Failure schema due to lack of progress.)	To detach, avoid vulnerability associated with schema activation (e.g., to avoid being hurt, rejected, overwhelmed, humiliated, losing control).	Detached Protector is mistaken for Healthy Adult mode. Therapist is insufficiently 'relentless' in bypassing this mode.

Angry Protector	Becomes annoyed if therapist suggests experiential work: 'Why do we have to do this stupid imagery work anyway?'	Hostile, annoyed, irritated. Implicit message 'I don't need you!'	Tension or 'hardening' of the upper and lower diaphragm area, neck, jaw. Holding breath. Urge to shut others out, withdraw.	Intimidated, with urge to comply by avoiding experiential work (may trigger therapist's Subjugation schema).	To avoid interactions which will lead to vulnerability due to fear of humiliation, rejection, abandonment etc.)	Therapist backs off and enables avoidance of vulnerability by sticking to 'safe' topics.
Complaining Protector	Gives details of perceived problem-issues or problem-people in a repetitive, detailed manner. Seeks 'solutions' but then rejects these: 'yes, but …' and/or 'that doesn't work'.	Complains in a relentless, detached manner.	Pulling shoulders up, arms and legs crossed or tucked close to the body, hunched posture. Chin pulled down. Eye gaze and expression may convey passive hostility.	Feeling trapped, stuck, frustrated, impotent. (May trigger therapist's Subjugation & Self-Sacrifice schemas.) May trigger therapist's Unrelenting Standards schema, leading to an urge to give advice, & 'fix' the problems.	As above.	Complaining Protector is mistaken for Vulnerable Child, so therapist responds with reparenting, whilst avoiding empathic confrontation.
Compliant Surrenderer	Agrees with everything that therapist suggests, goes along with suggestions, carries out homework diligently.	Smiley, pleasant, agreeable façade. May compliment therapist. Attempts to take care of therapist's needs by bringing gifts, and is overly accommodating.	Posture is overly accommodating, leans forward, allows others to invade personal space. Apologetic for taking up space.	Feeling stuck, frustration at inability to access client's true needs and feelings.	To avoid conflict & rejection.	Therapist reacts by making all decisions rather than accessing client needs and emotions.

Table 3.3 (cont.)

Modes	Verbal Content	Non-verbal Gestures, Behaviours and Tone	Typical Body Experience and Urges	Countertransference Reactions	Mode 'Agenda'	Therapist Pitfalls
Self-Aggrandiser	Describes self in grandiose or entitled way, and considers others as 'the problem'.	Values therapist only insofar as they provide gratification (recognition, approval).	Arms outstretched or elbows outward with hands behind head. Limbs open, taking up available space. Chin up, eye gaze may 'look down on' others.	Feels devalued, used, powerless.	To distance self from underlying sense of worthlessness, shame, loneliness. To be 'on top' of all interactions.	Therapist waits too long to use empathic confrontation and limit setting. Therapist colludes with recognition-seeking, and client does not learn how to tolerate nurturance as Vulnerable Child.
Overcontroller	Intellectualising, pontificating, overanalysing. Describing rules, and situations in excessive detail. Presents self as all-knowing, knowledgeable, well-read.	Denies vulnerability & compensates through engaging in intellectual debates or power struggles with others. Takes control of therapy, sets the agenda, prefers to focus on cognitive work & finding logical solutions.	Closed posture, rigid, tense. Furrowed brow. Narrowed gaze. Tense expression.	Compulsion to be drawn into power struggles and micro-level debates. Therapist feels scrutinised, powerless, controlled, under pressure to get things right, to avoid mistakes, to be effective and productive. Relationship is viewed as a transaction.	To distance self from vulnerability through perfectionism, knowledge, productivity, invincibility. May also use self-flagellation & deprivation used as mechanism to gain sense of control, safety, atonement, propitiation.	Therapist mistakes Overcontroller for Healthy Adult. Therapist engages in intellectualisation, debates, power struggles. Therapist allows Overcontroller to take control of sessions, and avoids empathic confrontation. Therapist fails to recognise self-flagellation as coping mechanism and assumes it is Punitive mode.

Mode					
Helpless Surrenderer/Victim mode.	Describes difficulties in intense, helpless, passive manner. Pays lip service to therapeutic goals, with underlying agenda of seeking a 'perfect' parent who will take care of & never abandon them.	Presents self as fragile and helpless (can include illness behaviour). Expresses vulnerability in slightly inauthentic manner, as a means of seeking 'rescue' & protection. Presents as helpless & dependent, but if confronted, may move into Victim stance: 'You don't care about me'.	Looks down, averts eye gaze. Hunched/ collapsed posture. Hugs legs to chest/torso.	Initially: urge to rescue, and take on role of 'saviour' (may trigger therapist's Self-Sacrifice schema with excessive responsibility; May trigger sense of grandiosity in therapist within 'rescuer' role). Later: irritation, trapped, powerless, manipulated, urge to refer on (may trigger therapist's Self-Sacrifice schema – therapist feels guilty about difficulties accessing empathy).	To legitimise needs through helplessness, illness, fragility. To provide Abandoned Child with a substitute parent to avoid underlying pain of unmet needs associated with abandonment dependency, emotional deprivation.	Therapist mistakes Helpless Surrenderer as Vulnerable Child mode and does not use empathic confrontation. Therapist gratifies the mode through reparenting, rather than trying to access underlying Abandoned Child. Therapist enables avoidance of responsibility and does not bring client's Healthy Adult into chair work and imagery rescripting early enough. Therapist allows boundaries to become blurred (offers longer sessions, high contact between sessions, avoids setting termination date).

Healthy Modes

Healthy Adult (Higher Self)	Client takes responsibility for change; sets realistic goals; takes healthy	Uses healthy emotional regulation strategies	Upright posture, open expression, openness of chest/torso area. Relaxed expression,	Feeling connected with client on an 'equal' adult basis. Can trust client to take care of themselves, to	To heal the child modes through developing self-compassion and	Therapist takes on role of Healthy Adult too much (or for too long) instead of coaching

Table 3.3 (cont.)

Modes	Verbal Content	Non-verbal Gestures, Behaviours and Tone	Typical Body Experience and Urges	Countertransference Reactions	Mode 'Agenda'	Therapist Pitfalls
	steps to access support; seeks healthy connections with others; takes steps to get emotional needs met in healthy relationships; focuses energy on areas of mastery/achievement to strengthen sense of self-expression; assertively and compassionately protects own boundaries (from others' demands, work, etc.); sense of self is 'embodied' – based on being in the body and in tune with body signals; seeks sense of self and meaning that is interconnected with all living beings.	(especially connection) to enable them to tolerate distress associated with trauma processing; takes care of self and body.	maintains healthy level of eye contact.	prioritise their own needs; to carry out homework tasks between sessions.	learning to get emotional needs met; to regulate emotions through top-down (mindful problem-solving) and bottom-up (embodiment) processes; to embrace and transform coping modes, to set limits on Parent (Inner Critic) modes and Angry/Impulsive/Undisciplined child modes. Developing a sense of meaning and connection based on 'inter-being' – understanding the connection between self and all living beings.	client to embody this role. Therapist stays too cognitive/rational, but lacks warmth, and attunement.

Contented Child	Client can have fun, be spontaneous, laugh and enjoy life; engages in activities for enjoyment and pleasure, rather than solely for achievement; expresses self in creative ways (e.g., through dance, music, art).	Uninhibited self-expression, laughs, cries, reacts in spontaneous manner.	Sensations in head, upper limbs, and torso, enhanced sensations all over the body.	Feels a sense of *connection* with playful spontaneous part of client.	To experience greater levels of joy, fun, spontaneity and contentment.	Therapist is striving due to their own Demanding Critic and places disproportionate energy into focusing on trauma processing without nurturing the Contented Child. Therapist is too stuck in their own Overcontroller mode, trying to get the therapy 'right', and follow the rules, but misses opportunities for emotional connection, and introducing fun and 'light' activities into therapy.

activation and its developmental antecedents. A useful starting point for this exercise is to ask the client to visualise a current trigger situation (e.g., an argument with a family member, a situation at work), noticing subsequent thoughts, feelings, and visceral felt sense. The client then focuses on the emotion (affect) to evoke childhood experiences (bridge) that generated similar feelings. This process is outlined in Box 3.5.

Box 3.5 Example Script: Imagery Affect Bridge for Assessment

<u>Start:</u> Choose a recent schema-triggering episode that the client would like to examine (e.g., triggered by a colleague at work).

Step 1. Close Eyes and Activate a Memory
Therapist: Close your eyes and take me back to this recent episode. What is happening in the image? Take some time to thicken out the image . . . What do you see (hear, smell)? Are there any characters involved in the image?

Step 2. 'Tune in' to the Client's Feelings, Specific Triggers, and Meaning Derived From the Image
Tune in to the specific feelings and felt reaction in the body.

How do you feel in this image . . . and where do you feel that in your body?

Tune in to what seems to be the main trigger in the image. What's happening for the client to feel this way? Make sure the client is immersed in the image as indicated by them speaking in the first person, using the present tense. For example: 'I'm in the lunchroom, he's over by the door laughing'. It is often quite powerful to identify the hotspot in the image:

Therapist: What is the moment here in the image that is most painful for you? . . . OK, it is the fact that he is laughing at you . . .'

Tune in to the meaning/takeaway that the client derived from the experience.

What does it mean to you that this is happening?

Step 3. Affect Bridge: Float Back From the Recent Experience and Connect to a Relevant Childhood Image
OK . . . now that you are connected to that feeling . . . and that feeling in your body . . . we can let that image wash away a little bit . . . but stay with that feeling . . . the feeling of xxxxx [insert feeling label/bodily sensation/schema theme/meaning].

. . . You know . . . I'm willing to bet it's not the first time you've felt this way . . . this feeling of (e.g., being not good enough, and that feeling in your throat) . . . now let's gently take that feeling . . . and take it all the way back to being a little boy/girl . . . (pause) . . . what is the first image that comes up for you connected to this feeling . . . (pause) . . . (pause) what do you see . . . ?

Step 4. Elaborate the Relevant Childhood Image
What is happening in the image . . . what's happening for little x? Take some time to thicken out the image . . . What do you see (hear, smell), are there any characters involved in the image? What does little x need in the image? How do any caregivers respond to those needs? How does that feel?

Step 5. Bring the Client Back into the Present Moment
OK . . . now let's slowly and gently . . . pan out of the image and floating back towards the present moment . . . and drifting towards the recent episode . . . just notice this recent episode as you float towards it . . . notice if there is any connection between this image and

that of the child . . . How might this image be similar to the childhood image? . . . How might it be different? (*optional: safe place imagery* . . .) and now when you are ready . . . can I get you to slowly and gently open your eyes and reorient yourself to the room . . .

Step 6. Debriefing the Exercise

Generally, the therapist will derive a lot of rich information from such an exercise directly by getting feedback from the client about their experience during the task. Some interesting reflective questions to debrief this task might include:

1. What was that like for you?
2. What did little x (the child) need in the childhood image?
3. Were your parents (or caregiver) available to meet those needs?
4. What did you need in the adult scenario?
5. Is there any connection between the two?
6. What might this say about your needs going forward?

Generally, what might ensue is an open discussion of how characteristic this kind of scenario was of their childhood experience, and how these needs and schema themes might relate to the kind of problems they experience these days. This information will go straight into any formulation.

Part II – Process Issues in Assessment

During the assessment phase, the main goal is to enable the client to describe their presenting issues and life history in their own way whilst observing how they communicate. As clients describe their difficulties, the schema therapist notices both the way in which they tell their story and the meanings they have derived from their experiences. The process of telling the story will also help to reveal the client's level of 'mindsight' – the capacity to reflect on one's own mind and that of others – or awareness, which is an indicator of the strength of a client's Healthy Adult mode. In later assessment sessions, the way in which the client has told their story can form points for discussion and shared observation, to stimulate the development of Healthy Adult mindsight, whilst providing preliminary education about schemas and modes (see Box 3.6 for examples of how to use observations of clients' in-session behaviour to identify schema therapy concepts).

Recent research indicates that coherence in retelling the details of childhood is a sign of secure attachment [31]. As the client tells their story, consider its coherence and completeness. These qualities may indicate the presence of EMS or problematic coping modes. What does the client include, and what is omitted? How much detail is given, and to what degree does the narrative sync with any expression of emotions? As schema therapists observe the client telling their narrative, they might hold in mind the following questions to guide the assessment and hypothesis testing process:

• Does the client describe their childhood in a chaotic manner (describing events disparately or haphazardly, with little use of sequence or themes of connection) or a rigid manner (describing events in an overly detailed way that is disconnected from emotion/ sensory experience)? For those with a pattern of disorganised attachment characterised by emotional/physical/sexual abuse and/or neglect, memory gaps may be linked to the child using dissociative coping as a survival mechanism. These patterns may be

Box 3.6 Clinical Examples of Incorporating Observations of Client Behaviour Into Schema Therapy Assessment

Therapist: I'm curious about something I noticed just now . . . I'm guessing that it must have felt traumatic for you to have been bullied at school, and yet when you describe this to me, your facial expression and tone of voice conveys a different message, almost as if it didn't affect you. I wonder what happened [or didn't happen] in your past for you to have learned to dismiss or shut off from those emotions . . . It's almost as if there is a part of you that operates as a protector, to keep your emotions at a distance . . . Does that resonate in any way for you?

s

I notice that, on the one hand, you describe your relationship with your parents as close, but on the other hand it sounds like your feelings and needs weren't really a topic of conversation in your family. I wonder if you can help me understand what 'closeness' means to you . . . how would I know you were close if I were a fly on the wall in your home?

or

I notice that as you are telling me your story, it feels a little bit like the memories and pieces of your life are a bit disjointed or chaotic. Does it ever feel like that to you as you are living day-to-day . . . as if life is a puzzle and it's hard to piece it together in a way that makes sense?

associated with a range of schemas, especially those from the Disconnection and Rejection domain, including Defectiveness, Mistrust/Abuse, Abandonment, and Emotional Deprivation.

- Does the client describe childhood from an overly positive stance in an attempt to gloss over any events that may cast parents or other family members in a negative light? (This may indicate that loyalty to others interferes with acknowledging negative emotions toward them.) This is commonly associated with modes such as Detached Protector ('I'm fine, my childhood was fine'); Compliant Surrenderer ('I must be what others want or expect me to be, and go along with their wishes'); Guilt-Inducing Critic ('If I get angry/upset with others, I'm a bad person'); and Punitive Critic/Flagellating Overcontroller ('It's better to be a bad kid in a good family than a good kid in a bad family'). Or are they able to describe both negative and positive experiences in a Healthy Adult balanced way (i.e., give examples both of needs that were met and needs that were not met)?

- To what degree does the individual focus on relationships amongst family members when they are describing events from childhood (as opposed to simply focusing on external life events)? This will provide information about the value that the client has learned to place on relationships. A person who grew up in an emotionally detached environment, in which their parents were emotionally inhibited and had limited capacity for connection, will learn to abandon their internal world and focus on the external world (events, achievements, appearances). They learn to connect with others through communicating concrete concepts and intellectualising, but lack capacity to communicate about their emotional experiences. Although they continue to experience emotions and sensations, these remain in the background, detached and minimised. Alternatively, individuals who have experienced a chaotic childhood environment where there are high levels of expressed emotion and/or instability can become highly preoccupied with interpersonal relationships as an adult, due to expectations that the past chaotic patterns (e.g., abandonment, loss, rejection, humiliation) will recur in present relationships (schema perpetuation). Thus, the degree to which discussion of others features in stories of early childhood may inform the development of hypotheses about the client's schemas and unmet needs.

- How connected is the client to their emotions as they talk about their difficulties and their childhood? Does the client describe difficult circumstances (e.g., traumas) in a way which is emotionally congruent, or in a detached manner? For example, a client with a strong Emotional Deprivation and/or Emotional Inhibition schema (linked to insufficient emotional attunement in childhood) may talk about their life in very concrete terms, and may be dismissive of the impact of childhood and/or describe their childhood memories in a vague manner that lacks sensory or emotional detail. A client with a significant Abandonment schema may tend to confuse past and present and be preoccupied by a constant fear that others will leave them in the here and now.

- It is easier to detect schemas in clients with a surrendering coping style; these clients are more in touch with the felt sense of their schemas. However, for clients with strong overcompensatory or avoidant coping styles, conscious awareness of schema-driven patterns will be limited, depending on how well their coping strategies work. For example, a client with a substance addiction may manage to keep their feelings of abandonment and defectiveness at bay through consistently ensuring they have access to their substance of choice. A client with bulimia nervosa may block activation of schemas through regular bingeing and purging. A client with relationship difficulties, who is a highly successful CEO with his own business, may keep the loneliness and shame associated with their Emotional Deprivation and Defectiveness/Shame schemas out of awareness through workaholism and an excessive focus on achievement. In these cases, the therapist will have to work harder to identify schemas by integrating both what the client says/doesn't say, their non-verbal communication, and the evolving countertransference.

- From a schema mode perspective, you might pay attention to whether the story is told from the viewpoint of a coping mode, a parent mode, or a child mode. From the Detached Protector mode, the client will tell their story in a numb, detached manner that may be out of sync with the content of their life story. Alternatively, they may just answer 'I don't know' to questions, with a blank expression. In relation to questions about childhood, they might say, 'Oh, I have already dealt with that stuff in the past. I just want to focus on the present now and don't want to go back there and talk about my parents.' A client with a strong Paranoid Overcontroller mode might withhold important information for fear of losing control (e.g., 'Why do you need to know that?') and might give suspicious or vague answers to questioning. A client in Angry Protector mode might become hostile when the therapist asks about childhood and deny any connection: for example, 'I really don't see what you're getting at. You therapists are so predictable, I don't see the point in this!' A person in Self-Aggrandiser mode might turn their focus back to the therapist, either in a charming way (e.g., 'I heard you were the best therapist in the area, and I thought that with your expertise you would really understand me'), or asking about the therapist's qualifications, and questioning the therapy model and/or the therapist's way of working. From the viewpoint of the Pollyanna mode, a client is likely to gloss over any negative details whilst producing an overly glossy or optimistic perspective of their childhood that is incongruent with their circumstances: for example, 'My parents are wonderful . . . just the best. I've had an ideal childhood, perfect in every way. All of my needs were met. I'm so fortunate.'

See Table 3.3 for further information about how schema modes may present in session.

Part III – Defining Treatment Goals and Gauging Client Motivation

It is important that the client's key problem areas can be translated into some clear treatment goals. Therapists should note the degree to which the client can articulate their treatment goals. Is the client able to describe in specific terms what they would like to be different in their life, and what they would like to work on from a personal perspective? Similarly, how motivated is the client to pursue these goals? The therapist should enquire about the client's fears and feelings (short-term and long-term) if they do versus do not work on these issues. What are the motivating factors? Did they decide to attend of their own volition, or has someone else in their life encouraged them or made an ultimatum to motivate them to attend therapy? Do any of their goals clash with those of other family members? Are the client's goals linked to their presenting issues? To what degree is the client exercising a sense of autonomy by engaging in therapy or considering change? Below are some key questions and considerations that might guide the schema therapist in understanding the client's treatment goals and motivation for change.

What Stage of Change Might the Client Be In?

In Figure 3.1 we have mapped schema therapy objectives and interventions onto the stages of change model [32]. How ready/able is the client to set long-term vs. short-term goals? Are their goals focused on short-term relief or on long-term contentment and fulfilment? Is the client seeking a 'quick fix', or do they require psychoeducation to help them recognise the

Stages of Change in Schema Therapy
(based on Prochaska & DiClemente, 1983)

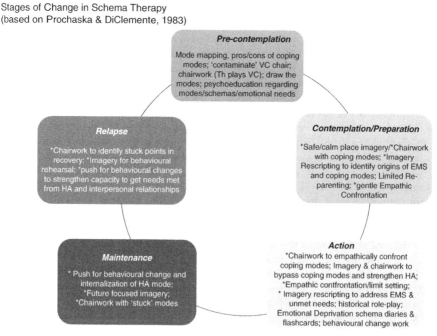

Figure 3.1 Stages of change model and schema therapy interventions [32]

intense work and commitment that comes with long-term therapeutic change? How willing are they to tolerate short-term stress or difficult emotions to achieve their longer-term goals? How might they envisage their life evolving in five and ten years' time if their goals were achieved? What barriers do they anticipate that might block their progress at this early stage? Is there anything that can be learned from previous therapy relationships about what might trigger blocks to treatment engagement, adherence, and progress (e.g., a tendency to be suspicious as soon as the therapist forgets to do something they had promised, whilst assuming that all therapists are just like everybody else and don't really care about them)?

Explore Client Treatment Goals That Relate to Presenting Issues

Over the course of treatment, the client's capacity to self-reflect and consider more possibilities may allow their goals to evolve. It can be useful to revisit and fine-tune goals to ensure that they cover a broad range of life domains. This might include relationships and connections (to self, others, nature), work, spirituality, bodily and mental well-being, or any domain that is significant to the client. Clients who are aware of their distress, such as those with BPD, are more likely to be able to describe their current difficulties in detail and to formulate goals linked to these. For those with Cluster C and NPD, the presence of strong coping modes can interfere with the person's capacity to recognise or describe their underlying suffering. These clients can easily lose sight of their reasons for attending therapy, increasing the risk that sessions will be dominated by 'downloading' details, general chatting, or a space for intellectual-ising or self-aggrandising (depending on dominant modes). With the ultimate goal of bypassing coping modes, it is therefore crucial to link treatment goals with the client's underlying (and sometimes hidden) experience of vulnerability. Treatment goals should to some extent be linked to these areas of vulnerability (e.g., to reduce feelings of suicidality or loneliness, and to learn healthy ways of getting needs met). For clients with narcissistic and highly avoidant presentations, the clear identification of difficulties and goals will later be a source of leverage to motivate the client to engage in experiential work that will mitigate their emotional suffering. For clients with more chaotic symptom presentations, the goals will serve as a compass to which both therapist and client can return, to ensure that working with crises and schema activation on a week-to-week basis remains consistent with the overarching goals. For those with more rigid and compulsive presenting issues, regularly revisiting the goals will serve as a beacon that brings hope and motivation to work on bypassing stuck – and seemingly impenetrable – coping modes, to facilitate healing work with the child modes.

What Length of Treatment Might Be Appropriate or Realistic?

Schema therapists must ensure that they are available to provide longer-term therapy, especially when working with clients who require extensive trauma-processing work. However, this may be flexible to some degree by incorporating phase-based schema therapy [33] and/or a combination of group and individual therapy. Short-term (~20 sessions) schema therapy has also been found to be effective for many client groups (see Chapter 1: From Core Emotional Needs, to Schemas, Coping Styles, and Schema Modes for details). Goal setting can then be planned around phases and/or length of treatment to ensure that it is realistic and achievable within this time frame.

Box 3.7 Clinical Examples of Feeding Back Hypotheses Formed During Assessment

(a)

Therapist: Could it be that this pattern of expecting that others will become ill or die might be linked to the early experience of suddenly losing your grandmother, the only person who really understood you and was there for you?

(b)

You mentioned that procrastination and turning up late is causing you stress at the moment . . . I wonder if when your boss sets a deadline that triggers old memories of your dad telling you what to do? And there is this part of you that pushes back against that feeling of being controlled?

(c)

I can see that it's so hard for you to confide in others about what you need and feel. I'm curious as to whether you might have learned to protect yourself by detaching from your feelings as a little girl, as neither of your parents really 'got' you, and your brother teased you incessantly . . . What do you think about this idea?

(d)

I wonder if your inability to switch off from your studies and relax might be related to your mum's high expectations in childhood . . . the way she would always act disappointed if you didn't get the top grade in your class?

Provision of Feedback in Assessment

The schema therapist tentatively links current problems with early patterns and unmet needs over the course of the entire assessment phase. Even at the end of session one or two, the experienced schema therapist can provide a basic mode map, which can be presented on paper, a white board, or via chair work, to introduce the client's main modes and link these to early experiences. This is collaboratively presented, as a summary of the most conceptualisation-relevant information obtained via the assessment to date. This can be a validating experience, by helping the client to consider possible origins of their difficulties and providing a developmental framework for understanding their presenting issues.

At this stage the therapist aims mainly to 'plant seeds' by introducing the notion that the client's presenting problems make good sense when they are considered in the context of the early environment in which they emerged. This can be highly liberating as the client starts to realise that their problems might not be due to an inherent flaw but be at least partly a side effect of their survival as a human being. Although therapists' suggested links are only tentative hypotheses at this early stage, they set the scene for the development of the more stable conceptualisation and therapeutic work that follows (see Box 3.7 for examples of how a therapist feeds back their assessment).

After approximately 4–8 sessions, once historical information has been gathered, questionnaires have been filled out and discussed, and early exploration and linking (of early experiences with current difficulties) has begun, the therapist can move into a more formal process of collaboratively constructing a case conceptualisation to guide therapy.

Concluding Remarks About the Assessment Phase

The assessment process in schema therapy requires a blend of determination and flexibility on the part of the therapist, to carry out the detective work that will enable them to piece together the puzzle of linking multiple presenting issues, childhood and adolescent experiences, and unmet needs and/or traumas. As much as possible, the schema therapist should be genuinely curious, open-minded, and attuned to the individual, whilst drawing on previous research and guidance, and should resist the urge to make assumptions based on diagnostic labels. At some level, the assessment process continues throughout the entire course of therapy, as more information is revealed and understood, allowing for re-conceptualisation and fine tuning. Throughout the assessment process, the schema therapist suggests possible links between current presenting issues and interpersonal patterns, early attachment processes and schema development. This process is aimed at building rapport through deep attunement and transparency whilst providing education about schema development, thereby gradually strengthening the client's capacity to self-reflect. Schemas and modes are gradually introduced into the conversation, integrating information gained from discussions about current presenting issues and early experiences. As the assessment proceeds, the focus gradually moves from addressing 'What's wrong with you?' to 'What happened in your life for you to have learned to think this way about yourself and to cope in this way?' Once there is enough preliminary information to piece together (at least provisionally) the factors that link early experiences with the onset and maintenance of schemas, modes, and presenting issues, the therapist can begin to tentatively verbalise these case conceptualisations, checking out how well these ideas resonate with or make sense to our clients. In some cases, the therapist will be wrong and need to return to the drawing board; in other cases, clients will immediately feel relieved that at last someone understands their world. On yet other occasions, clients might not be ready to focus on the truths that underlie their difficulties, and the therapist may need to revisit these in a gentle yet persistent way as they move forward with the early phase of treatment.

Even a tentative shared case conceptualisation provides the basis for schema therapy. It is therefore essential to spend sufficient time exploring childhood and adolescent issues to understand how these may be linked with presenting issues. However, the therapist must acknowledge that exploring unmet needs in childhood is often a painful process and find a way to work collaboratively with clients to help them understand their own truths and experiences. The therapist must resist any urge to prioritise the therapist's preconceptions, agendas, and internal timetables. At the end of the main phase of assessment, it can be helpful to feed back the therapist's assessment and case conceptualisation in a way that helps the client make sense of their own story. One way of doing this is in the form of telling a fairy-tale, as a way of 'bringing it all together'. For example: 'Once upon a time, there was a little child who went through A,B,C [experiences associated with parenting, and wider family]. The child felt X a lot of the time, and learned to cope by doing Y and Z. This helped some of the time but ended up creating more problems through . . .'.

This leads us to the next chapter, wherein we explore the schema therapy case conceptualisation in greater depth.

References

1. Siegel DJ. *Aware: The science and practice of presence – a complete guide to the groundbreaking Wheel of Awareness meditation practice.* Tarcherperigree; 2018.

2. Siegel DJ, Bryson TP. *The whole-brain child: 12 revolutionary strategies to nurture your child's developing mind.* Bantam Books; 2012.

3. Linehan M. *Skills training manual for treating borderline personality disorder.* Guilford Press; 1993.

4. Farrell JM, Shaw IA, Reiss N. *The schema therapy clinician's guide: A complete resource for building and delivering individual, group and integrated schema mode treatment programs.* Wiley; 2014.

5. Roediger E, Stevens BA, Brockman R. *Contextual schema therapy: An integrative approach to personality disorders, emotional dysregulation, and interpersonal functioning.* New Harbinger Publications; 2018.

6. Haugh JA, Miceli M, DeLorme J. Maladaptive parenting, temperament, early maladaptive schemas, and depression: a moderated mediation analysis. *Journal of Psychopathology and Behavioral Assessment.* 2017; **39** (1):103–16.

7. Young JE, Klosko JS, Weishaar ME. *Schema therapy.* Guilford; 2003.

8. Kennedy E. Orchids and dandelions: How some children are more susceptible to environmental influences for better or worse and the implications for child development. *Clinical Child Psychology & Psychiatry.* 2013; **18** (3):319–21.

9. Belsky M, Pluess J. Differential susceptibility to rearing experience: the case of childcare. *Child Psychology & Psychiatry.* 2009; **50**(4):396–404.

10. Rothbart MK, Dweck CS, Eisenberg N, Sameroff AJ, Bates JE. *Becoming who we are: Temperament and personality in development.* Guilford Press; 2011.

11. Cloninger CR, Svrakic DM, Przybeck TR. A psychobiological model of temperament and character. *Archives of General Psychiatry.* 1993; **50**: 975–90.

12. Fuchs T, Koch SC. Embodied affectivity: on moving and being moved. *Frontiers in Psychology.* 2014;**5**:508.

13. Arntz A, Rijkeboer M, Chan E et al. *Towards a reformulated theory underlying schema therapy: Position paper of an*

international workgroup. Cognitive Therapy and Research. 2021.

14. Windhorst E, Williams A. Growing up, naturally: The mental health legacy of early nature affiliation. *Ecopsychology.* 2015;**7**:115–25.

15. Groeger N. Meta needs in the context of schema therapy: Psychometric qualities of a new meta needs questionnaire and relationships with depression, anxiety and schemas. *Maastricht Student Journal of Psychology and Neuroscience.* 2012;**1**:65–79.

16. Renye D. We are the environment: Understanding how when we interpsychically and interpersonally take care and heal ourselves, we aid the evolution of the environment and planet. Presentation at The Annual Meeting of the California Sociological Association; 2007, 17 Nov.; Berkeley, California.

17. Pilkington P, Younan R, Bishop A. Early maladaptive schemas, suicidal ideation, and self-harm: a meta-analytic review. *Journal of Affective Disorders Reports.* 2021; **3**: 100051.

18. van der Mark W, van Oort N. The genogram as a tool to break free from Intergenerational Schema Transference in Present Relationships. A presentation at: International Society of Schema Therapy (ISST) Conference; 2014, 14 June; Istanbul, Turkey.

19. Siegel DJ. *The developing mind.* Guilford Press; 1999.

20. Young J, Brown G. (Eds.). *Young Schema Questionnaire – Long form 3.* Professional Resource Exchange; 2003.

21. Young J. *Young Schema Questionnaire-3.* Cognitive Therapy Center; 2005.

22. Yalcin O, Marais I, Lee C, Correia H. Revisions to the Young Schema Questionnaire using Rasch analysis: The YSQ-R. *Australian Psychologist.* 2022;**57**:8–20, DOI: 10.1080/00050067 .2021.1979885.

23. Kriston L, Schäfer J, Jacob GA, Härter M, Hölzel LP. *Reliability and validity of the*

German version of the Young Schema Questionnaire–Short Form 3 (YSQ-S3). *European Journal of Psychological Assessment.* 2013;29(3):205–12.

24. Bach B, Simonsen E, Christoffersen P, Kriston L. The Young Schema Questionnaire 3 Short Form (YSQ-S3): Psychometric properties and association with personality disorders in a Danish mixed sample. *European Journal of Psychological Assessment.* 2017; 33(2);134–43.

25. Young J. *Young parenting inventory.* Cognitive Therapy Center; 1994.

26. Louis JP, Wood, AM, Lockwood, G. Psychometric validation of the Young Parenting Inventory – Revised (YPI-R2): Replication and Extension of a commonly used parenting scale in Schema Therapy (ST) research and practice. *PloS One.* 2018;13(11):e0205605.

27. Young JE, Arntz A, Atkinson T, Lobbestael J, Weishaar ME, van Vreeswijk MF. *The Schema mode inventory.* Schema Therapy Institute; 2007.

28. Louis JP, Wood AM, Lockwood G, Ho MH, Ferguson E. Positive clinical psychology and schema therapy (ST): The development of the Young Positive Schema Questionnaire (YPSQ) to complement the Young Schema Questionnaire 3 Short Form (YSQ-S3). *Psychological Assessment.* 2018;30(9):1199–213.

29. Weathers FW, Blake DD, Schnurr PP et al. The Life Events Checklist for DSM-5 (LEC-5) [Internet]. National Center for PTSD; 2013. Available from: www.ptsd.va.gov/ professional/assessment/te-measures/life_ events_checklist.asp

30. Holmes EA, Mathews A. Mental imagery in emotion and emotional disorders. *Clinical Psychology Review.* 2010; 30 (3):349–362.

31. Siegel D, Hartzell M. *Parenting from the inside out.* Penguin; 2004.

32. Prochaska JO, DiClemente CC. Stages and processes of self-change of smoking: Toward an integrative model of change. *Journal of Consulting and Clinical Psychology.* 1983; 51(3),390–95.

33. Reubsaet R. *Schema therapy – A phase-oriented approach, targeting tasks and techniques in individual and group schema therapy.* Pavilion Publishing; 2021.

34. Simpson S, Smith E. *Schema therapy for eating disorders: Theory and practice for individual and group settings.* Routledge; 2019.

35. Edwards D. Self pity/victim: A surrender schema mode. *Schema Therapy Bulletin.* 2015;1(1):1–6.

36. Edwards DJ. An interpretative phenomenological analysis of schema modes in a single case of anorexia nervosa: Part 2. Coping modes, healthy adult mode, superordinate themes, and implications for research and practice. *Indo-Pacific Journal of Phenomenology.* 2017; 17(1):1–12.

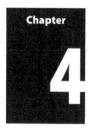

Case Conceptualisation and Mode Mapping in Schema Therapy

Introduction

Composing and communicating a clear and accurate case conceptualisation should occur before any treatment begins. The main purpose of the case conceptualisation is to aid the therapist and client in understanding how the client's presenting problems have been caused, and are now maintained, by the operation of schemas and modes. A therapist's treatment direction is always informed by this conceptualisation [1]. The case conceptualisation continues to be refined as the therapist learns more about the client. A second important function of a case conceptualisation is to help engage the client in therapy. An accurate conceptualisation, clearly communicated, helps the client feel heard and understood. It also helps the client to understand themselves better by increasing their *mode awareness*. By the end of the assessment phase, the schema therapist will document a full *schema therapy case conceptualisation* and then communicate a summary of its most important parts using a *schema therapy mode map*. In this chapter, we will provide an overview of the information schema therapists document as a part of their overall case conceptualisation before outlining how this information may be summarised and communicated to clients using schema therapy mode maps.

Documenting an Overall Case Conceptualisation

Using the assessment methods described in Chapter 3: Schema Therapy Assessment, the schema therapist will collect detailed information. The International Society for Schema Therapy (ISST) currently recommends the Schema Therapy Case Conceptualization form, 2nd Edition (Version 2.22) as a template for assembling the information that should be collected to form the case conceptualisation. This form has been developed and elaborated over time by an ISST workgroup led by Jeffrey Young [2]. An overview of the domains detailed in a comprehensive case conceptualisation based on this form are given in Table 4.1, and a case example using the template is provided in Box 4.1.

Developing and Sharing a Schema Mode Map With the Client

The full case conceptualisation, as described herein, is generally too dense for clients to benefit from. Instead, the central parts of the case conceptualisation are communicated to the client through a visual schema therapy mode map using a template such as the one in Figure 4.1. The mode map is completed with the client, and is written directly onto a paper template or drawn up on a whiteboard or similar. This process is intended to be educational and collaborative. It allows the schema therapist to convey their understanding of the client's presenting issues, but also provides an opportunity for the client to give feedback

Table 4.1 Schema therapy case conceptualisation: Key content

Client Background Information
Includes client name/ID, age, current relationship status/sexual orientation and children (if any), occupation/position, highest educational level, country of birth/religious affiliation/ethnic group (if relevant).

Key Problem Areas: Why Is the Client in Therapy?
What are the primary problems motivating the client to seek help? Examples of this are given in Chapter 3 on assessment under key problem areas (e.g., anger problems, self-harm behaviour, lack of intimacy in relationship, problems establishing boundaries with parents).

General Impressions of the Client
How does the client present in a global sense in therapy sessions? (e.g., reserved, hostile, eager to please, needy, articulate, unemotional).

Current Diagnostic Impression
A. Identify any relevant ICD-10-CM/DSM5 disorder(s).
B. Current level of functioning across five major life areas (includes occupational/school performance, intimate/romantic relationships, family relationships, friends and other social relationships, solitary functioning, and time alone. The Client's current function is rated on a 6-point scale (1=*Not Functional/Very Low*, 6=*Very Good or Excellent Functioning*) and elaborated via a more qualitative explanation.

Major Life Problems and/or Symptoms
Here we elaborate on central problems identified as key problem areas, describing the nature of the problem(s), and how they create difficulties in the client's daily life. A list of 1–5 is ideal.

Child and Adolescent Origins of Current Problems
A. General narrative of client's early history
B. Specific early core unmet needs (and linked to specific origins)
C. Possible temperamental/biological factors
D. Possible cultural, ethnic, and religious factors

Most Relevant Schemas
List of 1–5 of the EMS most relevant to the client's current problems, and a narrative description of common antecedents (triggers) and negative consequences the client experiences when this schema is triggered.

Most Relevant Schema Modes
List of 1–5 of the schema modes most relevant to the client's current problems, and a narrative description of common antecedents (triggers) and negative consequences the client experiences when this schema mode is triggered.
A. Child modes
B. Maladaptive coping modes
C. Dysfunctional Critic (Parent) modes
D. Other relevant modes
E. Healthy Adult mode (Summarise the client's positive values, resources, strengths and abilities)

The Therapy Relationship
Description of the therapist's positive and negative reactions to the client countertransference up until this point.

Reparenting Relationship and Bond
A. Description of the reparenting relationship and bond between the therapist and client up until this point.

Table 4.1 (cont.)

B. Reflection on how the reparenting relationship and bond between therapist and client might be improved.

Therapy Objectives: Progress & Obstacles

Create a list of 1–5 of the most important therapy objectives that are the focus of treatment. Be as specific as possible. For each objective, describe how the Healthy Adult mode could be changed to meet it. Then discuss the progress thus far. Also describe any obstacles and how they might be overcome.

Box 4.1 Full Case Conceptualisation Example (Initial Sessions): The Case of Samira

Client Background Information

Client Name/ID: Samira

Age: 38

Current Relationship Status/Sexual Orientation and Children: Married with two children (both boys, aged 6 & 9)

Occupation/Position: Full-time mother/homemaker

Highest Educational Level: MBA – Business

Country of Birth/Religious Affiliation/Ethnic Group (if relevant): India/Islam/N/A

Key Problem Areas

1. Chronic worry, perfectionism, and over-control
2. Chronic avoidance behaviour
3. Practical dependence and lack of assertiveness in relationships
4. Chronic loneliness

General Impressions of the Client

Client presents as anxious and needy, and 'in need of saving'. At times also presents as articulate, perhaps reflecting her high level of education.

Current Diagnostic Impression

1. Major depression
2. Generalised anxiety disorder (GAD)
3. Dependant personality disorder (with avoidant traits)

   Current level of functioning across five major life areas: client's current function is rated on a 6-point scale (1=*Not Functional/Very Low*, 6=*Very Good or Excellent Functioning*) and elaborated on via a more qualitative explanation.

1. **Occupational/school performance** (Rated 1/6). Client has avoided any activities related to competence and achievement since immigrating to the UK in 2010. Becomes panicked at the thought of working outside the house. Even household duties are generally avoided (e.g., cooking). The husband's solution to her lack of functioning has been to either do it himself or employ domestic help for just about all duties.

2. **Intimate/Romantic Relationships** (Rated 1/6). Client has struggled to feel valued in her marriage, more or less since having the two children. Partner has pulled away emotionally and physically and will not talk with her about the relationship. When pushed he has said that he doesn't love the client, but that he will fulfil his 'duties' as a father and husband and 'look after' the family. Client feels powerless in this situation as mostly unable to look after herself, feels dependent on her husband for practical needs (which he fulfils), but feels desperately alone and angry. Feels there is 'no point' and no solution to his behaviour towards her.

3. **Family Relationships** (Rated 3/6). A real strength is her relationship with her two young boys. Spends as much time as she can with them, tries to help them with their homework, plays with them as much as she can, and is there for them to take them to cricket. Bonds with them around this activity, although recently her avoidance behaviour is even interfering with this. Also feels isolated from her wider family in India. Has no other family in the UK.

4. **Friends and other Social Relationships** (Rated 3/6). Also somewhat of a strength, Samira has a small group of female friends (not from her culture) who she met at mothers' group after the birth of her second boy. Seems to interact well with them and feels supported when she makes time, but because of her depressed mood and avoidance seems not to make enough time for this. Client avoids engaging with other potential social connections from her culture for fear of judgement.

5. **Solitary Functioning and Time Alone** (Rated 2/6). Client is an avid reader and tries to read to relax when she can but struggles to really do this a lot of the time due to chronic worry. Personal hygiene is fine but struggles to do household chores, relying mainly on her husband and domestic helper to do the bulk of the household duties.

Major Life Problems and/or Symptoms (On Admission)

Problem 1: Worry, Perfectionism, and Over-Control
Life Pattern: Client is overly concerned with controlling her world to avoid potential disaster to the degree that she engages in several hours of worry per day resulting in a loss of functioning associated with axis I GAD (e.g., concentration, sleep problems, muscle tension, uncontrollable worry). Tends to worry mostly about her performance and potential failure and incompetence. This was the most prominent initial complaint that had sparked motivation to engage in therapy.

Problem 2: Low Self-Esteem and Related Chronic Avoidance Behaviour
Life Pattern: Client avoids and procrastinates doing just about anything that may result in a perceived failure/defectiveness experience and activating self-criticism and shame. This has become severe to the point that she is too scared to write forms or submit paperwork of any kind for fear of making a mistake. Client has recently also started avoiding leaving the house (including taking her kids out for activities and community engagement) for fear that others would judge her. This avoidance relieves her of having to confront her feeling of failure and defectiveness, but ultimately leaves her depressed and feeling like a failure as she is not engaging with key life goals (e.g., gaining meaningful employment, taking her kids to activities).

Problem 3: Sense of Incompetence, Practical Dependence, and Lack of Assertiveness in Relationships
Life Pattern: Perhaps her most pertinent problem. Client almost completely depends on her husband and domestic helpers for practical support, maintaining her feelings of incompetence and fears of failing these tasks. She also almost completely submits to her husband's

requests and demands. This is despite her husband's critical and stonewalling behaviour towards her. Feels unable to consider leaving given her practical dependence.

Problem 4: Chronic Loneliness and Lack of Intimacy
Life Pattern: Stays with her husband despite his critical and distant behaviour. Client feels very distant from him, feels that he does not care, does not meet her needs, except for practical needs (e.g., food, shelter etc.). Stays in the relationship because she feels that no one else would want her (Defectiveness/Shame), no one else would look after her practical needs (Dependence/Incompetence), and that divorce/separation would make her a bad person in the eyes of others in her cultural community (Defectiveness/Shame and Social Isolation).

Child and Adolescent Origins of Current Problems
Grew up in India to working-class but 'perfectionistic' parents. Parents had escaped extremely poor socioeconomic conditions through considerable hard work. Client had no siblings; parents overinvested in her, resulting in extreme pressure on her to succeed in achievement/academic domains. Set very high standards for academic performance and was sent to an expensive private school at great personal cost and sacrifice from her parents, a school where she felt she did not belong due to her lower 'social class'. Parents had a pattern of expecting her to be perfect at school, and when Samira returned home she was not taught anything practical (e.g., cooking, cleaning, etc.). Her 'duty' was to perform at school and gain entry into a top university. Any violation of these family rules or expectations resulted in harsh criticism/demands for better performance and threats of abandonment. Both parents appear to have had a similar distant relationship with her and presented a relatively united front when it came to these extreme demands.

Specific Early Core Unmet Needs
1. **Specific Early Unmet Need: Unconditional Acceptance**
   Parents' early and unrelenting focus on academic performance coupled with criticism and scolding when imperfect left her feeling like nothing she ever did was 'good enough'.
2. **Specific Early Unmet Need: Stability of Emotional Connection and Attachment**
   An early extreme and pressurising approach to academic performance was coupled with threats of abandonment if she did not perform or comply. On occasion, this materialised: her parents would stonewall her for days or even weeks if they were not 'happy' with her. The demanding nature of the relationship often left her feeling misunderstood and alone.
3. **Specific Early Unmet Need: Competence and Independence**
   Parents 'sacrificed everything' for her education, sending her to an expensive private school and 'relieving her' of any chores or domestic duties. While the client became academically quite proficient, she lagged behind at the basic skills required to be an adult (e.g., looking after herself, household chores, even the skills necessary for paying bills or using public transport). Parents would take her to and from school so she could be 'maximally' focused on her studies. She never learned the basics of everyday adult functioning as her parents took full responsibility for everyday functioning.
4. **Specific Early Unmet Need: Spontaneity and Play**
   In Samira's family of origin, there really was no time for fun and play. An unrelenting and demanding focus on studies and over-control of her behaviour meant that spontaneity and play was at best absent, and at worst – punished.

Possible Temperamental/Biological Factors

Reports being introverted and reserved as a child. Father seemed to suffer from undiagnosed depression. Client was clinically depressed on intake, was started on SSRI by her GP on admission and responded well in terms of overall mood.

Possible Cultural, Ethnic, and Religious Factors

Samira reported feeling that her Indian cultural heritage, particularly the culture of the state/city she was from in India, was highly competitive, thus reinforcing her parents' demanding approach to academics. She also felt considerable pressure from her family, religion, and culture to stay in her marriage and to suppress her needs in the relationship.

Most Relevant Schemas

List of 1–5 of the EMS most relevant to the client's current problems, and a narrative description of common antecedents (triggers) and negative consequences the client experiences when this schema is triggered.

1. **Unrelenting Standards**

   This is one of Samira's important EMS as it is linked to most of her other (core) schemas. Her central way of relating to her caregivers was through the lens of unrelenting standards and associated demands. This schema is triggered these days by just about any performance, or even everyday tasks (e.g., paying a bill, looking for work, getting together her CV). Such tasks trigger either intense anxiety and vulnerability and/or self-criticism or self-pressure that she needs to be 'perfect'. This typically leads to coping through episodes of worry and/or avoidance/withdrawal.

2. **Defectiveness/Shame and Failure**

   Her parents' early and unrelenting focus on academic performance coupled with criticism and scolding when imperfect left her often feeling like nothing she ever did was 'good enough'. In situations that are imperfect, or where she shows her imperfection or vulnerability, the client experiences considerable feelings of shame and self-criticism. When in this state, she readily identifies as 'feeling defective'.

3. **Emotional Deprivation and Abandonment**

   The client experiences chronic loneliness on a daily basis, particularly when home alone or when being isolated by her husband. On occasion, when he pulls away for several days or weeks, she experiences considerable anxiety and fears that he will leave her. This is partially because she will lose the relationship, and partially because she will lose access to practical 'support'. This often leads to some form of surrendering behaviour.

4. **Dependence/Incompetence**

   The client is greatly impaired with regards to her feelings of competence in everyday activities and tasks. Whenever she is pushed or asked or pushes herself to take responsibility for everyday tasks (e.g., cooking, paying the school fees), she becomes flooded by self-doubt and associated anxiety that she will 'make a mistake'.

Most Relevant Schema Modes

List of 1–5 of the schema modes most relevant to the client's current problems, and a narrative description of common antecedents (triggers) and negative consequences the client experiences when this schema mode is triggered.

Backstage Modes

Vulnerable Child mode: This mode is often triggered either in performance situations where she has a task to complete (predominant feeling of anxiety), or at times when she is isolated and alone for long periods or has been rejected by her partner (predominant feelings of loneliness and abandonment).

Angry Child mode: This mode is mostly suppressed in her daily life but is coming out more in therapy, especially when talking about her marital situation or times when she feels a 'lack of support' from her husband.

Demanding Critic mode: This is a very dominant mode for the client; it appears to be activated pretty much from the time she wakes up to some degree, commenting, and putting pressure on the client (e.g., 'you're lazy', etc.). However, this mode becomes very loud and dominant in any performance situations or situations where she notices she has made a mistake or been imperfect.

Front-Stage (Coping) Modes

Compliant/Helpless Surrenderer mode: The client's general way of operating around other people, especially those she is close to, is to surrender in one way or another. When she is in this mode the client is either submissive (to others' preferences or demands) or helpless (which seems to function to elicit help or 'support').

Overcontroller/Over-Analyser mode: When the client does push herself to engage in performance-related tasks she tends to approach them in a rigid and perfectionistic manner, aiming to 'get it perfect'. This mode also has an overanalysing aspect that looks like worry and rumination. When approaching tasks, Samira tends to overthink things, trying to anticipate and plan for everything that might go wrong. After engaging in such tasks, Samira tends to engage in post-event rumination, torturing herself about all the aspects that were not perfect.

Avoidant Protector mode: Ultimately, if Samira cannot master an approach perfectly, or rely on others to complete tasks, she will fall back on avoidance as a way of managing the feelings of being overwhelmed with anxiety and vulnerability that come with such tasks. When in this mode, she often becomes pessimistic, saying 'What's the point? Nothing ever works for me!'

Healthy Adult mode: The client is intelligent and psychologically minded, curious about her background and how they link to her current schema-based problems. She is also clear about her values and what matters to her (e.g., family, intimacy, competence, and independence) and is relatively motivated to tackle these issues. She is also ultimately a very social and easy to engage person who wants to connect, and is easy to connect with once she develops rapport.

The Therapy Relationship

I feel that a strong limited reparenting relationship has been established, especially given the early phase of the therapy. There is a warm and open candour to the relationship, and the client has been able to quickly develop trust in me and the therapy process. She responded well to the conceptualisation and was quick to engage in self-monitoring. There have been challenges, mainly in my understanding of her cultural and religious background and the influence of these on her schema patterns and sense of 'stuckness'. I want to be very helpful to the client. She has a very adolescent aura and approach to many issues that triggers my empathy and urge to be helpful and provide guidance. I feel I must be careful of this too, as my own urge perhaps to self-sacrifice, while perhaps somewhat helpful up to a certain point (the client feels my genuine care), risks thwarting development of her autonomy and competence.

Initial Therapy Objectives

Therapy Objective 1: Help the client to reduce her feelings of Defectiveness and set more realistic standards for herself; reduce the constant feeling of 'pressure' and increase self-compassion in the Healthy Adult mode. This seems to be an obvious initial target in the therapy as this problem often shows up in the therapy room and is central to her problems. This will involve targeting her Demanding Critic mode and its underlying themes of defectiveness and unrelenting standards and building her healthy compassionate side.

Therapy Objective 2: Build a sense of competence and mastery in everyday activities, and work/achievement strivings. This will involve working to reduce her reliance on her Surrender and Avoidant modes, and gradually encouraging her to build a (Healthy Adult) commitment in order to increase engagement with competence- and mastery-related tasks. This will of course involve negotiating a hierarchy that perhaps starts with everyday functioning (e.g., feeling confident enough to cook regular meals for the children), and eventually looking at higher-order tasks such as feeling confident enough to think about engaging in meaningful employment, which is a key medium- to long-term goal for her. It is likely that, as she reduces her reliance on these coping modes, she will need considerable therapy focus to help her manage and heal her Demanding Critic and Vulnerable Child modes.

Therapy Objective 3: Increasing independence and autonomy and asserting her needs. This will involve reducing her over-reliance on Avoidance and Surrender mode behaviour as a starting point, then starting to communicate more openly regarding her need for autonomy, independence, and competence, with significant others. Those around her will need to develop an understanding that, while they may be trying to help, by doing things for her they ultimately maintain her sense of incompetence. As the client is encouraged to express her needs more, and as she becomes stronger, it will be important also to support her to confront issues to do with verbal abuse and stonewalling in her relationship. This will involve helping her confront her fears of abandonment (Vulnerable Child mode) and Critic mode messages (that she is worth a better relationship).

to the therapist. The mode map can be conveyed in a number of ways, but we have found relaying it as a narrative can be particularly helpful, starting with the developmental origins. For example, 'From what I can understand, things were not easy for little Samira growing up. It was really hard for her to get her needs met in important ways . . . especially when it came to . . .'. The therapist finishes the narrative by explaining the presenting key problem areas as resulting from these developmental experiences and adaptations.

Once the mode map has been completed in collaboration with the client, the therapist encourages the client to familiarise themselves with the map. Mode awareness is a key attribute of the Healthy Adult mode, and reviewing the map develops mode awareness. Typically, early in treatment the sharing of the mode map is coupled with setting take-home tasks involving some form of self-monitoring or 'mode monitoring'.

Often, the final task in a mode-mapping session is to make some explicit links between the client's mode map and an initial set of planned treatment objectives. Clients will often ask directly at this stage 'OK, so now what? How do I fix this?'; you will need to be able to offer them some plausible and appropriate response about the initial plan and focus for

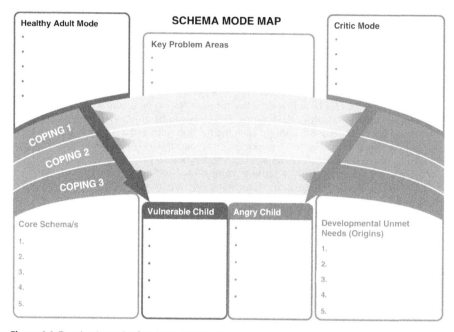

Figure 4.1 Template/example of a schema mode map

Box 4.2 Example of How to End a Mode Mapping Session

Therapist: So Samira, now that you are more aware of your modes, I wonder if you could try to use this awareness to try to understand when your modes get triggered and what mode(s) you are in when you are experiencing these problems? Perhaps it would be a good idea for you to take a photo of your mode map, and even put it on your phone as a screensaver, as a reminder of your map, and a prompt to think about your schemas and modes when things get triggered for you?

---

intervention based on the *Initial Therapy Objectives* identified in the full case conceptualisation. Figure 4.1 is an example of a template that can be used for mode mapping, but various formats have been used for this purpose. Figure 4.2 shows a completed mode map for Samira using a format devised by Simpson [3]. As you can see, there is considerable creative licence in generating these maps. The goal is to generate an engaging map of the client's predominant modes, their strength or dominance, and their relationships.

Concluding Remarks

This chapter has illustrated the two key tasks that bridge the transition from time focused mainly on assessment to time focused mainly on therapy. We have illustrated how detailed and comprehensive the therapist's conceptualisation should be, which provides a marked contrast to

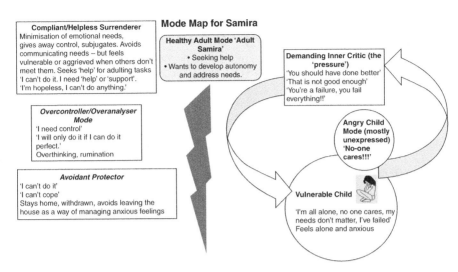

Figure 4.2 Example of a completed mode map

those usually developed in short-term psychotherapies. The therapist aims to identify the key targets of any psychotherapeutic assessment – presenting problems, client goals, possible psychological disorders and socio-occupational functioning – and the predisposing factors of temperament and early socialising and child-rearing experiences. The therapist then seeks to understand how problems are perpetuated and progress stymied by the operation of schemas and modes. The therapist collaborates with the client to produce a user-friendly, workable initial understanding of the client's progression from their early history to their current challenges, via a shared narrative and visual mode map. Care and attention during this mapping process are critical for ensuring that the client feels seen and heard, and to lend focus and direction to treatment. Schema therapy – as a long-term, multicomponent therapy – can be overwhelming for both client and therapist. The conceptualisation makes this manageable.

In the next chapter, we aim to help beginning (and more advanced) schema therapists try envision what a long treatment programme might entail, and explain in more detail how the conceptualisation guides therapy.

References

1. Young J, Klosko J, Weishaar M. *Schema therapy: A practitioner's guide.* Guilford Press; 2003.

2. Schema Therapy Case Conceptualisation form (2nd Ed., Version 2.22). International Society of Schema Therapy (ISST) Case Conceptualization Committee; 2018.

3. Simpson S. Schema therapy conceptualisation of eating disorders. In Simpson S, Smith E, eds. *Schema therapy for eating disorders: Theory and practice for individual and group settings.* Routledge; 2020. pp. 56–66.

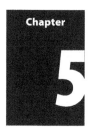

Envisioning the Road Ahead
A Model for the Course of Schema Therapy

Introduction

Many psychotherapists seeking to learn schema therapy will not have had experience in maintaining a structured therapy over such a long timeframe. It can take several years to experience a satisfactorily completed course of therapy, and thus it can be very difficult for the neophyte to envisage how a client's course of treatment will evolve over its journey. The purpose of this chapter is to sketch a model of how schema therapy might look at different points throughout its course and provide signposts to the clinician as to when to maintain or alter their focus and emphasis on different in-session schema therapy activities over time.

The Challenges of Long-Term Therapy

Those learning schema therapy often seek a model of how the treatment should unfold, step by step, from start to finish. Given the longer treatment orientation, complexity of individual cases, and transdiagnostic approach, it is difficult to illustrate a manualised, sequential schema therapy approach. Schema therapy is formulation-driven but not *formulaic*. It is a highly flexible and idiosyncratic approach, the true essence of which unfortunately resists a set of steps. Nonetheless, it is important to provide clinicians with general principles that will guide the therapy regardless of presentation. Specific techniques and methodologies are important in different stages in treatment. Knowledge of the core principles, processes, and treatment considerations can assist in therapeutic decision making and treatment planning.

Schema therapy was designed specifically to treat chronic and enduring psychological issues whose lineage can usually be traced to chronic unmet needs in childhood. Such clients often attract diagnostic labels of 'personality disorder' and are often experienced by therapists as the most difficult clients to treat. As a result, treatment typically involves an extended timeframe. The length of treatment can depend on several factors, such as the severity of the presenting issue, the strength of schema coping modes and styles, and the client's willingness to engage in experiential techniques.

Longer-term therapy with chronic clients can easily lose focus and efficacy due to common treatment roadblocks. One danger is that schema therapy sessions remain an intellectual process, with the clinician using schema therapy terminology without activating enough emotional experiencing in the sessions to promote deeper emotional change. In these cases, the therapy relationship remains at a surface level; core material central to the presenting problem is not examined. Second, practitioners may earnestly implement specific interventions rigidly when they are not indicated by the clinical situation. In these circumstances, the clinician becomes overly focused on using a 'schema technique' rather than considering the case conceptualisation and the predominant issues presenting in the session. For example, a therapist might plan some techniques for a client session to bypass Detached Protector but is unable to pivot to emotion-focused or limited reparenting techniques when the client attends in a vulnerable state. Fluctuation in a client's emotional state and the related verbal material communicated in session can confound treatment aims and objectives. Clients may suddenly disagree with a plan after previously having agreed to it. These kinds of rapid mode flips can derail the proposed treatment course of a session that would otherwise be clear.

Schema Interventions Are Guided by Clear Treatment Goals Linked to Agreed 'Key Problem Areas'

Chronic treatment-resistant clients most often present with several comorbid disorders and varying clinical problems [1]. Comorbidity is the rule rather than the exception. It is common for such clients to present with a complicated array of presenting issues. To manage the degree of complexity, it is very important to obtain specific goals for treatment that are linked to agreed *key problem areas* identified in the case conceptualisation.

The identification of key problem areas is a major component of a schema therapy case conceptualisation (see Chapter 4: Case Conceptualisation and Mode Mapping in Schema Therapy). The conceptualisation should be used to guide the treatment plan generally, as well as more micro-level in-session decisions regarding therapist responses. The key problem areas provide the client's motivation for attending treatment: 'Why am I here? What is the point of treatment?' The goals for treatment and the therapist's chosen interventions need to be broadly aligned. To use a metaphor, the client wants to drive to a destination (goals/problem focus); the therapist knows of several effective routes (schema therapy interventions) to reach this destination. For example, a client may present with chronic low mood (key problem area) and is seeking to reduce depressive symptoms (therapy goal); accordingly, the therapist will employ several treatment strategies based on the conceptualisation (e.g., chair dialogues, limit setting).

Therapists will choose or prioritise different therapeutic strategies depending on the stage of treatment. Such shorter-term objectives feed into the more general longer-term treatment aims. For example, the shorter-term objective of bypassing avoidance of experiential techniques is a necessary early step towards a longer-term aim of increasing self-compassion and self-care. Shorter-term objectives typically change over time, depending on the client's needs and the presenting problems that arise through the therapy process, and will generally support the longer-term objectives. Box 5.1 provides a useful metaphor to illustrate the unfolding schema therapy treatment as a 'journey'.

Box 5.1 The Schema Therapy Journey

'Navigating schema therapy is like sailing across a vast ocean, where currents, landmasses, and weather influence the journey. At the commencement of the trip (as the ship captain) you cannot see the destination ahead. You will be able to sketch a basic map (your case conceptualisation). You will also carry a compass to guide you (the schema therapy model), knowing that if you head northeast, you will reach your destination. You will need some necessary seafaring skills to manage where there's no breeze (these are your skills in bypassing problematic coping modes), or, if bad weather hits, you will have to ride out the storm (skills in helping clients manage their emotional arousal).'

Core Principles of Schema Therapy Practice

Several core principles within schema therapy are fundamental and help to distinguish the model from other psychotherapeutic treatments. Such concepts overarch the specific interventions used in the treatment and help the therapist guide the therapeutic process.

1. Develop a Safe Therapeutic Relationship and Treatment Alliance

A central vehicle of change within the schema therapy model is the therapy relationship [2]. The style of therapist interaction – termed *limited reparenting* – aims to go beyond 'standard therapist' caring and warmth, within the appropriate boundaries of the therapeutic relationship [3]. Here, the therapist seeks to meet the client's emotional needs directly in the therapy relationship, creating an environment of genuine care and empathy (see Chapter 6: Intervention Strategies for Schema Healing 1: Limited Reparenting). For many clients, bonding with the therapist in this way can trigger schemas related to safety and safe attachment. Without first having established this safe relationship, the chronic client may not be inclined to engage in other schema change procedures. It is thus a crucial first step in the process of schema therapy. Box 5.2 gives a clinical example of how this might unfold early in the treatment.

2. Bypass Coping Modes, Help Clients Connect to and Share Schema-Driven Cognitions and Emotions

Accessing emotion is central to schema therapy's design and its focus on providing *corrective emotional experiences*. Directly evoking emotional components of schemas and modes that are part of a client's presenting problems can facilitate change at cognitive, affective, and behavioural levels. The client's clinical conceptualisation determines which emotions are the specific focus.

Many clients remain stuck largely because their habitual ways of coping (e.g., Protector modes) severely limit awareness of their thoughts and emotions, resulting in neglect of their own core emotional needs. To change the schemas and modes that perpetuate their emotional and interpersonal problems, clients need to be able to access and share schema-relevant cognitions and feelings. This will be impossible when the client's coping modes are too dominant. Helping clients bypass maladaptive coping modes and access their emotions is therefore the next most important intervention priority, after establishing safety and bonding. Indeed, unless the client is spontaneously expressing their inner world, the therapist will be unable to accurately meet the client's needs (highest treatment priority) without first bypassing their coping modes. For therapy to be successful, the therapist must

---

Box 5.2 Clinical Example of Limited Reparenting Early in Schema Therapy

Greg had a childhood of neglect. His experience of caregiving was detached, unattuned, and withholding. The belief 'I don't matter, I'm not important' (Emotional Deprivation schema) was developed within this home environment. His therapist was direct in meeting his core needs and was genuine and straightforward in his caring responses: 'I care about you, Greg, I genuinely do. I can see how hard it is for you.' The therapist made a conscious effort to demonstrate care throughout therapy: for example, by acknowledging Greg's birthday or other significant events, such as wishing him luck for a job interview (via a message or within the session).

not collude with the client's coping modes that desire to remain detached, avoidant, or otherwise engaged in counterproductive activity.

Client emotional expression typically occurs naturally as a result of the therapist attuning to them. The therapist encourages healthy emotional expression in session because, historically, clients may have been punished for displaying emotions or suffered invalidation, rejection, or neglect. Such encouragement provides the client with an opportunity to not rely on their habitual methods of coping (within the therapy relationship or their lives in general) and experience healthy responses from others to their emotions.

Experiential exercises are used to evoke further emotion. The therapist then responds with limited reparenting, responding directly to the client's emotional needs as they become evident during these exercises. As the clinician notices the client struggling to access thoughts or emotions, they suggest an imagery or chair dialogue exercise likely to intensify schema or mode activation to a level at which thoughts or emotions are 'visible'. At the same time, the therapist takes care not to stimulate so much emotion that it overwhelms or 'floods' the client. Exercises are adjusted and adapted to allow clients to feel and identify emotions while being able to attend to the therapist's limited reparenting communications and understand them.

Accessing core emotions in treatment sessions also assists the therapy more directly. First, the client can be more aware of the emotions linked to their schemas and modes, rather than having just an 'intellectual' understanding of schemas and modes. Clients may be unaware of the origins of schemas and modes or have false narratives about why they feel things or act in particular ways. Discussing a schema or mode without emotion is analogous to a traveller who wants to experience a region they have never visited and seeking only to experience it via books or webpages in a library (rather than travelling there and exploring for themselves). Via techniques such as imagery rescripting, clients can gain a deeper understanding of the origins of their beliefs and experiences. Clients experiencing schema therapy describe this as a vital strength of the treatment [4].

Second, when emotion is activated in the session, the therapist can respond in a way that meets the client's emotional needs. Thus, emotion activation provides more opportunity for *corrective emotional experiences* [5]. These include the client experiencing feelings of comfort, validation, and care, which directly transform the expectancies associated with EMS. Through receiving corrective emotional experiences from the therapist, the client learns to adopt new ways of regulating their emotions [6]. The therapist aims to model how to respond to emotions and relate to themselves in healthy ways.

Evoking emotion will often also activate the client's coping modes. This is to be expected. Such modes can restrict engagement with the therapist and block meaningful change. Specifically, as a result of different forms of detachment, clients will often demonstrate poor emotion awareness and regulation. Emotions can signal when our needs and values are threatened. They can also communicate the effect of frustrated needs to others and help give other feedback about their impact. Furthermore, emotions can motivate clients to pursue meeting their needs and enacting their values. By blocking emotions, clients' physiological reactions and behavioural inertia may not make sense. For example, a client may be left with vague impressions that something is wrong but with no clear direction to correct the situation. Furthermore, interpersonal problems may ensue because their non-verbal communication is inconsistent with their words or behaviour or is disproportionate to the situation (i.e., they may come across as 'different' to others). It is thus crucially important that the client learns how to experience and share their feelings throughout the therapy. The therapist is initially there to help in this process and, over time, it is hoped that the client internalises this healthier way of approaching emotions.

Clients whose emotional dysregulation presents as a pattern of both extreme emotional arousal and extreme emotional avoidance can be challenging for therapists to manage. In these cases, clients may generally avoid affect; however, when they experience emotions, they are overwhelmed and in crisis. This pattern reinforces a 'black and white' experience of emotions as either present and unsafe or absent and safe. It is essential for the therapist not to collude with the emotional coping of the client. Instead, the therapist remains steadfast in pursuing emotional activation within a window of tolerance (i.e., not absent but not overwhelming). Use of the mode framework to bypass coping modes is exemplified in Box 5.3.

3. Help Clients Identify and Address Critic Mode Activation

Critical and punitive self-talk is likely to increase as the client's reliance on coping modes is reduced. It is important not to leave punitive messages unchallenged, and to instead repeatedly demonstrate to the client that these messages are not authoritative, accurate, or helpful. Messages generated from critic modes and schemas are often initially considered by clients to be central to their self-concept (i.e., ego-syntonic). A major aim within schema therapy is to help increase clients' awareness of punitive and critical messages and their origins. The next aim is to externalise the Critic so that self-criticism and self-blame become criticism and blame from another source [7]. The therapist aims to create separation between the client's self-concept and punitive, critical, and demanding messages so that these become ego-dystonic or defused from the self. In sessions, the therapist will refer to Critic messages as 'coming from the mode/schema', referring to the schema or mode in the third person (see Box 5.4 for an example). The use of experiential techniques such as mode

---

Box 5.3 Clinical Example of Bypassing a Coping Mode to Activate Emotion

Greg presented reporting 'no feelings' about what would appear to be an understandably challenging altercation with his partner. Greg denied that the interaction had 'bugged him' and seemingly spoke about the encounter in a matter-of-fact manner. The therapist could have taken Greg's position at face value and not probed more deeply into the altercation. Instead, the therapist attempted to bypass Greg's 'Numb Man' mode (Detached Protector coping mode) by asking how 'Vulnerable Greg' felt about his partner speaking to him this way. By doing so, Greg could access feelings of humiliation and shame (pervasive, deeply held feelings linked to the Defectiveness/Shame schema). The therapist was then able to respond to Greg's shame, providing corrective emotional experiences of acceptance, care, and validation. If the therapist had not probed for affect and bypassed coping, Greg would have missed a valuable therapeutic exchange.

Box 5.4 Clinical Example of Externalising Critical/Punitive Thoughts

Nikki presented in session with self-loathing, stating 'I'm a loser, what's wrong with me?' The therapist encouraged Nikki to view these sentiments as being derived from a Punitive Critic mode ('The Punisher'); 'Nikki, that's The Punisher talking, *she's* saying you're a loser, *that side* of you is taking things out on you.'

work or chair work can help with such separation (see Chapter 8: Intervention Strategies for Schema Healing 3: Experiential Techniques).

4. Strengthen Healthy Adult Functioning Over Time

The ultimate aim of schema therapy is to strengthen the client's Healthy Adult mode so that they can eventually self-regulate without the need for ongoing therapy. This mode acts as an 'executive' that healthily regulates different aspects of self (i.e., the other modes). The Healthy Adult mode is akin to an internalised 'healthy parent' who is compassionate, rational, encouraging, sets boundaries on their own behaviour, and is wise in decision making. As a result, the mode propagates healthy, logical cognitive processes, functional emotional expression, and adaptive behaviours. The Healthy Adult mode can rationalise and challenge negative core beliefs, underlying assumptions, and self-talk. At an emotional level, the Healthy Adult mode contains feelings of compassion, courage, indignation, strength, and a connection to personal values.

The Healthy Adult mode's strength can vary significantly from case to case, from very weak to largely resilient. In clients with poorer functioning, we would typically expect the Healthy Adult mode to be underdeveloped and/or less active, with the client's coping style governing their day-to-day functioning. In such cases, the therapist spends more time providing a model of the Healthy Adult mode (rather than expecting the client to have the internal resources). Opportunities to model healthy dialogues occur through experiential exercises (see Chapter 8: Intervention Strategies for Schema Healing 3: Experiential Techniques), limited reparenting (see Chapter 6: Intervention Strategies for Schema Healing 1: Limited Reparenting), and reviewing mode/schema diaries.

Wherever possible, it remains useful for the therapist to acknowledge the presence of the client's emerging Heathy Adult mode rather than assume it is not available. The treatment goal is to build upon the client's internal resources (no matter how weak they are), rather than the therapist being solely responsible for the clients' well-being. Just as in other cognitive-behavioural therapies, the schema therapist asks questions to elicit healthy perspectives and behavioural responses wherever the client is capable of generating them. Ultimately, the effective schema therapist balances providing direction, care, and guidance, encouraging the client to take greater responsibility over the course of the treatment.

Phases of Schema Therapy and Practice Guidelines

Knowledge of the therapeutic sequence within schema therapy can help treatment stay on course and inform the practitioner's decision making throughout. Across a course of schema therapy, several key phases are typically observed. Within each phase, several goals and objectives will drive the treatment process.

A common question we receive in trainings is 'How long should schema therapy go on for?' This really depends on a myriad of factors, some of which we consider here. A shorter-term treatment might be expected for clients that are higher functioning or whose problems do not have a chronic trajectory. For these clients, 12–20 sessions may be sufficient to address the presenting issues. Conversely, longer-term treatment will likely be required if the client's problems: (a) are chronic, perhaps based on longstanding issues related to childhood; (b) meet diagnostic criteria for a personality disorder; or (c) are related to chronic issues of attachment. Previous studies can also provide an indication of the expected duration of treatment needed based on diagnosis. For example, a 50-session treatment

Table 5.1 Treatment length in schema therapy treatment trials

Study	Clinical population	Treatment length
Bamelis et al. (2014) [8]	Avoidant/dependant/OCPD	50-session protocol
Malogiannis et al. (2014) [9]	Chronic depression	60-session protocol
Giesen-Bloo et al. (2006) [10]	BPD	3-year protocol
Bernstein et al. (2021) [11]	Forensic personality disorders	3-year protocol
Huntjens et al. (2021) [12]	Dissociative identity disorder	222-session protocol

protocol was effective with clients with Avoidant, Dependent, or Obsessive-Compulsive Personality Disorder [8]. Another factor that may determine the duration of treatment is the degree of deprivation of essential basic needs in childhood and adolescence. Typically, more entrenched and rigid coping responses as an adult can ensue from the severe and early frustration of needs. For example, extreme deprivation of safety (a very early and basic core emotional need) in childhood may require longer courses of therapy. In contrast, clients deprived of the opportunity to develop autonomy (a need that becomes more central later in the developmental process, e.g., in adolescence) may benefit from a shorter treatment duration. A guide to previous research and treatment length can be viewed in Table 5.1.

It can be helpful to think of a course of schema therapy as being divided into four phases. The first phase is a pre-treatment phase and consists of enough assessment, psychoeducation, and conceptualisation that the client can give informed consent to undertake a full course of schema therapy and the clinician can ascertain the client's ability to do so. Treatment itself can then be structured to have a beginning, middle, and end phase. By evaluating each stage on predetermined criteria, the therapy process can thus be closely monitored and possibly adjusted. Methods and techniques are used differently in each phase, and the therapist's attitude and reparenting approach also changes for each step. Although the overall expected duration of the treatment will be impacted by the client's needs and disorder-specific profile, the typical sequence of the sessions across time and within sessions is somewhat standardised. These are discussed in later sections in this chapter. One consideration of how the treatment unfolds is the focus across sessions, within a treatment phase, on particular treatment techniques: limited reparenting, cognitive techniques, experiential techniques, and behavioural pattern breaking. In the following sections, we describe how the distribution of these basic classes of therapeutic activity might vary during the different phases of schema therapy.

Phase 1: Pre-Treatment – Assessment, Education, and Case Conceptualisation

The main activities of this phase were described in Chapter 3: Schema Therapy Assessment and Chapter 4: Case Conceptualisation and Mode Mapping in Schema Therapy. The purpose is to gather enough information about the client to develop a case conceptualisation, which, in turn, is necessary for developing an initial treatment plan. The treatment plan will estimate how long the treatment will last, identify treatment goals, and state how the treatment will be structured. This plan also describes the most relevant treatment techniques and highlights any expected challenges or obstacles. The pre-treatment phase

is a period of undertaking enough assessment of the client and providing enough information about what schema therapy for the client would involve that the clinician and client can
make an informed decision about whether to undertake schema therapy together.

Phase 2: Beginning Treatment Phase – Connecting with the Client and Building Schema/Mode Awareness

Awareness of schemas and modes in daily life is an initial objective within the beginning
phase of therapy. Building such awareness will be an important step if the client is to benefit
from the full schema therapy package wherein the therapist aims to generate corrective
emotional experiences. Internalising such experiences will be an essential basis for strengthening the client's Healthy Adult mode.

The duration of the therapy's initial phase is strongly dependent on the therapy plan
drawn up during the case conceptualisation. The choice of duration for this initial phase is
often based on how best to distribute the available time. For example, a treatment plan of 50
sessions for a Dependent PD client can mean that the initial phase lasts 20 sessions, leaving
enough time for the middle phase (20 sessions) and the final treatment stage (10 low-
frequency sessions). Box 5.5 provides a framework for evaluating the client's readiness to
move into the middle phase of treatment.

Limited Reparenting (Healthy Relating). The therapeutic relationship is an important area
in which the client can gain new corrective experiences. In this initial phase, the client's
emotional development can often be best compared to that of a young child of primary
school age. As a result, the therapist takes a more active lead, taking the initiative in
recognising and clarifying feelings and patterns as a role model of a 'good enough parent'
[13]. The therapist also seeks to generate experiences that meet the client's unmet basic
emotional needs and helps the client internalise these experiences. The therapist can use
empathic confrontation to help the client gain more insight into the impact of coping and
critic modes on the therapy and the therapeutic relationship. However, the emphasis for
many clients in this early phase of treatment is on empathy, and the use of such confrontation is often limited.

Box 5.5 Evaluating Whether the Client Is Ready to Move Into the Middle Phase
of Treatment

It is advisable to schedule moments to evaluate the treatment plan and the progress made in
treatment. Planned informal evaluations can help the treatment be more focused. Some pre-
defined specific evaluation criteria can clarify whether the client does not achieve these
objectives.

Evaluation criteria after the initial phase of therapy can include:

- Does the client use schema concepts/language?
- Is it possible to use techniques (such as experiential exercises) essential to schema
  therapy?
- Is it possible to create corrective emotional experiences for the client via techniques such
  as imagery rescripting?
- Is the client able to retain such experiences, new insights, and skills between sessions?
- Is there any effect on assessment measures?

Cognitive Techniques (Healthy Thinking). Emotion-focused techniques aim to generate meaningful emotional experiences. Cognitive techniques provide rational responses to and understanding of such experiences. In the early phase of schema therapy, the therapist's role is to provide psychoeducation about basic needs, healthy child-rearing and upbringing, and schemas/modes. To assist, the therapist may use a flipchart or whiteboard to draw out the mode model. The therapist may also use audio recordings (ideally accessible via their mobile phone as a voice memo), whereby the therapist records important messages for the client. Triggering situations can be further documented and explored via schema diary forms with which clients practise recognising, monitoring, and challenging schemas/modes.

Experiential Techniques (Healthy Feelings). In this initial phase, emotion-focused techniques aim to link current problems to their origins and generate corrective emotional experiences. Mode dialogues can assist in helping the client build more awareness of different modes and to make such modes more 'ego-dystonic' ('a *part* of me doesn't want to talk about it' vs '*I* don't want to talk about it'). Imagery rescripting can help the client gain more insight into the origins of schemas and modes and allow the client to experience how genuine and appropriate care would have been in such experiences. The choice of methods – such as imagery rescripting or chair work (or any other emotional focused method) – will be partly determined by how the client responds to experiential work. If a client refuses to do imagery work, it is useful to use mode work and chairwork dialogues (see Chapter 8: Intervention Strategies for Schema Healing 3: Experiential Techniques) to explore the reluctance. It may be helpful to blend imagery and chairwork approaches to allow for more variation in therapeutic content.

Behavioural Techniques (Healthy Coping). There is typically less of a specific emphasis on behavioural change in this initial treatment phase; instead, there is usually a greater focus on feeling and thinking domains. Behavioural interventions within this phase may involve the therapist actively coaching the client in how to handle difficult situations. Just as a parent might provide instructional guidance to a young child, the therapist may also simply provide direct advice regarding client problems at work, in their studies, or in their relationships, more so at this point than in later phases. Influencing client behaviour in this way mainly aims to prevent or limit further problems in the client's life, while at the same time strengthening the therapeutic relationship.

Phase 3: Middle Treatment Phase – Titrating Therapist Involvement and the Client Taking More Responsibility

Overall Therapist Objective. Within this phase, the therapist seeks to elicit a greater level of responsibility and action from the client within the therapy exchange. The therapist's view of the client's role can be likened to how a parent's expectations change as their child moves into adolescence. The client contributes to setting the agenda, initiates formulating difficult situations and generating healthy perspectives and action plans, and takes the initiative in suggesting therapeutic exercises and activities. By now, the client is aware of the schemas, modes, and life patterns that perpetuate presenting issues. The middle phase's general aim is to strengthen the client's Healthy Adult mode and encourage the engagement and use of this functional mode in daily life (e.g., work, relationships).

Limited Reparenting. Within this phase, the therapist encourages the client to take more responsibility for their emotional and behavioural responses. The therapist may express to the client in sessions that they 'believe in them' and that they 'have their back', illustrating to the client that they have greater faith in their problem solving and self-care. The therapist is ultimately encouraging the client to place more significant levels of trust in themselves and their capacity. Empathic confrontation is also used increasingly in sessions, whereby the therapist starts to confront behaviour outside of session that perpetuates schema material. Box 5.6 provides a clinical example of limited reparenting during the middle phase. Box 5.7 provides a framework for evaluating the client's readiness to move into the final phase of treatment.

Experiential Interventions. Emotionally focused approaches in the middle phase increasingly seek to identify, strengthen, and utilise the client's Healthy Adult mode. Exercises such as historical role-play can help the client explore making a desired behaviour change in which they gain experience in standing up for their basic needs. Imagery exercises can help the client form a visual image of their Healthy Adult mode. Furthermore, in imagery rescripting, the therapist can encourage the client to visualise themselves as the Healthy Adult who stands up for the needs of the Vulnerable Child in the image. Within mode work and chairwork, the therapist may allocate a separate chair for the Healthy Adult and coach the client in how to respond from that chair. More specifically, the therapist may coach the client to express compassion to the Vulnerable Child part (represented by another chair) or read a warm letter to that child part, while seated in the Healthy Adult chair. Having the client complete the exercise while facing a mirror can further intensify the experience.

Box 5.6 Clinical Example of Limited Reparenting During the Middle Phase

Greg had been off work for 18 months. He had been employed as a gardener before his mental health declined and he was unable to work. His anxiety had improved over the last few months, and his therapist thought he could now work part time. The therapist encouraged Greg to compose a CV: 'I think you have so many great skills, people need to see it.' He used empathic confrontation, challenging Greg's reticence to submit his CV to employers: 'Part of me feels like backing off, accepting that you didn't get around to it this week, but my healthy side thinks, "Greg, you need to get this done ASAP".'

Box 5.7 Evaluating Whether the Client Is Ready to Move Into the Final Phase of Treatment

The following criteria can be used to help evaluate whether the objectives of the middle phase have been achieved:

- Can the client recognise schema modes in retrospect?
- Is the client able to visualise a Healthy Adult?
- Is the client capable of accessing and using elements of the Healthy Adult mode?
- Is the client able to have compassion for the Vulnerable Child mode?
- Is there a cognitive awareness of why critic and coping modes are maladaptive?
- Can the client show different, more adaptive behaviours in the session?

Cognitive Interventions. In the middle phase, the client's beliefs and assumptions about themselves, others, and the world should become increasingly more aligned with a Healthy Adult perspective. The main objective in this phase is that the client understands and remembers how a Healthy Adult mode functions and operates.

A framework for the function of the Healthy Adult mode in response to triggering events can be translated into three steps:

1) *Compassion*: First, the client should learn to look at their emotional reactions to problematic situations with understanding and compassion. Compassion is something many clients have not experienced in their upbringing. As a role model of a healthy caregiver, in the preceding therapy stages the therapist has demonstrated care and compassion to the client. Now, the therapist seeks to hand this skill over to the client. Compassion often means acknowledging that the emotions evoked are very understandable from the current problem situation, and certainly understandable from the past's emotional deficits.

2) *Cognitive Restructuring*: In this middle phase, beliefs and assumptions related to schemas and modes are more directly challenged and modified. Cognitive techniques such as reattribution of causal elements linked to schemas and modes (typically identified in the conceptualisation) are used. The therapist may look at ways of healthy, balanced thinking in the client's current life. Here, the therapist can educate the client about unhelpful thinking styles and impart skills to challenge unhelpful thoughts and provide a more balanced, Healthy Adult, logical response. In this phase, the client is increasingly responsible for filling in the cognitive diaries independently and examining whether automatic beliefs are realistic.

3) *Behavioural Modification*: Finally, the therapist encourages the client to respond to the problem situation in a healthy way. Specifically, clients are coached to develop solutions that are realistic and that meet their needs.

Behavioural Interventions. Therapy is a safe haven in which clients practise behaviour change. The therapist can coach the client to break through old behaviour patterns and try out new, healthier behaviour in session. The therapist can encourage the client to share more of what they feel or think, to be more active in bringing up meaningful topics, and to express positive self-reflections or receive compliments. Audio flashcards can be used to remember these experiences, in which the emphasis is increasingly on choosing a healthy way to handle problem situations.

Phase 4: Final Treatment Phase – Pushing for Change and Autonomy

General Concepts. The last phase of therapy aims to strengthen the client's Healthy Adult as preparation for the post-therapy period. The scheduling of such sessions is typically less frequent (e.g., once a month), to give the client enough time to apply the learned skills independently in their life. In the final phase, therapy focuses on helping clients achieve the practical goals they initially presented with at the start of therapy.

Limited Reparenting. Continuing the parallel with a child's developmental stage, the client is now starting to move more and more towards young adulthood. As a result, the therapist increasingly emphasises that the client applies the learned skills independently in their life. The therapeutic position changes from coaching to *insisting on* behavioural change. To this end, the tone and content of limited reparenting messages is more direct, as it would be when dealing with a young adult rather than a young child.

Experiential Interventions. The emotion-focused techniques now concentrate on strengthening the client's Healthy Adult side and enforcing the necessary behaviour change. For example, imagery rescripting in the final phase is more focused on future problematic situations; exercises enable the client to practise new behaviours and manage common challenges. In chairwork exercises, the therapist encourages the client to negotiate with the coping modes and combat critic modes. The therapist may also prepare the client for future challenges by articulating typical coping mode messages and encouraging the client to dispute them, generating alternative adaptive statements.

Cognitive Interventions. Cognitive interventions during the final stage become more and more like traditional cognitive therapy. Underlying assumptions and core beliefs are assessed and challenged using schema diary forms. There is also an increasing emphasis on behavioural experiments. The therapist encourages the client to test whether their assumptions are correct by trying them out and letting go of old coping styles.

Behavioural Interventions. In this final phase, the necessity of behaviour change is concertedly emphasised; without breaking old behavioural patterns, the risk of relapse is extremely high. All methods and techniques that can facilitate this behavioural change are permitted, including skills training, couple relation interviews, and self-monitoring procedures.

Termination Activities. In addition to seeing through the fulfilment of long-term therapy tasks, the therapist also must be aware of issues related to the conclusion of the therapy (see Chapter 12: Preparing for Termination and the End Phase of Schema Therapy for a full overview). Box 5.8 provides a framework to help evaluate and guide decisions about the conclusion of therapy. Box 5.9 provides a clinical example overviewing a complete course of treatment for clients 'Jack' respectively (see also Figures 5.1 and 5.2).

Schema Therapy Session Structure

Although schema therapy is rarely delivered with a prescribed session plan throughout the whole course of therapy, sessions should nevertheless be organised and strategic. It is easy for the therapist to be distracted from the client's core needs and issues that treatment could address. A balance between 'being with' the client's presenting concerns and providing change (or 'doing to') techniques needs to occur.

Frequently, a client's coping mode may impact the flow and focus of the session. For example, a rational and unemotional exchange may result from an unchallenged display of detachment and emotional avoidance in session. Here, the therapist needs to guide the structure of the session, focusing on critical issues that are most pertinent to the client's presenting problems and goals.

Box 5.8 Evaluating When to Conclude Therapy

The following criteria can help evaluate whether the objectives of therapy have been met:

- Can the client recognise modes in problem situations and switch back to the Healthy Adult mode?
- Can the client, looking back at trigger situations, independently bring in arguments against Coping and Critic modes?
- Is the client able to display different behaviour outside the sessions?

Box 5.9 Clinical Example Overviewing a Complete Course of Treatment for 'Jack'

Jack was a 43-year-old male referred for treatment of depression after losing his job. However, on initial presentation, he did not seem entirely depressed, but rather arrogant, intimidating, and irritated, which was palpable within seconds of meeting him. In initial sessions, the therapist could have attempted to extract information about his background and provide assessment questionnaires. However, such an approach would have resulted in Jack dismissing the treatment. Furthermore, the unaddressed and understood bullying and alienating behaviours in session may have resulted in the therapist ending the therapy.

Instead, the therapist immediately prioritised the use of a mode conceptualisation and provided this to Jack after three sessions. This case conceptualisation noted three central modes: the 'Top Dog Bully Mode' (Aggrandiser), the Detached Self-Stimulator (who used gaming and gambling to distract himself from painful emotions), and his 'vulnerable side' (primarily linked to Emotional Deprivation and Defectiveness/Shame schemas). Jack was open to the conceptualisation and how this linked to his presenting problem of not being able to hold down a job and be 'successful'.

The initial treatment plan primarily focused on helping Jack to become aware of his modes and understand that his 'top dog mode' was self-defeating, particularly because it alienated others and ultimately stopped him from being a 'success in his work'. In the proceeding sessions, Jack gained a better understanding of the origins and functions of his modes and schemas. It became apparent that Jack had been bullied a great deal in primary school about his weight, and his parents had been unavailable emotionally and practically. The therapist developed a way to manage Jack's in-session overcompensation modes using empathic confrontation, and Jack subsequently become much more forthcoming with information useful to building the case conceptualisation.

Over the next four months, the focus of the treatment moved to the use of two primary change strategies: (1) schema mode work and (2) limited reparenting, specifically empathic confrontation. Mode work typically was completed via the use of chairs. Chairwork was used to manage in-session 'Top Dog' behaviours, such as criticism of the therapist and others, bragging, and subtle contempt of other people's feelings. When Jack began to belittle or compete with the therapist, the therapist would ask Jack to speak briefly from the Top Dog Chair, whereafter the therapist would ask Jack to move out of this chair while he listened to the therapist empathically confront the Top Dog mode (see Chapter 6: Intervention Strategies for Schema Healing 1: Limited Reparenting).

The therapeutic relationship and limited reparenting was critical to Jack changing. Empathic confrontation was repeatedly used to challenge Jack's in-session behaviour, and link it to its childhood origins of inadequacy and neglect, to enable access to Jack's Vulnerable Child mode. The therapist focused on the prospect of Jack losing his professional standing as leverage in treatment. If he were to continue operating in Top Dog mode, it would limit his career success, a prospect that was sobering to Jack. Furthermore, it was made clear that the therapeutic relationship echoed relationships with others in his life outside of therapy. The take-home point was that if the therapist felt criticised and alienated, others would feel the same way. The therapist would continue to care and support; however, others would be more hostile and less accommodating of his needs. As a result, the therapist provided care and empathy to Jack's displays of vulnerability while at the same time providing strong confrontation of aggrandising behaviour.

Overall, Jack was impressed with how different this had been to other interventions with mental health professionals. Typically, other clinicians had not addressed in-session behaviour and had instead focused on supportive psychotherapy or offering cognitive change suggestions. After five months, Jack allowed himself to partake in an imagery rescripting exercise and became more aware of the origins of his 'Top Dog' behaviour. Rescripting by the therapist of the images of bullying and intimidation Jack experienced as a child resulted in him experiencing lower levels of shame and reduced his pervasive preoccupation with others 'doing better' or 'having a go' at him. Jack was then willing to proceed with more imagery rescripting, helping him to understand the origins of his reactions at work and experience corrective experiences of unconditional acceptance from the therapist. In this phase, most of the sessions were focused on chair work and imagery rescripting, with some time allocated to addressing Jack's aggrandising and status seeking in sessions where this was triggered. Overall, in-session Jack had become more reasonable and displayed less alienating behaviour towards the therapist.

Over the next four months, the therapist generally used two-thirds of each session to focus primarily on experiential exercises (such as imagery rescripting or chair work exercises), with one-third of each session focusing on in-session issues and mode activation and some more structured cognitive change work. Specifically, the therapist challenged beliefs encapsulating Jack's Unrelenting Standards schema (i.e., the inflexible, high demands he placed on others and himself). Also, beliefs about self-acceptance and his 'weaknesses' were addressed and restructured.

By session 30, Jack demonstrated greater self-awareness and was more willing to lead chair work and imagery rescripting experiential exercises. He had also entered a new intimate relationship, and the therapist spent time teaching him how he could express his needs to his new partner in a non-aggressive and non-demanding way. Here, the therapist provided didactic information, modelling, and coaching through role-plays in session. Behaviour change strategies also included prompting Jack to take specific time to consider his new partner's perspective (akin to practising empathy). Jack was initially resistant to the task as it was so alien to him. Consequently, the therapist used chair work to understand (conceptualise) the resistance to behaviour change.

After session 40, Jack sought to reduce the frequency of his sessions (with sessions being biweekly or monthly). He remained in stable employment and had managed to sustain a mostly healthy relationship. During the next ten sessions, Jack's Heathy Adult, 'The Wise Guy', was increasingly evident. He demonstrated awareness of problematic modes and, in particular, displayed a greater capacity to respond to his urge to aggrandise and 'dominate others' in and out of session. The therapist typically used 15–20 minutes of session time either in imagery rescripting or chair dialogues to help him become primed to use his 'Wise Guy' mode, practice Healthy Adult self-talk and make new healthy plans for the following weeks.

The session structure needs to be flexible enough to meet the client's core emotional needs at the time. A typical session can be viewed as having three phases, with 15–20 minutes of session time spent on each phase:

1. The Attunement Phase.
2. 'The Work'
3. 'The Wash Up'

The Attunement Phase (First Third of the Session)

In the first third of the session, the therapist actively attunes to the client's presentation 'in the room'. The therapist pays careful attention to gauging the client's current emotional state, looking for recent triggers and possibly reviewing homework assessments or following

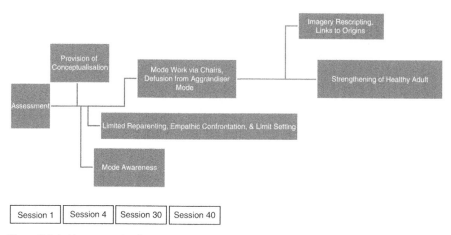

Figure 5.1 Jack's treatment timeline

up conversations from previous sessions. Limited reparenting is prominent in this section, with the therapist responding to the client's needs via empathy, validation, and attunement to verbal and non-verbal cues. The therapist may suggest focusing on one specific triggering event or topic and deeply attune to the emotions and meanings associated with the event. Furthermore, the therapist makes links between current triggers and emotions and past life events.

Ultimately, the aim is for the client to feel understood and attuned to at the beginning of the session. This allows for intervention targets to emerge, and for any interventions that ensue to accurately target the relevant underlying needs and schema themes. Such attunement to current emotional states typically takes precedence over homework assignment follow-up and evaluation. However, if there is no significant initial emotional presence in the session, the therapist can explore homework assignments set in previous sessions.

'The Work' (Second Third of the Session)

In this section of the session, the therapist may use specific strategies for change (such as experiential, cognitive, or behavioural techniques or discussion of the therapy relationship itself). A linking comment to this section may include 'So, what would be a good use of the time today? How would you feel about doing X'? Here, the therapist can provide some guidance on what could be useful and helpful to the client and, at the same time, be collaborative and attuned to core emotional needs. For example, the therapist may suggest a chairwork exercise (to explore feelings linked to a pertinent trigger discussed earlier in the session) or suggest time spent writing a flashcard to help with such triggers outside of the session. Here, the critical factor is that the therapist offers an invitation to do some 'work'. Rather than colluding with the client's Coping modes and providing empathy and care throughout the session, the therapist seeks to move into a change sequence.

The 'Wash Up' (Final Third of the Session)

In the final section of the session, the therapist aims to capitalise on insights and changes made in 'the work' section. The therapist may seek to highlight the 'take-home message' of the exchange or discuss further feelings and thoughts observed in the sequence and link these to overarching life patterns and goals. Within this sequence, the therapist may also encourage some self-reflection or 'assignments' outside of session. These can range from relatively general to more concrete. Suggested activities need to be meaningful to the client, and related to the current session's content and the overall therapeutic goals and needs (see Chapter 9: Intervention Strategies for Schema Healing 4: Behavioural Pattern-Breaking Techniques for a full overview of homework/take-home tasks in schema therapy). Box 5.10 provides a clinical example of the flow of a schema therapy session.

Tips to Encourage a Steady Direction in Schema Therapy

Be Aware of Client Coping Modes

Clients' habitual ways of coping are typically present in the session. When therapists collude with coping modes, treatment sessions have poorer focus, direction, and outcomes. In other words, therapists who fail to prompt the client to identify a coping mode in operation during the session allow the client to remain in habitual ways of ineffective interaction. For example, a therapist might not challenge the client's Self-Aggrandiser mode and associated behaviour in session, resulting in the exchange being dominated by the client bragging about their achievements and

---

Box 5.10 Clinical Example of Session Structure

Greg arrives in session to the therapist asking 'How has your week been?' Greg notes several issues linked to illness in the family and then indicates recent hostility with his girlfriend. One of Greg's therapy aims is to enter into and sustain a healthy relationship. The therapist appraises Greg as having limited awareness of his schemas and modes. With the conceptualisation in mind and knowing Greg's life pattern related to difficulties in relationships, the therapist slows down Greg's description of the events with his girlfriend and seeks to access emotional and cognitive components of the experience. Following this, the therapist empathises, validates, and meets Greg's emotional need related to the trigger, which in this case was understanding and care (the 'Attunement' section). Next, the therapist asks Greg, 'How would you feel about doing an imagery exercise to understand the feelings related to what happened with your girlfriend?' Greg agrees to complete an imagery rescripting exercise in which the therapist links the recent altercation between Greg and his girlfriend with an associated memory related to childhood deprivation (the 'Work' section). After completing the imagery exercise, the therapist discusses the links between past events and the present trigger. This increases Greg's awareness of schema activation. Greg is encouraged to write a small message from his 'Healthy Side' (Healthy Adult mode) to his 'Shut Down Avoider' (Detached Protector) highlighting the need to engage with his girlfriend rather than detach and withdraw (the 'Wash Up' section).

successes, topics that are unrelated to the presenting problem. Alternatively, the client might speak superficially about emotionally laden material while suppressing their emotional reactions (Detached Protector mode), and the therapist then misses an opportunity to provide understanding and care to the client. In such cases, the therapist should attempt to use mode work to bypass the coping mode and access the Vulnerable Child mode.

Conceptualisation as a Compass

The case conceptualisation and awareness of the client's core emotional needs can be akin to a therapy compass: a helpful reminder of the treatment direction and therapeutic objectives for the client. A useful conceptualisation should be able to remind the clinician of several specific elements of the case; these include the presenting problems, background of the client (including the experience of caregiving and traumatic events), central schemas/modes of coping, and therapeutic objectives and goals. Although it may not be pragmatic to have a large conceptualisation document in view every session, therapists can employ a basic mode conceptualisation diagram to refer to within each discussion, highlighting the reason for a suggested intervention or treatment objective and noting when particular modes are activated in session or by recent triggers.

Enhancing Client Motivation and Responsibility

The length of a course of schema therapy can affect the client's motivation to change, especially if phases are prolonged because of suboptimal responding to the client's presentation. Habitual use of coping modes and styles by the client can result in low motivation to change. Furthermore, clients may evade challenges when they find themselves within the 'titration phase' of treatment, and are expected to take more responsibility for self-care and healthy behaviours. Here, empathic confrontation can be used to encourage further client effort and heighten the emotional meaning of change. Also, mode dialogues can be employed to assist in localising and understanding the modes that are blocking change.

Concluding Remarks

Schema therapy requires more time than traditional cognitive-behavioural psychotherapies. It can be challenging to maintain adherence to the model's techniques over this extended timeframe. Furthermore, the choice of interventions and how they are used changes across the course of treatment. As a result, it is wise for the therapist to bear in mind specific three sources of direction:

1. Objectives/goals of the client: what is the client seeking help with? What do they want from therapy?
2. Primary schema therapy aims and principles: to identify and meet core emotional needs and provide schema- and mode-corrective emotional experiences.
3. The treatment phase in which the client is positioned: see the client as taking more responsibility and exercising more autonomy as the course of treatment progresses.

References

1. Zimmerman M, Rothschild L, Chelminski I. The Prevalence of DSM-IV Personality Disorders in Psychiatric Outpatients. *American Journal of Psychiatry*. 2005;**162**(10):1911–18.

2. Behary W, Dieckmann E. Schema therapy for pathological narcissism: The art of adaptive reparenting. In Ogrodniczuk J, ed., *Understanding and Treating Pathological Narcissism*. American Psychological Association; 2013. pp. 285–300.

3. Fassbinder E, Arntz A. Schema therapy with emotionally inhibited and fearful patients. *Journal of Contemporary Psychotherapy*. 2018;**49**(1):7–14.

4. Tan Y, Lee C, Averbeck L et al. Schema therapy for borderline personality disorder: A qualitative study of patients' perceptions. *PloS ONE*. 2018;**13**(11):e0206039.

5. Alexander F, French T. *Psychoanalytic therapy: Principles and application*. University of Nebraska Press; 1946.

6. Brockman R, Stevens. B, Roediger.E. *Contextual schema therapy: An integrative approach to personality disorders, emotional dysregulation, and interpersonal functioning*. New Harbinger Publications; 2018.

7. Kannan D, Levitt H. A review of client self-criticism in psychotherapy. *Journal of Psychotherapy Integration*. 2013;**23**(2):166–78.

8. Bamelis LL, Evers SM, Spinhoven P, Arntz A. Results of a multicenter randomized controlled trial of the clinical effectiveness of schema therapy for personality disorders. *American Journal of Psychiatry*. 2014, *171*(3), 305–22.

9. Malogiannis I, Arntz A, Spyropoulou A et al. Schema therapy for patients with chronic depression: A single case series study. *Journal of Behavior Therapy and Experimental Psychiatry*. 2014;**45**(3):319–29.

10. Giesen-Bloo J, van Dyck R, Spinhoven P et al. Outpatient psychotherapy for borderline personality disorder. *Archives of General Psychiatry*. 2006;**63**(6):649.

11. Bernstein DP, Keulen-de Vos M, Clercx M et al. Schema therapy for violent PD offenders: A randomized clinical trial. *Psychological medicine*. 2021 Jun. **15**:1–5.

12. Huntjens RJ, Rijkeboer MM, Arntz A. Schema therapy for dissociative identity disorder (DID): Rationale and study protocol. *European Journal of Psychotraumatology*. 2019 Dec. 31;**10**(1):1571377.

13. Bettelheim B. *A good enough parent*. Pan Books; 1987.

Intervention Strategies for Schema Healing 1
Limited Reparenting

Introduction

Schema therapy has a characteristic style of therapeutic relationship which likely differs from the style that most readers would have been trained in. The schema therapist consciously and intentionally provides a role model of a good parent. The therapist seeks to partially replace the child-rearing and socialising experiences the client actually received with healthier responses, healthier guidance, and healthier limits where necessary. Consequently, schema therapy has a more intensely personal flavour than most short-term therapies, and the therapist remains mindful of how each of their responses addresses or fails to address the client's core emotional needs. Over the course of therapy, the therapist adjusts their manner of interacting with the client analogously to changing from addressing a young child, to an adolescent, to, finally, a young adult. This chapter unpacks this style of interaction, called *limited reparenting*.

Limited Reparenting: An Overview

Helping clients discover (or rediscover) their core emotional needs and experience them being satisfied ('getting their needs met') is at the heart of schema therapy. Clients who experience their needs being met are likely to also experience a reduction in schema activation and then, over time, schema healing. We have observed that the emotional development of many chronic clients has been blocked through the chronic frustration of their core emotional needs as children. We have had many adult clients report feeling that their emotional maturity has been stunted, and that they function at a lower level than their same-age peers. Limited reparenting aims to provide limited but powerful doses of need-satisfying interpersonal experiences within the therapeutic relationship that had not been adequately experienced in childhood. It is hoped that in helping the client experience satisfaction of their core emotional needs, we 'kick start' the emotional development of the client.

Rather than allowing the therapeutic relationship to simply 'develop over time', limited reparenting provides a specific architecture that guides how the therapist can leverage the therapeutic relationship to provide *corrective emotional experiences*. Limited reparenting is both a method and an orientation; the therapist attends to the client's specific needs profile, and fosters a robust, authentic therapeutic relationship, idiosyncratic to their individual case conceptualisation. For example, the kind of therapeutic relationship that is fostered for a client suffering primarily with issues related to trust (e.g., Mistrust/Abuse schema) is likely to vary significantly from those whose problems emanate from fears of abandonment. In using the therapeutic relationship to directly meet needs, the schema therapist aims to go

Table 6.1 Therapeutic relationship themes and treatment

Therapy Model	Purpose of Therapeutic Relationship	Characteristic Therapist Responses
Cognitive Behaviour Therapy	• The client ought to be their 'own therapist' • Emphasises the client solving problems • Socratic questioning and guided discovery • The therapist often in coach/educator role	Let's look at that belief 'I don't have what it takes'. How have you come to that conclusion?' 'Is it 100% true that you can't do your job?' 'What's a more balanced view?'
Psychoanalytic Therapy	• 'Blank slate' • No self-disclosure • The therapist provides an open space for the client to explore and analyse meaningful experiences • Therapist withholds emotional reactions towards the client	'So, for you, it seems you consider yourself as not "having what it takes".'
Schema Therapy	• Appropriate self-disclosure • Therapist acts as a parent-like figure to meet some of the needs directly in the relationship • This role is modelled and gradually adopted by the client's own Healthy Adult side	'Listen, I see a person who is trying so hard … I believe in you, I really believe you can do it'

beyond a 'standard level' of therapist care (e.g., in warmth, therapeutic alliance, unconditional positive regard) to become a genuine source of support and understanding, within the appropriate boundaries of the therapeutic relationship [1].

Limited reparenting is not a focused intervention or technique in the traditional sense of 'doing' something 'to' a client in a series of steps or phases; rather, it is a therapeutic style interwoven throughout the treatment and therapeutic relationship. At times, however, the process of limited reparenting may be more overt in the session (such as when the therapist is providing nurturance to a distressed client, or when the therapist is directly challenging a client's dysfunctional behaviour). In our training programmes we often say that the essence of limited reparenting is to 'be with' the client rather than 'doing to'. The distinctiveness of this approach, in contrast with other psychotherapy models, is illustrated in Table 6.1.

Theoretical Change Process

Many clients grew up in environments where their core emotional needs were largely unmet. While they concentrated on coping with these harmful conditions, to some degree their emotional development as children stagnated; they did not learn to give words to feelings, understand and regulate their emotions, or employ adaptive coping repertoires. Limited reparenting, through directly meeting needs, aims to provide the client with corrective emotional experiences, directly modifying the EMS associated with specific needs. In the limited reparenting approach, the therapist acts as a model of the 'good parent' that the client should have received earlier in life. Throughout therapy, the schema therapist authentically models responses to the client's emotional needs. As a result, the client comes to internalise the therapist's example as a basis for new, healthy scripts for cognition (i.e., healthy schemas) and more functional behaviours (i.e., coping).

The Process of Providing Care in Limited Reparenting: Meeting Needs Directly Using the Therapy Relationship

Limited reparenting is a style of interacting with clients in which the therapist aims to give the client experiences of having their emotional needs *met directly* within the therapeutic relationship. As an example, imagine a client who might present with a Defectiveness EMS and an underlying unmet need for acceptance and praise. In other approaches, such as traditional cognitive therapy, the therapist may primarily seek to undermine or challenge the Defectiveness schema in an indirect, Socratic way: 'What has led you to see things that way? How have you come to that conclusion about yourself?' In a limited reparenting relationship, the maladaptive schema content could be corrected more directly: 'I want you to know there is nothing wrong with you, and I look forward to our sessions.' This style of response is akin to how a parent would respond to a child: directly meeting their needs with warmth and compassion, rather than approaching the situation from a logical position.

With chronic client, schema therapists do not assume that the client has had access to sufficient healthy parenting to be able to access healthy functional scripts for thought and behaviour without the therapist's direct input. For example, if a ten-year-old child presented in a distressed state to a parent, saying 'Dad, I have no friends, I feel like a loser', a Socratic way to challenge the belief would be: 'How have you come to this conclusion? Is it 100% true that you have no friends?' Clearly, a purely cognitive approach to parenting in this situation risks the parent failing to attune to the child's *attachment* need. A Socratic approach primarily engages the rational/cognitive capabilities. However, in clients with personality disorders or chronic emotional problems, this 'healthy' rational side can be underdeveloped or seemingly absent. Furthermore, the modelling of rational methods from caregivers without also responding to the child's emotional needs such as warmth/connection/acceptance (i.e., 'got the words and not the hug') results in the rational responses having less impact than they would if delivered with warmth and acceptance. So, in other words, what people with impoverished (compared with healthy) childhoods feel in response to 'healthy cognitive dialogues' can be quite different: the latter might feel comforted by rational words, but the former don't have the same positive emotional connotations and so are less likely to feel comfort or reassurance.

Qualities of a 'Good Enough Parent'

To understand what limited reparenting might look like in practice, we must first consider some of the core ingredients of 'good enough parenting' from the perspective of core emotional needs [1, 2, 3].

Care, Attunement, Nurturance

Above all else, a good parent provides adequate care, but beyond this they also offer safe and supportive involvement in a child's life. They are attuned to the emotions and needs of their child and can respond with compassion when their child suffers. Through attuning and attending to their child's needs and feelings, the good parent provides a healthy model of self-regulation to the child. Through their dependability and stability, a good parent signals safety to the child and provides a stable, 'safe base' from which the child can explore the world, supporting healthy development.

Guidance, Direction, Confidence, and the Support of Autonomy and Competence

A good parent provides guidance and direction. In infancy, the parent makes all decisions affecting their child. However, as the child develops, the parent balances encouraging their child to make healthy choices and decisions with allowing their child to increasingly exercise autonomy and develop their own individual identity. The healthy parent will also instil confidence and support the competence of the developing child directly with support and belief in the child's developing attributes, and through modelling confident and competent behaviours and attitudes.

Boundaries, Limits, and Respect for Others

So far, we have described the central behaviours of a good parent as those of a nurturer. But a good parent must also help the child understand limits and boundaries in the world and manage any unhelpful and destructive behaviour or feelings of frustration. A child that never learns how to deal with feelings of frustration and anger may go on to struggle with these feelings in adulthood. A good parent teaches their child to balance meeting their own needs with co-operating and respecting others. The good parent actively discourages their child from engaging in behaviour likely to damage their relationships and teaches them how immature coping will, in turn, lead them to miss out on having their own needs met. How the schema therapist embodies these 'good parent' qualities to the fullest extent possible within the boundaries of a psychotherapeutic relationship is the focus of the rest of this chapter.

The Practice of Limited Reparenting

Schema Attunement: The Foundation of a Limited Reparenting Relationship

Like a good parenting relationship, a successful limited reparenting therapeutic relationship rests upon a solid foundation of attunement. Schema attunement is itself a powerful schema change strategy – perhaps even 'the glue of schema therapy' (p. 36) [4]. A key skill of any therapist is the ability to listen and empathise, but in schema therapy we endeavour to go beyond a standard level of therapeutic listening skills to directly provide a high level of attunement within the session. Many client, through histories of emotional neglect and invalidation, have not received adequate levels of attunement from their caregivers. The schema therapist – by providing attunement directly, in vivo – creates an opportunity for correcting the client's negative expectations and schemas, particularly those involving emotional deprivation and emotional inhibition. The attuned therapist can communicate to the client a deep understanding of the client's own 'internal reality' [5].

In therapeutic contexts, attunement has been conceptualised as a two-part process that begins with (1) *empathising* – being sensitive to and experiencing an understanding of another person's sensations, needs, and/or feelings, and (2) *communicating that understanding* to the other person with the aim of creating the experience of *resonance* [6, 5]. Attunement has several important therapeutic effects:

1) **Bypasses Maladaptive Coping Modes** – Attuned moments in therapy, in which the therapist makes space for the client to share their feelings and needs related to triggering events, are the antithesis of the maladaptive coping modes implicated in the client's psychopathology. Creating these moments more frequently in sessions helps the therapist bypass coping modes and starts the process of pattern-breaking in vivo, using the therapeutic relationship.

2) **Provides in vivo Opportunities for Schema Healing** – Through communicating their understanding, the therapist directly validates the client's needs, feelings, and experiences, providing a *corrective experience* that contrasts with experiences from their family of origin. This kind of attuned understanding was likely missing from their childhood experience and very likely meets their core emotional needs in vivo.

3) **Socialises the Client to Experiential Work** – Attending to and seeking to understand the client's emotional experiences teaches the client to value emotions and reinforces the expectation promoted at the outset that therapy will be experiential. After a lifetime of experiential avoidance, clients are reintroduced to experiencing, sharing, and processing their emotions at a manageable pace.

4) **Enhances the Case Conceptualisation** – The process of attuning aids the therapist's conceptualisation of the specific underlying schemas and associated needs that are driving clinical problems. It is very important in schema therapy that the interventions are 'hitting the mark' by addressing the correct schema-related need. Higher levels of successful attunement (marked by clients indicating that they feel understood) in session increases the therapist's confidence in the case conceptualisation, and the likelihood that any interventions targeting specific needs will be successful. Without a high level of attunement, the therapist risks providing limited reparenting and experiential exercises haphazardly, with clients less likely to progress as a consequence. For example, the therapist may respond as though the core concern of the client is *defectiveness*, when in fact the core concern might be *abandonment*. Such misattunement is very likely to 'miss the mark', and the client may feel misunderstood.

As stated earlier, a high level of attunement is so important that it can be thought of as the 'glue' of schema therapy: a necessary skill that underpins the efficacy of all four broad schema therapy intervention strategies (limited reparenting, experiential, cognitive, behavioural) [5]. We have also noticed that persistent problems in the efficacy of experiential techniques can often be traced back to a poor capacity for attunement on behalf of the therapist and/or the client. We have come to understand that higher levels of within-session attunement between the therapist and client appear to be a good predictor of readiness for emotion-focused interventions. Attunement is thus a foundational skill for schema therapists.

A Process-Based Approach to Building Schema Attunement in Session

Background and Aim

We have found that clients who have not learned healthy ways of processing and expressing needs and emotions from their caregivers are also those who experience the most difficulties 'tuning in' to their emotional world [5]. Consequently, these clients are likely to have developed strong coping modes to deal with emotions when they are triggered. In trying to orient clients towards their emotions it is likely that, at times, therapists will face the client's coping modes. An initial goal of attunement is to make space with the client to share emotionally evocative material within the therapy relationship. The therapist aims to 'trigger' the client's schema-based experiences in a safe and contained way in the therapy room so that they can be understood, attuned to, and co-regulated. The easiest way to do this is to enquire about specific recent triggering episodes for the client.

1. Focus on Specific Episodes of Distress. A good portion of schema therapy sessions should generally focus on understanding the client's recent emotional experiences or 'triggers'. This process often flows naturally from homework tasks (e.g., mode awareness forms, attempts at pattern-breaking) which can prompt the client to recall recent relevant triggering experiences. For some clients who are extremely avoidant or detached, sharing information about triggers may be difficult as this information may be ordinarily avoided or pushed out of awareness. It is important in these cases to be client and assume that all emotional episodes generally have triggering antecedents. For example, many clients report that there is no trigger to their feelings of intense loneliness and that they experience them occurring 'out of the blue'. However, close inspection of the antecedents might reveal this feeling to most often be triggered late at night when alone at home.

We have found that obtaining specific and detailed information about the trigger situation is more likely to help bring emotions into the room than generalised, abstract, or broad 'stories' about an episode. Ask direct, probing questions such as 'What was the specific moment that really did it for you?' It is often something specific, such as a particular act, non-verbal event (disapproving look), or verbal communication from other people. At other times it may be a lack of stimulation or connection that eventually triggers feelings of disconnection and loneliness. In any case, specific descriptions of the triggering situations are generally more conducive to clients sharing their emotions, while broad narratives are generally more conducive to clients remaining in maladaptive coping states.

As discussed in Chapter 5, it is generally advisable to structure schema therapy sessions such that the first third of the session (say, 15–20 minutes) will be spent discussing any recent triggering experiences. This can often be combined with a review of any homework tasks, which often trigger strong emotions. Over time, the client becomes socialised to expect that the first third of the session provides a space for exploring recent triggering events (see Box 6.1 for an example).

2. Tune in to the Emotional Response. This should be done by exploring the nature of the emotional reaction to the triggering event by identifying appropriate emotion labels (e.g., 'I felt scared') and/or related bodily sensations (e.g., 'My heart started pounding'). Box 6.2 illustrates this process.

Box 6.1 Example Identifying a Triggering Experience During the First Third of The Session

THERAPIST: So Jenny, you were saying that you have been beating yourself up all week, can you tell me about a specific time this week when you were feeling this way?

JENNY: Yes, last Friday was the worst!

THERAPIST: Can you tell me about a specific moment on Friday, perhaps when you were most triggered that day?

JENNY: My boss was on my back all day!

THERAPIST: Can you focus on a specific moment with your boss, Jenny? What <u>exactly</u> was it that was so upsetting about the way he was treating you?

JENNY: It was the words, he kept saying … 'this is not good enough' … but it was also the frown … he was really angry.

THERAPIST: OK … it was the words … not good enough … but also his frown, and angry tone?

JENNY: Yes … like I'm in trouble.

Box 6.2 Example Identifying the Emotional Response to a Recent Triggering Experience

THERAPIST: And how did you feel in response to being treated that way?

JENNY: I felt anxious … like pressure.

THERAPIST: And where could you feel this pressure or anxiety building up *[therapist gestures towards her own body]* in your body?

JENNY: In my stomach … like a churning … and up into my chest.

THERAPIST: *[summarising the understanding so far, and empathising]* OK, so let's see if I am understanding this right so far … your boss was badgering you, and frowning, and generally acting in an angry manner, and this led to you feeling intense anxiety and a kind of pressure, felt in your stomach and chest?

JENNY: Yes.

THERAPIST: That sounds really hard for you … no one likes being treated like that in their place of work, and I know how much you have been trying in this job! *[Also communicating empathy with facial gesture.]*

JENNY: Yes.

---

3. **Uncover Underlying Schema/s and Needs.** In schema therapy, it is important to attune not only to the feelings, but also to the underlying schemas and needs driving the emotional distress. Thus, we can call this process *schema attunement*, to differentiate it from attunement that might be solely focused on a person's emotional experience. In most cases, we find that episodes of emotional distress can be understood in terms of the activation of specific schema themes and their underlying needs. Here, we use our knowledge of the eighteen schemas to understand the specific meanings behind a person's distress or emotional reaction. What did this event mean to them, in terms of specific schema themes? Take a curious stance of enquiry to continue questioning about the meaning of the trigger

---

Box 6.3 Example of Attuning to Underlying Schemas and Needs in a Recent Triggering Event

THERAPIST: OK ... Jenny, I could easily assume why you were feeling that way, but I'd like to check with you. What did it mean to you in that moment that your boss was treating you that way?

JENNY: I'm in trouble ... I've done something wrong.

THERAPIST: Right ... and what would that mean to you if you were in trouble for doing something wrong?

JENNY: It's my fault. *[Activation of emotions becomes evident.]*

THERAPIST: OK ... [pause] ... and if it was your fault, what would that mean about you?

JENNY: I'm not good enough.

THERAPIST: Ah .... OK, I think I'm starting to get it. It was that 'not good enough' theme again? *[Therapist checks the emerging understanding in terms of one of the eighteen schema themes.]*

JENNY: Yes, of course ... I always feel that way when others criticise or are angry with me.

THERAPIST: That feeling of 'not good enough' ... does it capture all of that anxious-pressured feeling or is there something else too? *[Therapist checks to see if there are other schemas at play; sometimes there are multiple schemas triggered.]*

JENNY: No that is it, I just feel worthless, like nothing I do is ever good enough!

THERAPIST: It sounds to me like you really needed your boss to show more respect in that moment, even if he had to give constructive feedback. *[Therapist validates the under-lying need for validation and basic respect.]*

JENNY: Yes! That would have been nice!

---

and feeling for them, using cognitive techniques such as downward arrowing and Socratic questioning. Uncovering specific schema themes deepens the therapist's understanding and helps to pinpoint specific underlying needs. See Box 6.3 for an example.

4. Summarise and Check Your Understanding, Empathise, and Link to Historical Origins. At this stage, the client has really opened up about their inner feelings, their antecedents, and the schema themes that have been activated. They are much more likely to be 'in' their emotional experience. Tentatively summarise your understanding of what the client has communicated about their experience so far. The goal is to create a resonance between the client and therapist such that the client, in that moment, understands and can acknowledge that the therapist accurately comprehends their experience. This kind of attuned understanding is often a powerful antidote for clients with Emotional Deprivation EMS who often feel that 'no one gets me'. You may need to repeat steps 1–3 as necessary to fine-tune your understanding based on the client's feedback until the client reports a high degree of resonance. Once the client communicates this resonance, offer some empathic statements and look for opportunities to link to relevant childhood experiences, making such links explicit (see Box 6.4).

5. Bridge into Intervention Strategies – 'The Work'. Higher levels of within-session attunement, 'being with' the client in this way, will on most occasions be experienced as need-satisfying. However, now that the client is more in touch with their feelings and related

---

Box 6.4 Example of Summarising Recent Triggering Events and Linking to Historical Origins

THERAPIST: OK, so I think I'm starting to get it now: you were at work trying your best as usual, when your boss scolded you in a way that was invalidating and aggressive, making you feel like YOU were not good enough as a person. Is that right?

JENNY: Yes.

THERAPIST: Is it fair to say that this triggered off your own Punitive Critic, like YOU started believing it was true?' *[Therapist links to Punitive Critic in shared case conceptualisation.]*

JENNY: Yes . . . there it goes again . . . I always do this!

THERAPIST: Look, Jenny . . . this makes a lot of sense to me that you would react so strongly, you know . . . it's not the first time you have been treated this way by people in authority. In a way this is kind of like other times when you basically got the message you weren't good enough from someone in authority . . . It's a little similar to the kind of pressure, and message that mum would give you . . .?

JENNY: Yes . . . I can see that . . . I can't handle that . . . it's so hard . . .

THERAPIST: I'm really sorry to hear this Jenny because I don't think you deserve this from the people that you work with. I know you are always trying your best at work and you deserve more respect than that. At the same time, I'm really glad that you shared this with me. I feel like I understand you a lot more, particularly about the relationship with your boss and how he triggers off that old 'not good enough' critic feeling so easily.

Box 6.5 Example of Segue from Attunement Portion of Session to Intervention

THERAPIST: This issue of feeling 'not good enough' seems really important for you at the moment, Jenny; you've had this critic on your back all week *[reference to the prominent activated mode]*. I'm wondering if it would be a good use of our time today if we focus on this theme of 'not good enough' and put it on a chair *[for some chair work]*?

---

schemas and needs, schema therapists will capitalise by becoming more active in the session and skilfully bridge into intervention techniques (see Box 6.5).

Therapist Tips for Successful Attunement

It is usually helpful to slow things down during your attempts at attunement. Slowing down seems more conducive to emotional processing, while a faster pace of sharing seems to be more conducive to a 'cognitive' level of processing. Sometimes it may be necessary to heighten the experience by asking the client to close their eyes during this process. This may be particularly necessary in cases where the coping mode is strong, blocking emotional processing. For clients who are more easily able to process and share their emotional experiences, this may not be necessary. For those who are easily overwhelmed by their emotions, this kind of heightening is usually not desirable, so be guided by the client's 'window of tolerance'.

The Central Task of Limited Reparenting: Balancing Nurturance and Boundaries

In limited reparenting there is a balance between two 'poles' of client interaction that are always in some state of tension: (a) nurturance and support, whereby the therapist attends to the vulnerabilities of the client's emotional state by directly providing nurturance and care; and (b) boundaries and confrontation, whereby the therapist seeks to provide healthy boundaries and challenge the client to express themselves in healthy ways. Figure 6.1 depicts the four central types of limited reparenting interactions that lie on a spectrum from care, guidance and empathic confrontation through to outright limit setting. Throughout therapy, the therapist considers the overarching core emotional needs and presenting issues of the client. On some occasions, the therapist may need primarily to provide nurturance and attuned care to the client. However, as in real parenting, at other times the therapist may need to challenge behaviour and take a more assertive stance. For example, the therapist may need to set limits and challenge the client in managing unhelpful or inappropriate requests. Although care and nurturance are crucial aspects of limited reparenting, the therapeutic relationship needs to operate within secure, appropriate therapeutic boundaries. These therapeutic and ethical boundaries aid the client and protect the therapist. For example, a client may want extra out-of-session contact and care. However, the therapist needs to balance their own needs for personal privacy and professional boundaries (see Table 6.2). Attunement to the client's particular needs in the moment provides a guide as to which 'leg' the therapist needs to stand on: care or boundaries. Many vulnerable clients tend to require many more nurturance and care tasks. Overcompensating and aggressive clients often require more of a focus on boundaries and limits. Box 6.6 provides a clinical example of finding this balance.

Providing Guidance and Direction

The provision of developmentally appropriate guidance and direction is an important facet of the limited reparenting approach. Just as a good parent would not leave important decisions to a child without guidance, the schema therapist seeks also to 'have an opinion', particularly about client behaviours or decisions that seem to be driven by schemas or modes. This is most important for clients that appear to be operating from a low (emotional) developmental age and is less important for clients with a strong Healthy Adult self.

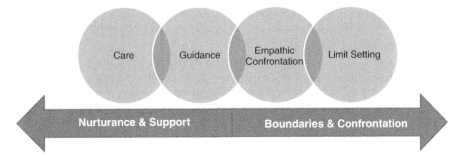

Figure 6.1 Core elements of limited reparenting

Table 6.2 Examples of healthy limit setting vs problematic boundary violations

Situation	Healthy Limited Reparenting	Problematic Boundaries
Client seeking more support out of session	Contacting client for a brief solution-focused discussion out of session (e.g., 10 minutes)	Regularly spending significant time on the phone (outside normal work role)
Client asking how a holiday was for the therapist	General noting of how the trip was for the therapist	Discussing very personal account of holiday
Client noting some romantic feelings for the therapist	Empathic confrontation and limit setting 'I'm your therapist, and it's important that it is clear to you that it's no more than that'	Validating and being 'too kind' to the client and refraining from setting a limit in a strong way out of 'fear I would hurt their feelings'

Box 6.6 Clinical Example of Balancing Nurturance and Support with Setting Limits and Boundaries

Therapist Ben likes aspects of the limited reparenting approach. He is a warm and nurturing clinician and finds that validating and affirming fits with his natural inclinations as a therapist. His client, Mary, is at first very detached and challenging for Ben to engage. He provides appropriate care and tries hard to demonstrate his willingness to support Mary. He allows for some email contact out of session and contacts Mary when she was expecting news from the family court about her son. In the proceeding months, Mary becomes more invested in the relationship. Ben notices that Mary drops into the clinic, wanting to pass on four long letters to Ben out of session. She then lingers around the clinic waiting room for an hour, seemingly hoping that she may have contact with Ben. In the following weeks, Ben avoids bringing these events up with Mary even though he feels unnerved by the communication. In the following weeks, Mary starts to initiate contact with him on his personal Facebook account. Similarly, Ben is uncomfortable in confronting Mary about these transgressions, feeling that it may 'trigger her defectiveness'.

Supervision Response

Although Ben is demonstrating good care and nurturance, he needs to set limits and boundaries on Mary's attempts to make contact outside of sessions. Understandably, Ben is worried about upsetting Mary; however, he needs to model good, healthy boundaries and limits to the therapeutic relationship. The supervisor suggests identifying specific schemas that are blocking Ben in asserting the boundary. Ben and his supervisor practise a way to communicate his concerns via empathic confrontation and role played this in his supervision meeting:

> Mary, I know it's not your intention, but I need to talk to you about your contact with me out of session and online. A part of me is saying 'just let this go', but my Wise Therapist side is saying I really need to discuss this with you. Outside of sessions I need to be able to sign off and be human, and it doesn't really feel right for me as your therapist to be friends on Facebook. Another thing I wanted to mention is that I know that one thing that enables me to ensure that I am the best therapist I can be for you is through keeping some kind of boundary between my personal and work life. It's important for me to take care of our relationship by protecting it from these sorts of confusions.

Such an approach contrasts with schools of therapy that refrain from 'giving advice' to the client. The schema therapist is encouraged to play an active role, at least at the beginning of therapy, in guiding clients' decisions in essential areas of life, such as study, work, relationships, and friendships. However, this is also done in a way which is mindful of the unmet needs that underlie the client's schemas. For example, a client whose Dependence EMS developed due to not getting enough direction or guidance will need more guidance at first, before transitioning to more independent functioning. In contrast, a client whose Dependence EMS arose from overprotective parenting which failed to meet their need for autonomy will need earlier opportunities and encouragement to make their own decisions to enable them to develop a sense of competence and self-reliance.

Authentic limited reparenting includes directly expressing genuine concern for the client and their needs. For example, 'I don't want you to re-enter into a relationship in which your needs aren't taken into account; I want you to live a life in which you feel loved and in which you feel safe with someone close.' Note that such advice and direction is not solely based on the values of the therapist but also on an understanding of the needs of the client. Therapists may offer direct opinions if this will encourage clients to take better care of their own needs. We have noticed that, in the early stages of practice, many schema therapists need to work on incorporating more expressions along the lines of 'I want you to . . . ', 'I think it could be a bad idea to . . . '. This guiding language illustrates the therapist's desire to play an essential role in the client's life and provide a role model for the client's emerging Healthy Adult self. Such a stance can unnerve beginner schema therapists into thinking that their clients might become 'dependent' on them. The 'dependence paradox' [7], can help illustrate the role of the schema therapist: a level of healthy dependence in close relationships when needed is associated with increased self-sufficiency and autonomous functioning. Accepting one's attachment needs paradoxically enables more independent engagement with the wider world over time. In line with this idea, schema therapy views a temporary hierarchical relationship as necessary for some clients to internalise the qualities of a healthy adult. The ultimate aim is an autonomously functioning adult so, over time, more responsibility is given to the client to drive change. Just as the schema therapist meets the client's dependency needs early in the therapy, they also push for the client's Healthy Adult to 'take over', thereby promoting autonomy in the latter stages of therapy. Box 6.7 provides more detail on how guidance may be provided by the therapist in regards to the client's relationships.

Box 6.7 Guidance in Relationships

A client may not yet have learned how to establish healthy relationships or partnering. Many clients become accustomed to neglectful or abusive relationships because that is all they have known as a child. Clients like this are often attracted to repeat these patents in their current relationships, a phenomenon called *schema chemistry*. Acting as a role model of a 'good parent', the therapist can interrupt this 'path of least resistance' by educating and supporting the client when they are entering into a new relationship, to look out for their needs. To what degree does a potential partner represent a good fit in terms of their core emotional needs? Such an approach can include providing the client with simple principles such as 'Does this potential new partner apologise if they have done something wrong?', 'Are they interested in your feelings?', 'Do they let you speak out and have a voice?', 'Are they attentive/responsive to what you tell them?'

Empathic Confrontation

It is clear that the nurturing qualities of care, compassion, and guidance are elements of 'good parental care'. However, a good parent is also required to manage and set boundaries on a child's unhelpful or disruptive impulses. Empathic confrontation is one of the most important therapeutic tools within schema therapy [1]. Within this approach, the therapist, in an empathic and non-punitive manner, challenges unhealthy behaviours that are typically mode- or schema-driven and which seem to perpetuate the client's presenting problems. Empathy grows from the therapist establishing an understanding of how the client's basic core emotional needs were neglected in childhood: 'What happened to you that you have to be this way (to survive)?'

Empathic confrontation is analogous to a faucet with two taps: (1) confrontation, which can feel painfully cold, and (2) empathy, which can heat the cold to a bearable temperature. How 'warm' or 'cold' the empathic confrontation is can depend on factors such as the stage of therapy and the emotional capacity of the client. Typically, in the early stages of treatment the therapeutic relationship is developing and the client's emotion regulation skills may not be sufficiently developed. As a result, a relatively high level of empathy may be required within the empathic confrontation. Towards the end of the therapy, however, the intention is to encourage more behavioural change, which leads to more confrontation compared to the beginning of treatment. The schema therapist is likely to begin with more 'gentle' or 'warm' empathic confrontation with a client with borderline personality disorder, compared to working with a client with narcissistic patterns, who may require a more direct approach earlier on in therapy.

When the therapist judges that the client's within-session behaviour is impeding therapeutic progress, the therapist typically confronts the client in a personal way, describing the dysfunctional pattern and the effect on the therapist. Often, confrontation is mitigated and defused by naming these patterns based on the mode conceptualisation of the client. For example, the therapist may note the impact of a coping mode on the session: 'That dominating part (mode) of you makes it very difficult for me to be there for you and to care for you the way you need'.

There are many ways in which empathic confrontation can be initiated. Often, therapists are more naturally adept in providing care and guidance to clients but find empathic confrontation challenging. Beginning schema therapists may benefit from some guidelines or 'scaffolding statements' that can serve as a guideline for conducting this intervention (see Box 6.8).

Limit Setting

Limit setting, just like empathic confrontation, aims to change interpersonally challenging client behavioural patterns which are impeding progress both within therapy and in daily life. Where empathic confrontation aims to achieve this change through clients developing insight and awareness, limit setting aims to stop the problematic behaviour immediately through responses designed to act as direct natural consequences of the client's actions. Typically, this means empathic confrontation is preferable to limit setting if the circumstances allow for it. Limit setting should be the final stage of a process in which various 'softer' interventions have been applied to change dysfunctional patterns without success, including attempts at empathic confrontation, or when the behaviour being addressed requires a strong boundary (e.g., aggression).

Box 6.8 Guidelines for Empathic Confrontation

Before the Session

- Identify the problematic behaviour that needs to be addressed.
- Check whether it is an appropriate time for this intervention. Is the client sufficiently emotionally stable in the session to hear feedback? Are there particular presenting issues that should take precedence? (e.g., a relationship breakup, very recent suicide attempt).
- Identify the primary emotional response you experience when confronted with this behaviour.
- Identify your immediate behavioural response when faced with this behaviour.

During the Session

- Indicate that you want to discuss what is happening in the relationship.
- Identify the behaviour in a concrete and specific way and check whether the client recognises it as an issue.
- Describe how it affects you emotionally and what your behavioural response would be if this behavioural pattern does not change: 'When you criticise me in that way, it's hard for me to be there for you, a part of me wants to disengage; I don't want that for you.'
- Use the relationship to extrapolate to other aspects of the client's life; 'I'm your therapist, I understand why you act this way, but other people don't have the training that I do and will just distance themselves from you.'
- Ask how the client feels; what is their reaction to your comments?
- Describe this behaviour as a 'schema' or a 'mode' (i.e., a pattern) in the client's life. Discuss this behaviour as part of a 'mode' of the client. Initiate the confrontation in a non-personal way: 'It is the bully mode that is attacking me' vs 'You are attacking me'.
- Identify the background in this mode – the basic needs that were neglected in the past.
- Indicate what could become a healthy alternative for the client, a healthy way of handling feelings and interpersonal relationships.

Example

THERAPIST: Mary, I need to speak with you about how you talk with me sometimes, particularly last session. A part of me wants to let this slide, but another side (my Healthy Therapist mode) thinks it's really important for you to know how it comes across. When you get angry at me in the way that you did last session, it makes me want to shut down. It's hard for me to take. Can you see what I'm saying?

MARY: Yeah, okay I messed up again [looking defensive].

THERAPIST: Well, I don't see you messing up. I think if you act in this way with me, then I am assuming that you do this with others too. But I'm a psychologist. I understand what's happening for you and where it's coming from, but others out there don't, and they will just back away from you. I want to be there for you, to help you. But it's hard for me to do that when you're speaking harshly to me. What do you think about what I'm saying?

MARY: Look, I was having a bad day, ok! [looks away, less defensive tone].

THERAPIST: I know it's not your intention to be harsh, but I'm a human, I have feelings too. I think it's your Fireball Mode [Angry Child mode], I think it comes out when you're feeling that others are not tuned in to you . . . when you're not feeling considered or understood. This reminds me of how things were in your family – people didn't take the time to hear you. Am I right?

MARY: Yeah. It just comes out sometimes. Yeah, I'm not rational.

THERAPIST: I know it's not easy, but we have to find a way to speak to each other where we both feel safe and ok. Can we spend a little bit of time today working out a way to understand your anger last week?

Setting a limit to curtail a specific behaviour is like taking a one-way street; there is no turning back once you have taken it. The therapist should ask themselves 'if this client behaviour does not change, is it important enough to interrupt the therapy by trying to limit it?' For example, forms of client aggression will have to be immediately limited to guarantee the safety of the therapist and/or the client. With many other behavioural patterns, however, there is no urgent need to set limits. Examples of these 'mild' forms of unacceptable behaviour can include such things as the client arriving late, the client asking too many personal questions, and the client regularly interrupting therapy. These are generally best managed using empathic confrontation.

Prolonged acceptance of mild forms of inappropriate behaviour can lead to the therapist losing sight of the conversations or becoming otherwise demoralised, or even abused, in the therapy. Although most therapists would agree with the importance of limiting aggression, limits on milder forms of inappropriate behaviour will vary from one therapist to another. It is up to the therapist to decide when a limit should be set. However, with the freedom to determine the right timing comes the responsibility to observe proper boundaries as a therapist. This is not an evident skill for many therapists as they often focus more on the needs and feelings of their client and less on recognising their own needs and boundaries. Like all aspects of limited reparenting, limit setting should be carried out in a personal way (see Box 6.9 for an example). The therapist explains what the boundary is and why it is important, just as a good parent would.

Inseparable from setting limits is specifying the consequences of any further crossing of these limits. The consequences should be related to the nature of the inappropriate behaviour (e.g., no extra session time for those that are late) and must not be conveyed in a punitive or rigid way. The therapist may consider consequences such as the shortening of the session or therapy, or asking the client to apologise (if they have not already done so) or to make an extra effort to repair the 'damage' caused by crossing the limit, for example by engaging in additional forms of journaling or similar activities.

Therapeutic Stance of the Therapist

Authentic Therapist, Appropriate Self-Disclosure, 'Realness'

Authentic, genuine responses and appropriate self-disclosure from the therapist are central qualities of limited reparenting [8]. Such 'realness' contrasts with a therapist appearing to be

---

Box 6.9 Example of Limit Setting

THERAPIST: I've explained to you that I don't want you to be so rude. I want you to stop doing this. But if it happens again, I want you to apologise and let me know you really understand why it's not ok to treat me this way.

'just doing their job' or robotically following manualised procedures. Being 'real' may involve the client knowing some small but meaningful elements of the therapist's life (such as if they have a family or if they enjoyed their holiday). It also means that the therapist does not attempt to appear 'perfect' or free from any personal troubles or difficulties. Being authentic often involves sharing honest personal reactions (both positive and negative) about the effects of the client's behaviour (such as criticism or anger) in session.

Therapists might sometimes wonder whether a potential disclosure would be authentic or wonder exactly how authentic to be. Three key questions the therapist should consider in guiding their decisions to self-disclose are:

(1) Will my disclosure strengthen the therapeutic relationship?

(2) Is my disclosure generated from my Healthy Adult/Therapist mode? Or is it being driven by a Vulnerable Child mode or maladaptive coping mode?

(3) How would such a disclosure be therapeutic, meeting the needs of the client?

Box 6.10 provides an illustration of how a therapist might weigh up whether or not to make a self-disclosure.

Disclosures about personal reactions or experiences could be driven by a therapist's maladaptive coping mode or reveal a deep vulnerability (an activated Vulnerable Child mode). For example, a client may be critical and hostile to the therapist for being late to a session. Suppose the therapist was to respond via their Healthy Adult. In that case, they might take a moment to compose themselves and respond (rather than react) to the client's grievances: 'To be honest, a part of me did feel criticised when you reacted like that. I don't think it was your intention, but if you did this with others it would be very tough for them to hear.' The resultant disclosure allows the client to understand the impact of their behaviour, healthily empathise with the therapist's experience, and understand how this interaction relates to more general difficulties they might have interacting with other people. In contrast, a therapist in Vulnerable Child mode may struggle to hold back tears, feel belittled and anxious, and disclose that they 'didn't like the way you were speaking to me!'. Here, the client could feel responsible for the therapist's emotional state or distrust the therapist's ability to assist them. Alternatively, a therapist driven by an avoidant coping mode may simply fail to address the client's behaviour, depriving the client of a valuable learning opportunity and delaying the client's recovery. An assumption of the schema therapy model is that the therapist has a well-developed Healthy Adult mode, enabling them to deal with a range of behaviours and schema patterns. For this reason, self-therapy and/or self-practice and self-reflection is highly encouraged for schema therapists [9].

Limited Reparenting Informed by the Background and Formulation

Attunement describes the process by which the therapist improves their understanding of the client's inner experience by a combination of careful listening, observation, and

---

Box 6.10 Clinical Illustration of Therapist Choosing Whether to Disclose

Greg is accessing treatment for alcoholism from therapist Ben. Greg presents to session following an alcohol relapse and is hungover and unwell in session. Ben empathises with his client's predicament; he had a large 40th birthday party two nights before and was very hungover himself the day before. He notes to his client, 'Yeah, I know how bad hangovers are, I had a horrible one yesterday'. In this case, would this therapist disclosure work to strengthen the therapeutic alliance? It would be very likely that the disclosure would result in the client feeling invalidated or that his struggle was being trivialised.

Furthermore, the client may feel unsure whether Ben is trustworthy or reliable enough to help support him. In contrast, if Ben was in recovery from addiction with a substantial period of sobriety behind him, self-disclosure could enhance the therapeutic bond. For example, a disclosure such as 'I know how hard hangovers and relapses are, I was there too ten years ago, and it will get easier, you can get through this' could convey a great depth of understanding.

---

checking in. This process of the therapist attuning to the client directly meets a need for understanding, but also models to the client how they can better understand themselves.

The schema therapist goes beyond basic empathic counselling by recognising past as well as current influences on the client's emotional reactions. For example, both a counsellor and a schema therapist might say 'Of course you are feeling this way (anxious, angry, sad); this is a difficult situation. Anyone in this situation would feel sad or anxious', but only the schema therapist is likely to go on to say 'And I want you to know that you matter here. I care about you, especially knowing what you have experienced in the past. I understand why this is a difficult situation for you! I can understand, you are feeling this upset not only because of this situation but also because when you felt this way as a child. It was because you thought it meant that you would never be able to rely on anyone to care for you, and it's hard not to believe that now.'

Having demonstrated attuned understanding, the schema therapist then aims to correct the EMS and meet the unmet need (e.g., in the above example, recognising the client's Emotional Deprivation EMS and past unmet need for nurturance and care). The most useful therapist disclosures depend on which schema predominates at that moment and which schemas are pertinent in the client's formulation. Table 6.3 lists examples of statements that could be useful depending on which schema is active in the context of specific unmet needs.

What If?

In some cases, the direct style involved in limited reparenting can be challenging for the therapist trained in traditional notions of therapeutic 'boundaries', and they may fear being judged by other therapists for impropriety. Genuine care may entail the therapist being more aware of meaningful events within the client's life (specific meetings, exams, job interviews). It may involve writing the client a birthday message or encouraging their treatment progress. Transitional objects can be utilised within the therapy relationship to promote and strengthen the therapist–client bond. For example, the therapist may give the client a symbolic object (such as a rock or a keyring) and suggest that they remind themselves (when looking at the item) that the therapist cares about them, 'has their

Table 6.3 Schemas, unmet need, and therapist limited reparenting sentiments

SCHEMA	UNMET NEED	POSSIBLE LIMITED REPARENTING SENTIMENT
MISTRUST/ABUSE	Safety	'I can guarantee you that I won't intentionally hurt you or mess you around, I will make this a safe place for you.'
EMOTIONAL DEPRIVATION	Nurturance, attunement, care	'I care about you; this is a space where we can talk about anything.'
ABANDONMENT	Secure and reliable connection	'I'm here; I'm not going anywhere, we are going to figure this out together, regardless of what is happening in your life.'
DEFECTIVENESS/ SHAME	Acceptance, praise	'I really think you're a good person; you are fine the way you are.'
SOCIAL ISOLATION/ EXCLUSION	Belonging, acceptance	'You are a cool and interesting person. I wish you would let others see that side of you the way I know you.'
FAILURE	Praise, encouragement	'I believe in you; you can do this!'
DEPENDENCE/ INCOMPETENCE	Autonomy, guidance	'You know what to do, and I have faith that you will make the right decision.'
VULNERABILITY TO HARM	Security, safety	'Everything is going to be ok'; 'You can manage and handle whatever comes your way.'
ENMESHMENT/ UNDEVELOPED SELF	Autonomy	'You have different needs and feelings to your parents, and you're not responsible for their feelings.'
SUBJUGATION	Autonomy, safety	'You can do what you want, and you are stronger than you think.'
SELF-SACRIFICE	Autonomy, realistic responsibility	'It's ok to think of yourself; you have needs too.'
APPROVAL SEEKING	Acceptance in expressing views/ emotions	'It's good to have your opinion'; 'Trust in your views and ideas.'
EMOTIONAL INHIBITION	Modelling of emotional expression	'Emotions are normal; I like it when you are more open about how you feel.'
UNRELENTING STANDARDS	Realistic expectations/ demands	'It's ok to take time out'; 'It's ok not to get it right all the time.'
NEGATIVITY/ PESSIMISM	Joy, fun, play	'There are also good things in life; it doesn't go all wrong. Look at how successful we've been working together already.'

Table 6.3 (cont.)

SCHEMA	UNMET NEED	POSSIBLE LIMITED REPARENTING SENTIMENT
PUNITIVENESS	Self-forgiveness	'I don't think you deserve to be punished that way, I would like to see you be more kind to yourself.'
ENTITLEMENT	Limits, awareness of other's needs	'Other people have needs too; you're not special and better.'
INSUFFICIENT SELF-CONTROL	Self-directed limits	'You need to say "no" to yourself sometimes, and sit with any frustration.'

back', and wants to help. Such symbols of care and therapist thoughtfulness can deepen the therapeutic bond between the client and the therapist and is particularly meaningful for clients with schemas within the Disconnection and Rejection domain, whereby their emotional needs centre around care, stability, safety, and attunement. Box 6.11 provides guidance on some classical clinical dilemmas therapists might experience trying to provide limited reparenting.

Limited Reparenting of Strong Within-Session Activation of Angry Child Mode

The Angry Child mode typically is linked to a client's perception of some threat to their core emotional needs. Clients can present as irritated and hostile towards the therapist (and often surrounding staff). The tone of the Angry Child is typically akin to a child throwing a tantrum.

In limited reparenting, the therapist needs to strike a balance between tolerating the activation and ventilation of the Angry Child mode and empathically confronting and reality-testing the expression of the mode. The therapist demonstrates that it's okay to be angry; however, the expression of the anger needs to occur healthily. This means that the therapist will balance their attunement stance with the need to potentially set some boundaries or communicate the maladaptive or disproportionate nature of their reaction in the here and now.

Whilst the interaction can at times be abusive, critical, and attacking to the therapist, the function of the Angry Child mode is not to dominate, humiliate, or attack (like some overcompensation modes, such as Bully and Attack mode). Instead, the mode is mostly viewed as a child-like attempt to get their needs met.

Often tied to feelings of hostility, frustration, and anger (within the Angry Child mode) is the pain and distress associated with the Vulnerable Child mode. The interplay of these two Child modes is akin to two sides of a coin. The therapist may experience the Angry Child mode as incensed and angry. However, tied to this is the Vulnerable Child mode that feels overlooked, uncared for, criticised, or unsupported. Clients who are in touch with their Angry Child mode within sessions will most likely benefit from attunement (discussed earlier in this chapter). However, for clients who present as overwhelmed by the Angry

---

Box 6.11 Clinical Dilemmas in Limited Reparenting

Supervision Question: What if your care and nurturance results in the client having sexual feelings towards the therapist? I'm worried that my care may encourage the client.

Answer: Appropriate care and nurturance provided by the therapist is not considered problematic. Instead, problems may reside in how the client interprets the care and nurturance. It would be useful for the therapist to understand what modes and schemas in the client may be involved. In some cases, clients with high levels of emotional neglect may have romantic feelings for the therapist. When the therapist meets the client's need for care, this can function as a trigger, putting the client in touch with their longstanding (but buried) longing for closeness. In contrast, a client may flirt with the therapist as part of an overcompensation coping mode to manage deeper feelings of vulnerability and insecurity. In any case, the therapist needs to acknowledge appropriate therapeutic boundaries and use empathic confrontation and limit setting to address such issues.

Supervision Question: What if my care is 'too much', too awkward for the client? I worry that they will react negatively to my caring sentiments.

Answer: Some clients may not be accustomed to appropriate attention, direct care, and nurturance. Here, the therapist could validate the difficulty, understand the problem in schema and mode terms, and possibly tailor their method of care to the client. Specifically, the therapist may need to adapt their tone and language. The therapist may use an empty chair and provide reparenting to the Vulnerable Child in the chair, allowing for the care to be indirectly received. The overall goal is to help the client accept care, compassion, and nurturance and learn to adapt to such new experiences. Further, when the client is in touch with their Vulnerable Child side, attuned therapeutic care and nurturance will resonate for them. On the other hand, if the client is in a coping mode, this care is likely to be rejected, treated with disdain, or dismissed. The therapist must also be alert to the fact that sometimes a Complaining Protector, Helpless Surrenderer, or Self-Pity/Victim coping mode can present in a similar way to the Vulnerable Child mode. In this case, the therapist should use empathic confrontation to bypass the coping mode and reach the authentic Vulnerable Child, to carry out reparenting. Reparenting of these coping modes can strengthen them, which is, of course, counter-therapeutic.

Child mode within the session, the following three-step model can be useful for therapists to implement. The aim is to allow for ventilation, care, and attunement, followed by some opportunity for empathic confrontation or reality testing.

A Three-Step Model of Working with Angry Child Mode in Session

The central aim is to build the Healthy Adult mode's capacity to regulate, modify, and functionally express underlying anger. Accessing the Vulnerable Child mode and understanding the associated frustration of needs is also central to helping the client manage their expression of anger.

Step 1: Ventilate. Here, the therapist takes a neutral and fact-finding approach, allowing for anger to be fully vented. The therapist asks the client 'So you're angry about X, is there anything else?' The therapist also reflects the list of complaints to the client: 'So let me get it right, you're angry about X, Y, and Z. Is there anything else? I want to make sure I understand it all.' Overall, the therapist remains *neutral*, refraining from empathy or validation. The primary reason for this position of neutrality is that the therapist's provision of care can sometimes curb the expression of anger without addressing its source, so it becomes reactivated later in the session. Such sessions can become derailed by intermittent activation of anger.

Step 2: Attune, Empathise, and Validate. Once the client has fully ventilated, the therapist typically experiences the client as having fully aired their grievances (e.g., Client: 'No, that's it, it's been a hard day, okay.'). The therapist then provides care and empathy and validates the client's emotional reaction and underlying needs (although the therapist does not necessarily need to agree with all aspects of the client's original complaint). The provision of attunement, empathy, and validation in this context typically results in some connection to the core emotional needs, and even some activation of the Vulnerable Child mode. For example, the client may then speak about the hurt and sadness tied to their anger, and their experience of the therapist's care.

Step 3: Empathically Confront the Anger and Look for Opportunities to Reality-Test. Once the client has been empathised with and has had their needs for care and understanding met, they may be more receptive to some empathic confrontation and/or reality testing. Here, underlying assumptions driving the reaction can be reality tested: 'I know you wanted to see me this morning, but do you really think that I don't care about you at all?' The therapist can challenge distorted assumptions and black-and-white thinking that may be driving the distress using the therapy relationship (e.g., Therapist: 'I know it was painful for you when I did not respond right away, of course I understand that, but also, it is only realistic that this might happen from time to time. Either with me, or with other relationships in your life.'). The therapist then considers whether they need to empathically confront the way in which the client expressed their anger. For example, the therapist can highlight that anger expressed in this way alienates others and prevents others from providing understanding and care. The core notion is that anger is not a 'problem', but how anger is expressed may not be consistent with getting their needs met via healthy means.

Pushing for the Expression of (Suppressed) Anger Using the Therapy Relationship

Where people with Cluster B personality disorders can be characterised as exhibiting occasional excessive expressions of anger, people with Cluster C presentations, such as Avoidant Personality Disorder and Dependent Personality Disorder, are primarily characterised by an absence of anger and suppression of the Angry Child mode. For these clients, shutting down all expressions of anger robs them of the ability to also be assertive and to communicate early signs of dissatisfaction in their relationships. In schema therapy, the anger of the Angry Child mode is seen as a natural source of strength that underpins more healthy expressions of strength and assertion in the Healthy Adult mode. One of the therapy objectives in the treatment of these clients is thus to stimulate the acknowledgement and expression of anger. Work is carried out to achieve this goal during each phase of treatment. The goal is to induce and communicate Healthy Adult expressions of anger and/or dissatisfaction as a way of asserting one's needs. This process is described here as it might unfold across phases.

The Case Conceptualisation Phase. The therapist places anger in the mode model, including for clients who say they never get angry. Clients are taught that anger is a natural emotional response that can serve as a source of strength and healthy self-protection, which, in turn, is necessary for the change processes that therapy involves. Even though such clients report that they never experience anger, the ('missing') Angry Child mode is still included on the mode map, and the therapist begins reminding the client they need to hear from the Angry Child mode too.

Start Phase. In this phase, the therapist acts as a role model for expressing healthy forms of anger (e.g., when confronting the Punitive Critic mode).

Middle Phase. In this phase, negative assumptions about anger are questioned and more realistic cognitive ideas about anger are formulated, using mainly cognitive techniques as is necessary (see Box 6.12).

End Phase. In this final phase, the client is stimulated to learn how to express anger in a more regulated and safe way. Learning to express anger can be done in a playful way by using a 'complaining exercise' (see Box 6.13).

Box 6.12 Clinical Example of Addressing Suppressed Anger in the Middle Phase of Schema Therapy

THERAPIST: We have talked about anger before and, as you know, I would like you to become better at expressing different forms of anger.

CLIENT: Yes, but I don't understand why that's necessary. I always find it very unpleasant when people get angry.

THERAPIST: I know that you see all kinds of reasons why anger is a negative thing, especially when it's expressed in unhealthy ways. But there are also a lot of good things about anger. So, let's take a moment to reflect on that question: 'What are the advantages of anger?'

CLIENT: I really have no idea.

[The therapist goes to the flip chart and writes at the top of it the following question: 'What is good about anger?' and then takes the lead in listing positive aspects of anger.]

THERAPIST: Your Protector complies with the needs of others, but because of that you sometimes do things that you would rather not do, don't you?

CLIENT: Yes.

THERAPIST: Exactly, anger helps to establish boundaries so that you do not have to do the things that you don't want to do.

[The therapist writes this down as an advantage: 'Helps establish boundaries'.]

Together, the therapist and the client draw up a list of the advantages of anger, including things such as:
- anger gives energy
- it clears the air to address what does not feel good
- anger helps to express needs
- by showing more clearly what your needs are and are not, you can connect better with others
- anger is also fun; just think about the comedians you laugh at when they get worked up about injustices in their life/society

Box 6.13 The 'Complaining' Exercise

THERAPIST: We're now in the end phase of the therapy and I'm impressed by everything you have already achieved during this course of treatment. But anger is still pretty difficult for you. You still have a hard time expressing it, is that right?

CLIENT: Yeah, that's something I'm not really comfortable with . . . no.

THERAPIST: Although I can see that in some ways you have come to think differently about anger, haven't you? What exactly are the advantages of anger again?

[Some of the advantages are briefly discussed with the aim of activating the client's Healthy Adult.]

THERAPIST: Great! And don't forget that anger can also be fun!

CLIENT: Euh . . . well . . .

THERAPIST: Let's improve your ability to express anger but then in a more enjoyable way. Anger doesn't just have to be heavy and upsetting. In a moment, we'll sit opposite each other and take turns expressing what made us angry last week.

CLIENT: But I never get angry.

THERAPIST: Well, you are a human being so you are bound to get angry, but maybe 'anger' is too strong a word for you, and it is more of a feeling 'of not really liking the fact that . . . '. I'll start.

[The therapist places a chair opposite the client and talks about a few minor irritations in their life.]

THERAPIST: The alarm clock woke me up early this morning and I honestly didn't like that, it was really a feeling of 'Bleugh!' Okay, now you!

CLIENT: . . . Yes, I know the feeling, I also had something like that this morning – 'noooo . . . '

THERAPIST: Yes, exactly, I notice you frowning with your forehead, what else did you feel apart from that feeling of 'don't like that . . . '?

CLIENT: Well . . . it kind of feels heavy, and tired as well . . .?

THERAPIST: Yes, I'm familiar with that feeling, I also had it the other day when I got stuck in a traffic jam, then I really thought 'Nooooo!' and felt heavy and tired as well as some tension in my hands *[the therapist clenches their fists for a moment]*.

In this way, voicing life's minor irritations is stimulated by becoming aware of the various aspects involved in how you experience anger and irritation. The next step is learning to vent your frustrations about other people.

A final step is to ask the client about any irritations they may have regarding the therapy and/or the therapist. This last step is the hardest for a lot of clients but is a good way to prepare for the expression of anger in everyday life.

Concluding Remarks

Limited reparenting is a foundational component of schema therapy. The frustration of core emotional needs underpins the development and perpetuation of schemas, coping styles, and modes. The schema therapist looks for any opportunities to meet these needs directly within the bounds of the therapy relationship. The aim is to provide corrective experiences that 'kick start' the emotional development of the client [1]. The therapist aims to provide a healthy model or template of caring, self-control, and guidance that can be internalised by the client over time into their own Healthy Adult mode. Based on a thorough assessment and formulation, limited reparenting offers a specific roadmap to leveraging the power of the therapeutic alliance to promote schema change.

References

1. Young J, Klosko J, Weishaar M. *Schema therapy: A practitioner's guide.* Guilford Press; 2003.

2. Louis J, Louis K. *Good enough parenting.* Morgan James Publishing; 2015.

3. Louis J, Wood A, Lockwood G. Development and validation of the Positive Parenting Schema Inventory (PPSI) to complement the Young Parenting Inventory (YPI) for Schema Therapy (ST). *Assessment.* 2018;27(4):766–86.

4. Roediger E, Stevens B, Brockman R *Contextual schema therapy: An integrative approach to personality disorders, emotional dysregulation, and interpersonal functioning.* New Harbinger Publications; 2018.

5. Brockman R, Stavropoulos A. Repetitive negative thinking in eating disorders: Identifying and bypassing overanalysing coping modes and building schema attunement. In Simpson S, Smith E, eds. *Schema therapy for eating disorders:*

Identifying and bypassing overanalysing coping modes and building schema attunement. 1st ed. Routledge; 2019. pp. 69–81.

6. Erskine R. Attunement and involvement: therapeutic responses to relational needs. In *Relational Patterns, Therapeutic Presence.* Routledge; 2018. pp. 43–55.

7. Feeney B. The dependency paradox in close relationships: Accepting dependence promotes independence. *Journal of Personality and Social Psychology.* 2007;**92**(2):268–85.

8. van Vreeswijk M. Authenticity and personal openness in schema therapy. In Heath G, Startup H, eds. *Creative methods in schema therapy: Advances and innovation in clinical practice.* 1st ed. Taylor & Francis; 2020, pp. 237–252.

9. Farrell J, Shaw I. *Experiencing schema therapy from the inside out: A self-practice/self-reflection workbook for therapists.* Guilford Publications; 2018.

Chapter 7

Intervention Strategies for Schema Healing 2
Cognitive Strategies

Introduction

The concept of schemas has been central to cognitive models of psychopathology now for more than half a century [1]. Core beliefs, underlying assumptions, and negative automatic thoughts constitute cognitive aspects of schemas and modes. The cognitive elements of EMS provide various layers of meaning for the client, structuring how they view themselves, others, and the world. Schema therapy aims to change this cognitive architecture, resulting in more functional, flexible, adaptive, and ultimately 'healthier' patterns of thinking. In this chapter, we describe when and how interventions targeting cognitive change are deployed in schema therapy.

Cognitive Elements of Schemas and Modes

Before administering cognitive interventions in schema therapy, it is crucial to identify and clarify the specific cognitive aspects of schemas and modes in the case conceptualisation. Fennell [2] describes three levels of cognition: (1) core beliefs or 'bottom lines'; (2) underlying assumptions; and (3) self-talk or negative automatic thoughts. These different levels of cognition can be thought of like the parts of a large, old tree. Beneath the ground, there is a root network, akin to the themes of core beliefs of a schema or the 'bottom lines' (e.g., Defectiveness/Shame schema: 'I am worthless, pathetic, unwanted'). These roots may not be observable or accessible to the onlooker but hold up the tree. Above the ground, there is the tree's trunk; this is more noticeable to the onlooker. The tree's trunk represents underlying assumptions. Underlying assumptions are typical 'if–then' assumptions linked to core beliefs (e.g., 'If I open up to someone, then they will reject me'). Finally, there are the tree's branches and leaves, which are its most noticeable features. These represent the self-talk and automatic thoughts which are accessible to conscious awareness (e.g., 'They don't like me; they prefer to talk to their ex-boyfriend'). Although all three levels of cognition are important in schema therapy, it is the core beliefs, or 'bottom lines' that are most synonymous with the EMS. When initially learning the 18-schema model, it is useful for trainee schema therapists to conceptualise the schemas via their associated core beliefs.

Cognitive interventions in schema therapy overlap substantially with those used in mainstream cognitive-behavioural therapy (CBT). CBT provides a wealth of effective strategies designed to challenge the assumptions created through activated schemas and adjust these into more realistic, adaptive thoughts. However, schema therapy differs significantly from CBT in how able it assumes clients are to change perspectives at the beginning of therapy. Therefore, CBT methods are often not viable for use in schema therapy in exactly the same way as in traditional CBT.

Beckian cognitive therapy relies heavily on Socratic philosophical principles [3, 4]. Socrates assumed that people have the capacity to become aware of their beliefs and reflect on them; they already have the answers to life's questions and merely need help to find these answers within themselves. Therefore, Socrates described his questioning style as a 'midwife technique' [5], in which questions are utilised to help the person 'give birth' to their answers and responses. This principle forms the basis of many cognitive techniques used within a traditional CBT framework [6]. In schema therapy terms, CBT would assume that the client has a sufficiently developed Healthy Adult mode to be aware of their beliefs, reflect on them, and draw realistic conclusions in response to the therapist's questions. For example, suppose a client with a social anxiety disorder is afraid of being laughed at when making a mistake. The underlying assumption appears to be that 'making a mistake will lead to social ridicule'. When the assumption is stated in this form, logically this would mean that when other people make mistakes, they will also experience social ridicule. Following this line of argument, the therapist can then ask if this is true: 'Does ridicule for making a mistake also apply to other people? Would it apply to me too, for example?' If the client denies this, there must be a logical explanation for why the rule applies to him but not to others. The process of concretising, logical reasoning, and questioning these assumptions begins anew.

CBT would also assume that all clients have been exposed to enough working models of a Healthy Adult to have access to healthy scripts across all domains of functioning. However, in many clients with chronic problems, this adaptive and rational mode is not sufficiently developed, and there are large gaps in their experience of healthy role models. As a result, clients often experience their activated schemas as reality and are not able to distance themselves from these schemas or adopt alternative healthy, adaptive perspectives. Therefore, a purely Socratic or 'guided discovery' approach to changing cognitive aspects of schemas and modes may be less effective, especially in cases with more severe or chronic problems. For example, messages and beliefs linked to severe childhood abuse or neglect can overpower the client's efforts to identify counter-messages. Open Socratic questions and dialogue intended to encourage the client to be aware of these convictions and examine them critically may end up confirming the negative self-image when the client is unable to put schema-driven messages aside. For example, the therapist may offer 'So, you believe you are worthless. Is it 100% true that you are worthless?' and the client may respond 'I don't know; I'm not doing this right, am I?'

In severe cases, schema-driven cognitions often seem ego-syntonic; core beliefs seem like truths – rigid and 'fused' to the client. In such cases, the client has a limited reservoir of healthy knowledge to draw on, which is inconsistent with the assumption of the Socratic principle.

Schema therapists view a client's capacity for reasoning and cognitive change in relation to their level of overall psychological developmental. The strength of the client's Healthy Adult mode influences the amount of cognitive intervention employed at the commencement of treatment. For clients with a severely weak Healthy Adult mode, the schema therapist approaches sessions as if working with a young child. Young children are 'fused' with their convictions, not yet fully capable of defusing themselves from these beliefs or thinking in nuanced or realistic ways, and typically need active support from attachment figures. Typical childhood thinking styles are also often found in adults presenting with chronic and enduring psychological problems. Such clients may think in very black-and-white terms ('no one cares', 'all of me hates this') or have difficulty taking the perspective of others. Also, they may have a pattern of internalising ('they don't like me, I'm bad') or externalising ('they made me angry') explanations for why they are unhappy. Later in development, a child's capacity for rational and reasoned thinking increases and such resources can be more actively utilised. For example, people correctly expect adolescents to be more able to draw independent and realistic conclusions than younger children. The final phase of schema therapy can be characterised by the therapist expecting the client to have the reasoning capacity of an adolescent. Cognitive interventions used during this final phase of schema therapy will most closely resemble cognitive interventions as described in the mainstream CBT literature. Early in schema therapy, cognitive interventions should be adjusted to the client's capacity for rational thought.

The stage of treatment and its immediate therapeutic aims also need to be considered in selecting cognitive interventions. Rational thinking can function to divert attention from emotional experience. It can be easier for therapists to utilise more familiar cognitive interventions and avoid experiential interventions, thereby colluding with coping styles and modes. It may be helpful for the therapist to consider: (a) 'Is using a cognitive intervention going to result in collusion with a coping mode?'; and (b) 'Does the client prefer cognitive interventions because they can experience less emotion in session?'

Therapists should also keep in mind that exploring cognition and meaning *without trying to change it* is an important part of schema therapy. For example, a therapist's knowledge and understanding of a client's experience can be clarified and refined via understanding cognitions about triggering events. Understanding the particular meaning behind schema and mode activation helps the therapist to attune to the client [7]. Attunement to meaning is often achieved by the therapist clarifying the cognitive aspects of triggering events and cognitions linked to emotions (e.g., Therapist: 'If the sadness could talk, what would it say?'; Client: 'I don't matter, like I'm nothing to him', suggesting the client's Emotional Deprivation EMS was activated).

Application of a Socratic Approach in Schema Therapy

The Socratic dialogue can help question the protective coping modes. The goal of schema therapy is for the therapist to bypass the client's protective modes and increasingly interact with their emotion-experiencing parts. The strategy used is often a form of negotiation with that coping mode. Coping modes are akin to gatekeepers guarding a fortress. The Socratic dialogue can be appropriate in this negotiation because it is a more open questioning method that gives the client space to make their own decisions instead of feeling pressured to change something (see Box 7.1 for an example).

Beginning the Process of Cognitive Change in Schema Therapy: The Psychoeducation Phase – Building Schema/Mode Awareness

Positive cognitive change can begin to develop when the client gains knowledge about normal human emotional needs, child development, and schemas and modes. At the commencement of treatment, the client, just like a young child, needs explanation and guidance to become more aware of schemas and modes, and to relate them to their own specific set of problems. As clients learn to recognise them, they become able to label their emotional experiences when schemas or modes are activated. At the

Box 7.1 Example Using Socratic Dialogue to Bypass Coping Modes

THERAPIST: OK, it sounds like you're stuck in an experience where it's better to feel nothing, is that right?

CLIENT: Yes, I don't see how feeling more will help me, I'm busy, and I have to keep functioning.

THERAPIST: Can you be that protector mode who is now keeping the gate closed, convinced that it's best not to feel. As a protector, I'd like to ask you a few questions, OK?

CLIENT: Sure.

THERAPIST: You may be right; it might be best not to feel anything right now, but why are you so sure that things would go wrong today if I would be able to connect more with your feelings?

CLIENT: Well, I always feel bad when I start feeling.

THERAPIST: But if that's the case, then things should have always gone wrong here as well, although I remember that you felt better last time when we talked about your feelings.

CLIENT: Yes, OK, that's true . . .

THERAPIST: But if you didn't feel worse and, in fact, felt better, how do you know that you'll feel worse now? I understand that you, as a protector, want to make sure things don't go wrong, but it also sounds like you're not sure that that will happen.

Box 7.2 Example of Ad Hoc Psychoeducation: Healthy Care Giving

During a session with Nicole (client), the therapist receives a call from his young daughter. After asking Nicole for permission, the therapist quickly takes the call to see if there is an emergency. He hangs up after a brief interaction of 10 to 20 seconds, after which Nicole asks him incredulously: 'Is this always how you talk to your children? Words like "sweet" and "I love you" really made me feel sick . . . ' The therapist uses the client's question to explain what a normal upbringing involves; children need explicit appreciation and care, and that this is what Nicole lacked during her childhood.

beginning of therapy, the therapist explains basic human needs, optimal child-rearing practices and family life, and how deficiencies and disruptions lead to schema and mode development. This will culminate also in at least one session focused on communicating the case conceptualisation, usually by way of a mode map (see Chapter 4: Case Conceptualisation and Mode Mapping in Schema Therapy), which will also help the client to understand and conceptualise their problems from a more distanced and, hopefully, rational standpoint. This process of *schema/mode education* – educating the client about the universality of human needs – begins a process of depathologising the client's experiences in a way that starts to also challenge many of the common schemas (e.g., Defectiveness: 'You are broken and defective'; 'There's something wrong with you'). Such psychoeducation can be more formal (such as involving an overview of their mode map) or more spontaneous and ad hoc, as the opportunities present (see Box 7.2).

Box 7.3 Whiteboard Summary

THERAPIST: So, you have two different sides. Firstly, there's an emotional Nicole. When you are in that mode, you feel sad.

The therapist draws a circle on the board containing the words 'Little Nicole' and adds the words 'alone', 'unseen', and 'sadness' – words Nicole used earlier in the dialogue to describe how she felt – and 'This side believes she doesn't matter, that she's a burden.'

THERAPIST: To survive this pain, you've learned to withdraw yourself, to close yourself off from your feelings, almost like closing a gate in a wall which allows you to numb these feelings to some degree.

The therapist now draws a wall around the small Nicole circle and adds the words 'Protector' and 'withdrawing, not feeling'.

Identifying Cognitive Components of Schema- or Mode-Driven Experiences During Psychoeducation

The psychoeducation phase of treatment aims to help clients learn to become aware of the schemas and modes within their case conceptualisation. Specific cognitions and emotions associated with each mode can be attuned to and clarified (e.g., Therapist: 'So, if your Detached Protector mode could talk, what would it say about speaking with me more?'; Client: 'What's the point? If I open up, I will be overwhelmed, I won't cope.').

Drawing a Diagram of a Specific Instance of Schema/Mode Activation

Emotional experiences activated by schemas and modes can be so overwhelming that a client's understanding of, insight into, and awareness of these experiences can be drowned out at the time of activation. A therapist can walk through and map out triggering events in a session, constructing a visual representation of the client's schema and mode activation via a whiteboard or work pad. This post-hoc analysis of a trigger is an essential tool for consolidating cognitive insights, allowing the client to internalise and better understand the model. A copy of the visual depiction can then be provided to the client to be reviewed for homework (see Box 7.3).

Use of Specific Cognitive Interventions

Beyond taking a generally educative approach, certain specific interventions may help to change the cognitive component of schemas. Therapists can apply any cognitive techniques typically used in cognitive therapy within schema therapy, although they may need to provide more active assistance and support than in traditional cognitive therapy.

Downward Arrow Technique

The Downward Arrow technique [8, 9] uses Socratic questioning to reveal and understand core beliefs and meanings linked to events. The therapist explores the

Box 7.4 Example of the Downward Arrow Technique

(NB: In the following example, the client has a Subjugation schema)

CLIENT: I really don't want to be late for the meeting.

THERAPIST: Well, if that was true, and you were late, what would that mean?

CLIENT: Well, I would be disrespecting my colleagues.

THERAPIST: And say if that was true, what would be so bad about that?

CLIENT: They would get irritated and angry.

THERAPIST: And if they did get angry, what does that mean?

CLIENT: I don't like it when people are like that.

THERAPIST: So, if you're late, others will get angry, and you couldn't manage it?

meaning of events via asking questions such as 'If this was true, what would that mean to you? What would that say about you? What would be so bad about that?' Following the client's response, the therapist continues to inquire about the meaning of the belief, using the questions mentioned earlier, until a core meaning is revealed. The therapist can continue with this process until an absolute and conclusive statement is reached. In schema therapy, these bottom lines are usually understood to be one or more EMS themes (see Box 7.4 for an example).

Schema/Mode Monitoring Forms

A helpful set of tools for increasing awareness of schemas and modes are the various schema/mode monitoring forms, or what used to be called cognitive diaries. Schema/mode monitoring forms allow the client to reflect on a meaningful event and learn to recognise which schemas or modes were activated during it. Monitoring forms typically start by describing the triggering situation, followed by the client describing emotions, thoughts, and behaviours related to the event. The therapist asks the client to reflect on the beliefs/assumptions and self-talk involved in schema or mode activation associated with a triggering event. The idea is to use the initial information to help the client become aware of their schema or mode pattern being activated. Such a technique has two broad aims: (1) to help the client become aware of their schema/mode patterns as early as possible, thus inducing a Healthy Adult mode of self-reflection; and (2) to give the client an opportunity to identify a healthier attitude or response to a given situation. Depending on the therapy phase, the client will require a different degree of support to complete diary forms. During the initial phase of treatment, the therapist may take more of a leading role in recognising and labelling schemas and modes. During the therapy's middle and final phases, there is a greater expectation that the client will complete the diary independently.

A commonly used type of monitoring form is the schema/mode circle diary [10] (see Figure 7.1). This diary follows a more circular investigation process wherein the initial recognition of thoughts, feelings, and behaviour expands into the underlying basic needs. Furthermore, the process reflects how the client can act to better connect to their core emotional needs in a given situation.

SCHEMA DIARY

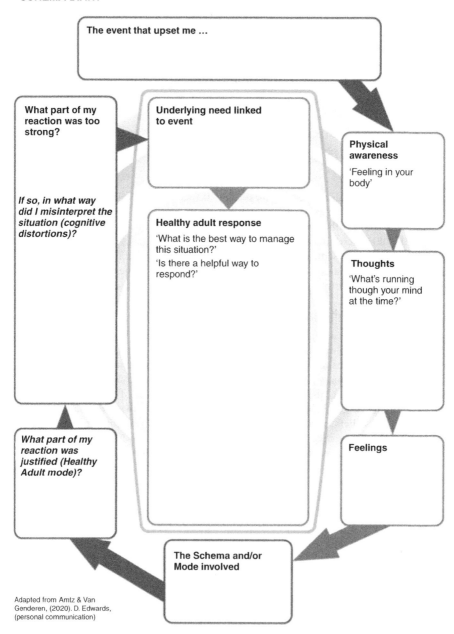

Figure 7.1 Schema diary example

The event that upset me …

What part of my reaction was too strong?

If so, in what way did I misinterpret the situation (cognitive distortions)?

Underlying need linked to event

Physical awareness
'Feeling in your body'

Healthy adult response
'What is the best way to manage this situation?'
'Is there a helpful way to respond?'

Thoughts
'What's running though your mind at the time?'

What part of my reaction was justified (Healthy Adult mode)?

Feelings

The Schema and/or Mode involved

Adapted from Amtz & Van Genderen, (2020). D. Edwards, (personal communication)

Schema Flashcard Outline

Right now, you feel _____
(note central emotions)

Because_____
(state specific triggering event)

This is really about your _____Schema(s)
(note related schemas)

This Schema came about from _____
(background events that effected development)

This Schema(s) leads you to exaggerate the degree to which_____
(state cognitive distortions)

Even if you think _____
(central state beliefs, self-talk)

The reality is _____
(note adaptive/healthy beliefs/self-talk)

This is backed and supported by the fact that _____
(note the evidence refuting)

So even though you feel like doing _____
(note the typical way of reacting behaviourally)

You need to instead _____
(describe healthy alternative behaviour)

Figure 7.2 Flashcard outline

Box 7.5 Example of a Schema Flashcard

'Right now, you're feeling tense and anxious because you are about to assert yourself with someone; this is your Subjugation schema that developed when you were bullied at school. This Subjugation schema leads you to overestimate the extent that others will be hostile and underestimate your ability to manage conflict. Even if you believe that others may get angry, the reality is that conflict is a part of life, and you can handle someone being displeased with you. In the past, you have spoken your view at work, asked for what you need, and managers have responded well. So even if you want to avoid the conversation or go along with things, you need to hold your head up high and assert what you need.'

Schema and Mode Flashcards

Clients can prepare for specific triggering events or themes linked to schemas and modes via schema and mode flashcards (see Figure 7.2) [11]. Here, the therapist works with the client to develop a statement that outlines a schema's or a mode's effect and provides a rational, healthy response that the client can rehearse when triggered. This prepared message also guides healthy behavioural responses. The therapist can then record the flashcard statement on a client's smartphone to be listened to out of session (see Box 7.5 for an example). As a result, the cognitive intervention can act as a quasi-transitional object encouraging a greater therapeutic connection between the therapist and client.

Evidence for and Against a Core Belief of a Schema

The therapist can look for evidence supporting and refuting a core belief linked to a schema or mode (both in childhood and adulthood), and could introduce the exercise as follows:

Box 7.6 Case Example of Exploring Evidence for and Against the Core Belief of a Schema

Nicky presented describing strong anxiety and inadequacy related to some work challenges. The therapist identified her Failure schema as being central to this distress. The therapist identified the core belief that she was 'stupid and intellectually inferior' and suggested that they look at the evidence for and against the core belief (both as an adult and a child). They came up with the following grid:

Belief 'I am stupid, intellectually inferior'
Evidence for (as a child)
Did poorly academically in primarily school
Stayed down a year in year 3
Parents called into school to discuss learning difficulties
Had to do extra tutoring

Evidence for (as an adult)
Peers are in more senior jobs, have degrees
Management have been slower to promote me
And old colleague (three years ago) said I 'shouldn't be doing this sort of work'

Evidence against (as a child)
My teachers were encouraging
No teacher ever said I was 'stupid'

Evidence against (as an adult)
Management wants me to study and be promoted
I passed my university entry course
I recently got a B for my first assignment

'Let's look at the evidence that supports and argues against the idea that you're unintelligent'. See Box 7.6 for an example.

Undermining and Reattributing Supporting Evidence

Reattribution of supporting evidence can be employed to help undermine a negative core belief. See Box 7.7.

Cognitive Techniques for Self-Blame and Negative Self-View

It is beyond the scope of this book to extensively discuss all existing cognitive techniques. To further explain the available techniques and methods, we refer the reader to the current literature [12, 13]. However, included in the following sections are several helpful cognitive techniques related to personal responsibility and guilt or calculating risk or danger.

Responsibility Pie Graphs. Responsibility pie graphs [14, 15] are particularly useful in cases where client difficulties are exacerbated by an overinflated sense of personal responsibility. A core negative belief is defined (e.g., 'It's all my fault that the project failed'), and the client is asked to rate the strength of their belief in the statement (e.g., 85%). The therapist asks the

Box 7.7 Example of Undermining and Reattributing Supporting Evidence for a Negative Core Belief

THERAPIST: So, you're saying that your school grades in primary school are evidence that you're stupid. I'm wondering how domestic violence at home during that time affected your schoolwork. I would say that the violence and chaos at home wasn't conducive to doing well at school.

client to identify all the factors that may have played a role in causing the adverse event. Each factor is then added into a pie graph, with each pie segment reflecting the client's estimation of how much it was responsible for the outcome (i.e., what percentage of all causes of the event was due to this factor). Importantly, the client's attribution for their own involvement is left until all other factors have been accounted for, leaving the client less responsible for the outcome.

Dimensional Evaluation or 'Continua'. In the continua technique [9, 13, 14, 16], the therapist asks the client to list specific traits, qualities, or factors that contribute to a 'final verdict' or core belief about themselves or others. This technique is mainly suitable for editing a strong negative self-image – for example, when the client believes they are 'unacceptable' – and hence is a helpful cognitive method for investigating and challenging assumptions derived from a Punishing Critic mode.

This technique begins by identifying a specific belief linked to a schema or mode. The therapist then writes this core belief (often on a whiteboard), for example, 'I'm a bad mother', and to rate the belief's strength (typically, using a percentage or a visual analogue scale). The therapist then has two options:

1. List several traits that make up a global evaluation. For example, for the core belief 'I'm a bad mother', the traits 'abusive', 'harsh', 'neglectful', and 'unsupportive' might be listed. The client rates their level of each trait (e.g., from 0 to 10). The therapist then makes an average score from the chosen traits. Because clients' global evaluations are usually unduly influenced by a single dimension, the average usually prompts the client to consider that, overall, they do not embody their negative global evaluation in most respects.

2. Several traits that make up a global evaluation are drawn as bipolar 'sub-continua' via a visual analogue scale. The client then marks where they 'lie'. NB: it is essential to ensure these sub-continua are bipolar: from the most negative extreme of the trait to the most positive (e.g., Emotionally Abusive vs Emotionally Nurturing/Caring). Clients then look at their visual profile across the sub-continua and re-evaluate their original belief.

Continua methods broaden the client's perspective to re-evaluate the severity of their human foibles in proper proportion.

The Courtroom Method. The courtroom method [17] is an experiential cognitive technique that uses forms of drama therapy to investigate and adjust assumptions regarding guilt and responsibility. It is mainly suitable for clients who often feel guilty because of alleged mistakes or shortcomings. The cognitions regarding guilt should first be investigated using one or more of the methods discussed previously – for example, using a pie chart or discussing the definition of guilt as responsibility (the fact of having deliberately and intentionally caused harm or difficulty) and questioning whether the client meets this definition. If this does not lead to sufficient change, the therapist can propose investigating how a court of law would view *feelings* of guilt. The rationale for imitating a court of law is that the court is an institution with centuries of experience in establishing whether a person is guilty or not.

After the usefulness of investigating the clients's actual guilt (as responsibility) is established, the therapist stands up and invites the client to set up a court of law in the therapy room. A decision on where the judge, the prosecutor, and the lawyer will sit is made, with the client given a defence lawyer's role.

The therapist opens the role-playing game by standing up as seriously as possible and turning to the imaginary judge to announce the charge. For example: 'Your honour, we are gathered here today because the accused is depressed and therefore causes others around him unacceptable suffering' or 'The accused is depressed, and therefore it is his fault that his spouse has a bad life.' The therapist now asks the client to stand up, turn to the judge and explain why the accused (the client) is not guilty and should not be convicted. By assigning the client the role of a defence lawyer, the client must critically assess their automatic assumptions. Moreover, this role-playing game capitalises on a phenomenon known in social psychology that speaking arguments out loud leads to them having greater credibility than if they had been only heard or read. The therapist notes both the charge and the defence and finally asks the client to sit on the judge's chair and deliver a verdict: guilty or not guilty. The therapist can also ask the client to repeat this verdict in the first person, so instead of 'the accused is not guilty because . . .', they can ask the client to say, 'I'm not guilty because . . .'.

Concluding Remarks

Cognitive change in schema therapy aims to help the client develop a capacity to reason and challenge beliefs and assumptions. Cognitive approaches can help the therapist develop greater attunement and understanding of the client's experience. Furthermore, cognitive change can work synergistically with experiential methods, allowing for change at both the 'head' and the 'heart' levels of knowing. Therapists need to be aware of the client's level of emotional functioning and tailor cognitive interventions to their needs. Furthermore, it is essential not to use cognitive techniques to detract from the treatment's overall aims and goals by focusing on cognitive interventions at the expense of emotions and colluding with client coping strategies.

References

1. Beck A. Thinking and depression: Idiosyncratic content and cognitive distortions. *Archives of General Psychiatry.* 1963;9(4):324–33.

2. Fennell M. Low self-esteem: A cognitive perspective. *Behavioural and Cognitive Psychotherapy.* 1997;25(1):1–26.

3. Padesky C. Socratic questioning: Changing minds or guiding discovery. A keynote address delivered at the European Congress of Behavioural and Cognitive Therapies, London. 24 Sep., 1993 (Vol. 24).

4. Clark G, Egan S. The Socratic method in cognitive behavioural therapy: A narrative review. *Cognitive Therapy and Research.* 2015;39(6):863–79.

5. Overholser J. *The Socratic method of psychotherapy.* Columbia University Press; 2018.

6. Beck J, Beck A. *Cognitive behaviour therapy. Basics and beyond.* Guilford Publication; 2011.

7. Roediger E, Stevens B, Brockman R. *Contextual schema therapy: An integrative approach to personality disorders, emotional dysregulation, and interpersonal functioning.* New Harbinger Publications.

8. Beck A. *Cognitive therapy and the emotional disorders.* Penguin; 1979.

9. Leahy R. *Cognitive therapy techniques: A practitioner's guide.* Guilford Publications; 2017.

10. Arntz A, Van Genderen H, *Schema therapy for borderline personality disorder.* Wiley-Blackwell; 2020.

11. Young J, Klosko J, Weishaar M. *Schema therapy: A practitioner's guide.* Guilford Press; 2003.

12. Beck A, Davis D, Freeman A. *Cognitive therapy of personality disorders.* Guilford Publications; 2016.

13. Beck J, *Cognitive behaviour therapy. Basics and beyond.* Guilford Publication; 2020.

14. Greenberger D, Padesky C. *Mind over mood: A cognitive therapy treatment manual for clients.* Guilford Press; 1995.

15. Davis D. Cognitive therapy for personality disorders. In: Leahy R, Abramson L, Alloy L, Arntz A, Beck A, eds. *Science and practice in cognitive therapy: Foundations, mechanisms, and applications.* 1st ed. Guildford Press; 2018, pp. 376–402.

16. Padesky C. Schema change processes in cognitive therapy. *Clinical Psychology & Psychotherapy.* 1994;1(5):267–78.

17. Bögels SM, van Oppen PC. *Cognitieve therapie: theorie en praktijk.* 3rd ed. Bohn Stafleu van Loghum, 2019.

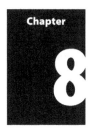

Chapter

8

Intervention Strategies for Schema Healing 3
Experiential Techniques

Introduction

Part of the impetus for the development of schema therapy was the insight that although cognitive interventions might alter people's rational conviction in schema-driven beliefs, they very often didn't *feel* different. Even after developing intellectual insight, people with EMS still frequently experience intense unwanted schema-driven emotions. Experiential – or emotion-focused – techniques in schema therapy have been selected to take away the emotional power of EMS. Schema therapy characteristically uses imagery, chair dialogues, and psychodrama to activate and alter EMS within and between sessions. This chapter describes why, how, and when to use experiential techniques in schema therapy.

The Importance of Experiential or Emotion-Focused Interventions

Experiential techniques in schema therapy aim to directly focus on the emotional elements of a client's presenting issues. Experiential techniques can be synergetic to changes within cognitive or behavioural domains or within the therapy relationship. A fundamental objective of experiential approaches is for the therapist to provide corrective emotional experiences to the client [1]. Experiential techniques aim to provide the client with real experiences that correct maladaptive schemas and modes.

Despite such techniques contributing to the effectiveness of therapy, they are often challenging for the therapist to use, or omitted. Some experiential techniques can be demanding for the client. For example, clients may have a shallow threshold for feeling vulnerable or exposed. It is also common for many schema therapists in training to delay or avoid using experiential techniques. Such avoidance typically is driven by two factors: (1) a lack of confidence in using such approaches, with the therapist preferring to use more familiar techniques (commonly cognitive, behavioural, or supportive psychotherapy); and (2) fear that accessing emotion will destabilise or make clients feel 'worse'. Therapist avoidance can limit the client's progress and prevent the therapist from developing valuable skills. This chapter will present ways to increase therapist confidence.

There are several reasons why it is necessary to activate the client's emotional responses in session. First, the therapist can respond to the emotional needs of the client. For example, the therapist can provide care, protection, and nurturance to the client who might be deprived of these experiences. Second, the therapist can provide a new model or 'template' for the client to internalise; they can demonstrate how to experience emotions without avoiding them, listening to learn what deprived needs their emotions may be signalling. The therapist provides a model of a Healthy Adult that the client can emulate. Third, schema

150

therapy's experiential techniques are consistent with Lang's theory of emotion [2] and other eminent information processing models (summarised in [3, 4]) which suggest that there are two systems to process information. One is a 'rational' system accessible and mediated via verbal/linguistic means and a second is a parallel 'experiential' system wherein behaviour is governed by directly experienced emotional consequences. In schema therapy, cognitive approaches are thought to target the 'head', and experiential methods target the 'heart'. Finally, even if the theories for why it is essential to experience affect in session prove ultimately to be incorrect, affective processing in session nevertheless remains correlated with successful therapeutic outcomes [5]. Experiential methods in schema therapy aim to bypass coping modes that block emotions, cognitions, and behaviours, revealing the interplay and impact of modes on the client, and the emotional needs that are otherwise obscured.

When Do We Target Emotion?

Typically, the therapist's initial goal is to bypass coping modes so that the client can identify their child modes and associated EMS when active. The longer the client spends in a coping mode during a treatment phase session, the more time is wasted and the longer the delay to recovery. Therefore, the use of experiential techniques is encouraged early in the treatment phase. The intensity of focus on the emotional aspects of difficulties can be titrated based on the client's capacity. For example, suppose a client declines the option of an imagery exercise; in that case, the therapist could use a chairwork exercise to understand the motives of the part of the client – typically, a coping mode – blocking the intervention.

Rationales That Can Be Provided to Clients for Targeting Emotions

As in all schema therapy interventions, the case conceptualisation will guide the therapist's use of experiential techniques. The therapist should consider what they are trying to achieve from an experiential exercise and educate the client with a rationale. Possible specific aims include to: (1) access emotions obscured by coping modes; (2) increase understanding of the impact and origins of problems; (3) help clients experience corrective emotions (such as empowerment, compassion, care, and nurturance).

Experiential Mode Modification Exercises

Mode dialogues are a central element of schema therapy. The ultimate aim of schema therapy is to strengthen the client's Healthy Adult mode so it can respond to their child modes, coping modes, and critic modes. The use of experiential techniques such as imagery rescripting, chairwork, therapeutic letter writing, and forms of psychodrama can fit within a spectrum of intervention (see Figure 8.1).

The model suggests five stages that can be implemented, depending on the needs of the client:

1) Imagery rescripting of images or memories linked to schemas and/or unprocessed trauma memories.
2) Mode dialogues in an imagery context: Modes are visualised in imagery and dialogues conducted between them (e.g., modes visualised around an imaginary table).

Schema Mode Work and Experiential Exercises

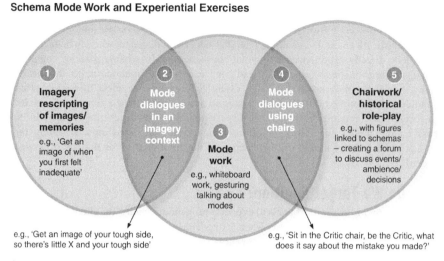

Figure 8.1 Mode work and experiential techniques

3) Informal mode work discussion and dialogues: Modes may be discussed informally, referring to modes on a whiteboard, and the use of gesturing to build and trigger a client's awareness of modes.
4) Mode dialogues using chairs: Use of chairs to represent the modes (e.g., chairwork with the Punitive Critic).
5) Chairwork or historical role-plays with figures and issues related to schemas and/or problems (e.g., chairs represent people involved in schema formation, or chairs provide a forum for expressing feelings or weighing decisions typically blocked by coping).

Imagery Work in Schema Therapy

Imagery has been a central feature of schema therapy since its formation [6]. Imagery has long been utilised to access and 'amplify' emotion and is particularly useful in providing adaptive/corrective experiences, counteracting the messages of EMS [7]. The use of imagery work is broad and its applications are wide ranging. However, several different variants of imagery used in schema theory include:

1. Safe place and 'container' imagery
2. Mode dialogues via imagery
3. Imagery rescripting for schema change
4. Imagery that strengthens the Healthy Adult

Safe Place or Container Imagery

Therapists can use safe place imagery to create positive experiences that promote a sense of safety and calmness for the client [8]. Safe place imagery can also be used at the end of sessions when there are high levels of emotion. A general principle is to let the client

---

Box 8.1 Safe Place Script

Can you close your eyes and get an image of a place where you feel safe and at ease? It may be somewhere you have been, somewhere you want to be. Get a sense of being there. What do you see? What is happening around you to feel at ease?

What can you hear around you? There may be sounds close and far from you. Just notice this, notice the feeling of being calm and at ease and safe.

What can you smell around you? Just notice that experience, feeling safe, feeling OK.

What can you feel? Pay attention to where your body makes contact with the ground, the effect of gravity, your feet or hands touching the ground. Just take a moment to stay with these safe feelings in your safe place. A place you can come back to when you need to.

Box 8.2 The 'Vault' Imagery

Close your eyes and get an image of a bank vault, like the vaults you see in James Bond, where you can walk inside. See if you can get an image of standing outside it. What do you see? Now I want you to imagine you have a trolley full of old files; these are old memories, distressing events from long ago. Can you get a sense of this? Now, I want you to get an image of you walking into the vault, pushing the trolley with the old memories and moving inside. What do you see? What colour are the walls? Is there furniture? Are there deposit boxes? Shelving? Now, I want you to imagine leaving these files in the vault; place them where you want. Where do you put them? Now, get an image of you leaving the vault. What do you see when you go, what kind of door is there, how does it close? Now, close that door, can you see yourself doing so, knowing that the door opens when you choose to open when we meet next? How does that feel? What's that like knowing that these things are sorted away and we can open the vault if you want next time?

Adapted from [9]

---

immerse themselves in the image and for the therapist to enrich the experience by prompting the client to attend to sensory components (such as visual, tactile, olfactory, and auditory). See Box 8.1 for an example script.

Imagery can also be used to 'contain' and restrict memories and painful experiences. For example, in trauma work the client may have difficult memories or experiences that cause them distress between sessions and overwhelm them. The therapist can ask the client to envisage a sealed and secure container that can hold and restrict painful destabilising memories (see Box 8.2). Such a skill can also be an example of 'healthy distancing', where the client learns to distance themselves from distress via helpful means.

It is essential to note, however, that many clients may not require the frequent use of safe place imagery. Since these exercises can be used by clients to detach from, avoid, and disconnect from feelings, the unnecessary use of safe-place and containment exercises risks delaying access to more important experiences. The use of these exercises should be limited to helping clients keep' emotional arousal levels within a window of tolerance.

Mode Dialogues via Imagery

In early schema therapy texts [10] there was little mention of 'chairwork' in interventions targeting schema modes; instead, mode work often occurred within imagery

---

Box 8.3 Example of Mode Dialogues via Imagery

THERAPIST: Can you close your eyes and get an image of the fight with your boyfriend you just mentioned

KATIE: [eyes closed] I can't seem to get anything.

THERAPIST: Is a part of you not wanting to get too close to those feelings?

KATIE: Yeah, I'm not sure I see the point.

THERAPIST: Can you get an image of your tough side, the side that wants to keep others away and shut down feelings? Can you get a sense of that? Can you be that side, stand in front of the side that is hurting and alone after your partner yelled at you.

KATIE: Yeah, I can do that.

THERAPIST: Can you be 'Tough Katie'? Step in her shoes. I'm going to ask her some questions: 'I know you're trying to help but what will happen if I get close to Vulnerable Katie? Why not let her get some help with what happened?' ... Be that tough side. What does she say back? [attempting to create a mode dialogue]

KATIE: She will get upset, so what's the point?

THERAPIST: [continuing the dialogue] 'I know you're trying to protect and support her; She has needed you for such a long time. But I know she also needs some understanding and care right now. Last night was very tough for her, and I want her to know that I'm here for her. ' ... What's happening?

KATIE: Tough Side isn't sure about the idea; it's wanting to disengage from talking.

THERAPIST: Tough Side, I'm not here to upset Katie. If you're always around, I can't help her in the way she needs. I feel that this was really hard for her. I want to help her with her emotions, not to make it worse.' ... How is she responding?

KATIE: I don't want to be difficult, but I have to go to work afterwards. It will just make me upset.

THERAPIST: Tough Katie, I know it's not easy, but if you're always around in our sessions, I can't help Katie the way she needs it. I'll help Katie to settle things, so she's not overwhelmed, so she can go to work settled and feel supported too.

KATIE: Yeah, I get it, it's just not easy to think about, but I see your point.

THERAPIST: So, can you get an image of the argument now?

KATIE: Yes, I'm walking in from work, and he's sitting watching TV. He doesn't even respond or acknowledge me. It's like I'm invisible.

---

rescripting. In imaginal mode work, the client is encouraged to embody specific modes (e.g., Therapist: 'Be the detached side of you') and construct dialogues with the therapist's assistance. This approach can be advantageous when an imagery rescripting exercise is 'blocked' midway by a coping mode (see Box 8.3).

Imagery Rescripting

Imagery Rescripting is a powerful experiential method and a central change mechanism in schema therapy. The technique aims to change the legacy of childhood experiences, images, and memories linked to the development of schemas and modes. Rescripting results in the formation of new adaptive meanings and access to feelings and insights. Rescripting can take different forms; this chapter will discuss the protocols noted by Weertman and Arntz [11] and De Haan and colleagues [12].

Selecting Meaningful Images for Rescripting

Imagery rescripting requires the therapist to access images linked to the development of schemas and modes. The therapist privately poses the question 'What happened to you' (to have such schemas and modes) as a way to conceptualise schema and mode development. Accessing meaningful images to rescript can be achieved in different ways.

1. **'Affect Bridge' Imagery.** Clients often experience emotional responses to events during daily life that seem objectively 'out of proportion' to what happened. These events often contain stimulus elements that overlap with the conditions that established their schemas and modes. We can capitalise on how emotions organise associated memories by using recent episodes of disturbing emotions to improve recall of events that led to schema or mode establishment. Attunement to emotion and the cognitive meaning of current life triggers can link current events with the past. Here, the therapist aims to understand the coordinates of emotion (longitude) and meaning/cognition (latitude) associated with triggers before vaulting to past events. The sequence is summarised in Box 8.4.

2. **Assessment, 'Google Image Technique', Young Parenting Inventory and the use of Photos.** The therapist can access childhood imagery via experiences noted during assessment. Specific touchstone events or examples of parental care (obtained in a developmental history-taking) can be good targets to rescript. The Young Parenting Inventory [13] can provide a detailed stimulus to help the therapist obtain examples of caregivers not meeting core emotional needs (e.g., Therapist: 'Give me an example of mum treating you as if you were younger than you really were'). An alternative option is the 'Google Image Technique' [14]; this technique is typically used in eye movement description and reprocessing [EMDR] therapy. Here, the client is asked to think of memories linked to schemas as being akin to completing a Google image search. For example, as a homework exercise, clients can be asked to record five images representing memories that may be linked to a particular schema (e.g., 'I am defective'), thereby priming the client for imagery in the next session.

Box 8.4 The Sequence in Imagery Rescripting Incorporating an Affect Bridge

A) Access an image of a recent triggering event. Therapist: 'What do you see, where are you?'

B) Attune to feelings and thoughts related to the event. Therapist: 'How are you feeling? What's running through your mind?'

C) Focus on emotion and physical elements and the idea of X (thoughts/meaning) related to the recent trigger and ask the client to let go of the current trigger and access an image when they felt the same as a child.

D) Access childhood image and proceed with the rescript.

Imagery Rescripting – Phase 1 (Therapist Rescripts)

The initial phase of imagery rescripting typically focuses on the therapist entering the image, meeting the child's needs, specifically responding to antagonists in the image, and comforting the child. It is important that the therapist rescripts before the client attempts to do so, for two reasons. First, the therapist models how to respond to antagonists and provides appropriate care and nurturance. In many cases, clients have had limited exposure to models of healthy caregiving. The therapist has more influence over adverse experiences when they are an active part of the image. For example, if the client becomes overwhelmed by parental actions, the therapist can enter the image and provide tailored responses. Second, by entering the image and giving care, the therapist aims to create a secure therapeutic attachment and meet the client's attachment needs via limited reparenting (see Chapter 6).

Initially, the therapist's primary objective is to provide safety within the image. The therapist can position themselves between the client (as a child) and any antagonist figure. Alternatively, the therapist can use fantasy to increase the perceived power and strength of themselves as the 'helper' figure, thereby increasing the client's feelings of protection. For example, the therapist can increase their size (Therapist: 'Make me bigger, so I'm standing over him') or use some form of barrier ('Place a bulletproof screen with you and me standing on one side and your mother on the other side'). Other fantasy elements can also be used, such as using 'child protectors' or helpers to provide a sense of safety.

The therapist is asked to enter and intervene close to the 'hot spot' of the imagery. Here, the client has some emotional activation towards the antagonist (e.g., when the critical parent is demanding towards the child). However, in the case of violence, abuse, or trauma, the therapist enters and intervenes before the abusive act takes place, protecting and meeting the needs of the child in the image [15]. The steps of imagery rescripting by the therapist are outlined in Box 8.5, and an example of its application is provided in Box 8.6.

Highlighting Mastery and Communicating a Purpose

It can be helpful for the therapist to state the 'purpose' for imagery rescripting and communicate this to the client. For example, the therapist may aim to increase the client's self-compassion or empowerment, validate the client's needs, or provide safety. Making the rationale clear will help clients accept the value of imagery rescripting and be more willing to continue to participate. It is also essential to inform the client that the ultimate goal of the imagery process is for them to respond to antagonists and meet their child self's needs in the image. When clients understand and see the value of achieving this, they may be more likely to actively engage in the exercises, rather than take a more passive role in the imagery. Such a process is similar to a chef modelling how to cook a meal to an apprentice. The chef may highlight to the apprentice that even though they may prefer to watch, they should be involved in cooking the meal because they will be preparing the meal on their own in the future.

Imagery Rescripting: Phase 2 (Client Rescripts)

The second phase of imagery rescripting begins during the middle and later stages of treatment. Here, the client's Healthy Adult mode has developed; the client has become

Box 8.5 Imagery Rescripting Script

Imagery Rescripting Script
Stage 1: Therapist Rescripts

Therapist Instructions
1) Discuss imagery and gain consent to do imagery rescripting
2) Ask the client to get an image of the childhood event ('Can you get an image where you felt really vulnerable?')

Identify a Memory
3) What do you see (hear, smell)? What's happening for you to feel this way?
   Please note: make sure the client is immersed in the image (using first 1st person present tense – e.g., 'I'm in the lounge room and he's across the room . . .')
4) What are you feeling?
5) What are you thinking to yourself?
6) What do you need? What would help right now?

Therapist Rescripts
7) Therapist enters the image and provides what the client needs
   (e.g., stand up to the perpetrator, call the police, speak to the parents, etc.)
8) How does the antagonist respond?
   Continue with meeting the need
9) How does the client feel as a result?
   'What's it like, me speaking to mum that way?'
10) Return to step 6 and see if anything else is needed
    (check on affect as a result of your intervention)
11) If possible, focus on a corrective emotional experience
    (i.e., feeling supported, safe, cared for) and ask the client to open their eyes

   - Please note: there is no need to 'play out' the extent of the trauma – the therapist enters the image and stops the abuse/protects the client
   - Get client into 1st person, present tense
   - Focus on the 'corrective emotional experience'.

more insightful and has had some modelling of how to respond to antagonists. In addition, emotions such as fear and shame should have subsided due to rescripting in phase 1.

In the imagery, the therapist asks the client-as-adult to enter the image and meet the client-as-child's needs (i.e., stand up against antagonists, provide care to the child in the image). One way to facilitate development of the client's Healthy Adult mode is through 'priming': starting the imagery exercise by having the client visualise their healthy side. The exercise then consists of three segments:

1. A description of the memory (often from an observer perspective), especially the events before the scene's most emotive part.
2. The client, as an adult (as they are now) entering the image and rescripting.

Box 8.6 Example of Phase 1: The Therapist Rescripts the Image

THERAPIST: Now, get an image of you as a child when you felt the same way, when you felt unloved and rejected.

CLIENT: My dad is angry at me; I've dropped a can of soft drink in the car, and it's made a mess.

THERAPIST: Where are you? What do you see?

CLIENT: I'm coming into the house from being in the car. Dad is in front of me as we walk up the path.

THERAPIST: What's happening?

CLIENT: He's angry and saying I'm a stupid child, he has the can of drink in his hand, he's so angry.

THERAPIST: How are you feeling?

CLIENT: I just feel like he hates me [tearful].

THERAPIST: What do you need?

CLIENT: I wish he would be less mean.

THERAPIST: You just want someone to be nice to you, protect you?

CLIENT: Yes.

THERAPIST: Bring me into the image. Can you get a sense of me there, standing between you and your dad?

CLIENT: Yes, I can see you.

THERAPIST: I'm standing tall and strong between you and your father. I'm going to talk to your dad [Greg]: 'Greg, you are going to stop right there, this is unacceptable. I'm not going to let you carry on like this. You are dealing with me now.' What happens next?

CLIENT: Dad isn't happy, he's saying, 'Who are you?!', and that he can parent how he likes.

THERAPIST: [continuing with the exchange] 'Greg, I don't care for this, I'm right, and your parenting is unacceptable. You need to leave, I'm not putting up with this.' Can you see me taking dad away?

CLIENT: [tearful] Yes.

THERAPIST: What's that like having someone there for you, standing up for you?

CLIENT: It feels good. No one has spoken to dad like that.

THERAPIST: [To the client in imagery] 'You're a good kid, a lovely kid, and dad is intolerant and mean. He's the one with the problem.' How does that feel?

CLIENT: Better, like someone cares.

THERAPIST: [in imagery] 'How about we get out of here? Do something nice, something you like doing?'

CLIENT: I loved climbing the tree out the front.

THERAPIST: Great, can you see yourself there? 'Can I come too? I like to watch you climb.' What do you see?

CLIENT: I'm up the tree. You're down the bottom looking up at me.

THERAPIST: I'm smiling, 'You're a brilliant climber!' How is it? What is it like being up the tree with someone kind there?

CLIENT: It's a nice feeling.

THERAPIST: Hold on to that nicer, cared-for feeling and let the image dissolve away; become aware of the room's sounds, and slowly open your eyes.

Cartoon 8.1 Imagery Rescripting with the Punitive Critic

3. The client taking the child's perspective and observing their self-as-adult providing care and meeting their needs.

As a result, the client can experience two levels of emotion: advocating for the child (such as healthy indignation, self-compassion) and feelings related to receiving care and protection. An example of a client rescripting their own image is provided in Box 8.7. Some tips for how to deal with common roadblocks in providing imagery interventions are provided in Box 8.8.

Chairwork in Schema Therapy

Chairwork has a long history in psychotherapy, particularly in the Gestalt Therapy tradition [18]. Chairwork has been used both as a stand-alone psychotherapeutic approach [19] and

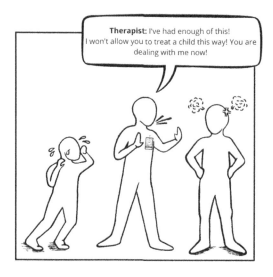

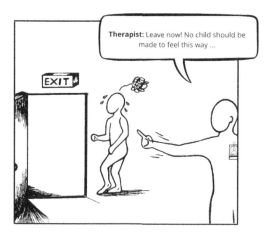

Cartoon 8.1 (cont.)

integrated into cognitive-behavioural therapy [20]. Chairwork is a very useful vehicle for delivering and enhancing schema mode therapy [21]. First, mode chair dialogues can illustrate mode interplay clearly and vividly to the client. Second, it facilitates the client's defusion from dysfunctional modes and schemas and viewing them as ego-dystonic. For example, the therapist can confront an empty chair representing a problematic mode, with the client sitting alongside. Here, the chairwork helps the client see that the therapist is speaking to the mode rather than confronting the client.

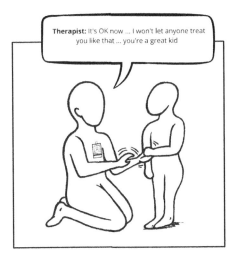

Cartoon 8.1 (cont.)

Box 8.7 Example of Phase 2 in Which the Client Rescripts the Image

THERAPIST: Bring up that image of you with dad being angry at you. What do you see?

CLIENT: We're coming into the house after I've dropped the can of drink in the car. Dad's angry ... really angry. He's yelling at me, saying I'm stupid.

THERAPIST: OK, bring yourself into the image as an adult, as you are now. Maybe place yourself between little Nicky and your dad. How do you feel about what's happening, how he's treating little Nicky?

CLIENT: It's pathetic. It's wrong. She's just a kid.

THERAPIST: Can you bring yourself in, an adult, as you are now, feeling angry that this is happening?

CLIENT: OK, I'm there standing next to him.

THERAPIST: Be that strong, healthy adult. What do you want to say to dad?

CLIENT: [in a defiant tone] 'Leave her alone, you're a bully, and I'm sick of it.'

THERAPIST: [coaching the client] ' ... and I'm not afraid of you'.

CLIENT: [to the father in defiance] 'I am not afraid of you; you're dealing with me'.

THERAPIST: How does he respond?

CLIENT: He looks stunned. No one questions him.

THERAPIST: What happens next? What do you say or do?

CLIENT: I take him by the shoulder, out of the room. I say, 'Don't ever do that again. She's a good kid'.

THERAPIST: Who's in the scene now?

CLIENT: It's just little Nicky and me.

THERAPIST: How are you feeling? What do you say?

CLIENT: 'Hey, little one, it's not your fault, your dad has problems, and I'm not going to let him do that anymore.'

THERAPIST: How does she respond?

CLIENT: She looks a bit uncertain but happier.

THERAPIST: What do you want to say to her?

CLIENT: 'I'm here for you, don't be afraid, you're a good kid'.

THERAPIST: How does she respond?

CLIENT: She smiles. It's good to see her safer and at ease.

THERAPIST: OK, notice that good feeling and the smile on little Nicky. Now, I want you to rewind the tape to the start of the imagery, to the moment that 'adult you' arrives in the image. Now, I want you to be little Nicky. Being little Nicky, what do you see?

CLIENT: I can see adult me coming into the room. She's standing between dad and me.

THERAPIST: What's happening?

CLIENT: She's [Adult Nicky] saying to my dad to back off, that he's a bully and she's not going to take it anymore.

THERAPIST: How does he respond?

CLIENT: He's surprised and tries to respond, but Big Me is having none of that! She says 'I've heard enough!', and she's not afraid of him.

THERAPIST: How does that feel?

CLIENT: Feels good. Someone is there to protect me. Stand up for me.

THERAPIST: What is happening now?

CLIENT: She leads him out of the room, sort of pushing him out.

THERAPIST: What happens next?

CLIENT: He's gone, it's just me and Big Me. She's saying I'm a good kid and that dad's a bully. She says that she will take care of things.

THERAPIST: How does that feel? What do you need?

CLIENT: Feels good to have someone on my side who cares. I need a hug.

THERAPIST: Can you ask Big You, say it out loud? 'I need a hug.'

CLIENT: 'Adult Me, can I have a hug?'

THERAPIST: How does she respond?

CLIENT: She says 'Absolutely!' and gives me a big hug. It feels great.

In addition to mode dialogues, chairwork can also provide a 'forum' for clients to explore mixed feelings, dilemmas, or decision making. Exploration of associated emotions and beliefs may typically be blocked or obstructed by coping modes. For example, if a client needs to decide on the future of a relationship but avoided thinking about the issue because of a coping mode, the therapist could construct a decision-making chair dialogue between the side of the client that wanted to pursue the relationship and the part that wanted to leave [19].

Box 8.8 Imagery Tips and Troubleshooting

What If the Client Becomes Overwhelmed?

Therapists are often concerned about clients becoming overwhelmed during imagery exercises. It is essential to demonstrate to the client that you have confidence in the technique and are confident that you can manage their emotions accessed via imagery. Clients are often anxious about affect and have beliefs related to not coping with emotion. The therapist can use their influence within the image to modulate the client's emotional arousal (this is preferable to asking the client to suddenly open their eyes and end the exercise). For example, the therapist can enter the image and provide safety and reassurance. Alternatively, the therapist can remove the antagonist from the image and focus on reparenting and care. To elaborate on feeling connected to the therapist (and grounded in the here and now), a shawl or rug can be held between the client and therapist [16]. The therapist gently can gently tug on the fabric, reminding the client that they are safe and connected with the therapist.

Do I Have to Start with a Highly Distressing Memory or Image?

Less distressing imagery can be initially used if the client is fearful of the process: for example, rescripting an image of the child alone focusing on care and safety. However, including the more aversive elements of the memory enhances the effectiveness of the imagery rescripting [17].

What Do I Do If the Client Jumps into the Abusive Act of the Trauma?

It is helpful to note to the client that there is no need to replay traumatic events in their entirety. If the client does jump into abusive content, the therapist can ask the client to pause and then 'rewind' the memory to a point just before the abusive act.

What If My Client Is Very Apprehensive or Doesn't Want to Close Their Eyes?

The therapist can assure the client that they have control over the process. The client may wish to look at the floor or away from the therapist. Alternatively, the therapist can talk through what they envisage would happen in the image. Describing the proposed imagery and possible helpful outcomes can provide less aversive expectancies.

What If the Client Fears Retribution from an Abusive Figure After the Session?

During the latter parts of imagery exercises, the client may fear retribution from antagonists. Here, the therapist can ask the client to imagine having a pager or 'magic phone' that, once pressed, brings the therapist into the image to protect and stand up for the client. The therapist conveys a sense of confidence in dealing with the antagonist.

What If the Client Says, 'I Can't Do Imagery' or 'I Don't Remember My Childhood?'

There are several reasons for such client statements. Clients' coping modes can typically block access to images or memories. At the same time, they may assume that the therapist is seeking vivid and clear experiences via imagery. Therapists can ask the client to visually describe a neutral place or situation drawing upon a mental image: 'What is your daughter doing right now? Paint me a picture of what she is up to at school. Where is she and what is she doing?' Regarding not having a clear recollection of childhood, the therapist can ask the client to 'get a sense' of themselves as a child feeling sad, anxious, or distressed. Here, it is essential that the client leads with the experience (primarily to prevent the therapist from being involved in suggestive actions).

Chairwork mode dialogues are an opportunity for the schema therapist to be creative. Chairwork can also help provide an active and energising element to therapy sessions that might otherwise feel flat and disconnected. Several principles can help guide more effective chairwork within schema therapy.

Separation of Modes Using Chairs

A specific chair can be allocated for each mode. The client then speaks with the 'voice' or sentiment of this mode only from this chair, which anchors the mode to that location. For example, a client's self-blaming for an error is ascribed to the Punitive Critic and a chair is allocated to this mode, more playfully labelled 'the Punisher'. If the client were to resume self-critical statements within the session, the therapist might gesture to the 'Punisher chair' (Therapist: 'That's coming from the Punisher mode', gesturing to the empty seat), or they might ask them to move to the prescribed chair and continue speaking. This is an attempt to contain punishing sentiments to a specific chair. The therapist may also assign a chair to the Vulnerable Child mode ('the Punished'), ascribing the thoughts, feelings, and sensations of being criticised to this seat.

Mode separation (or mode de-contamination) has several aims. First, the therapist aims to alleviate chaotic psychological processes associated with 'mode flipping'. Separating the modes makes the motives, associated emotional states, and ideas of each mode clearer, which in turn makes the impact of their interplay clearer. Second, the client can defuse from the ideas (beliefs, rules, and assumptions) of problematic modes and more easily adopt a healthier perspective. As a result, the therapist can help the client strengthen their Healthy Adult mode.

Once the client can reliably discriminate modes, the therapist can gesture towards the chair representing a particular mode, rather than having clients moving rapidly from chair to chair. For example, while gesturing to the Punitive Critic seat the therapist may say 'The Punisher mode is saying that you're a "loser", just like your brother did, just like the bullies did, and it's been internalised in you. We have to stand up to this side of you and say (*looking at the chair*) back off!'

Embodying and Personalising the Mode

When sitting in a chair during chairwork exercises, the client is encouraged to embody the mode and take the mode's perspective, giving the mode a 'voice' [19]. On these occasions, the client is supported to *speak from* the mode, expressing its thoughts, feelings, and sentiments. At other times, the client can be encouraged to look at an empty chair representing a mode and be asked how they 'see' the mode, so as to humanise the mode – for example, 'when you look over to the chair that takes the role of the punitive side of you, what do you see, what does it look like to you?' On some occasions, it may be helpful for the client to envisage specific antagonists from their life that helped form the mode and whose voice and messages the client may have internalised. For example, the therapist can ask the client to imagine their punitive father sitting in the seat, to access punitive messages.

Anchoring to a Context

It is usually helpful to provide a specific context or 'anchor' when initiating chairwork, rather than just saying 'Move into the Punisher seat, what does that side say?' The therapist

> **Box 8.9** Example of Anchoring Chairwork to a Specific Context
>
> THERAPIST: So, from the Punisher seat, what does that side say about your friendships and reaching out to your friends?
>
> [NB: The therapist does not simply say 'Move to the Punisher seat, what does that side say?']
>
> CLIENT: *[in the Punitive Critic chair]* 'What's the point? They don't really like you. They put up with you'.

might anchor the exercise using a recent triggering situation, by referring to a behavioural pattern that the client wants to break, or by analysing an instance of a mode being activated within the session. For example, with a client who has noticed a pattern of retreating from his friends, the therapist could anchor a chairwork exercise to a recent opportunity to socialise with friends. The therapist might ask the client to move to a chair representing the Punitive Critic mode (see Box 8.9).

Physical Location of and Number of Chairs

The physical location of the chairs can symbolically facilitate the quality and intensity of emotional activation, perspective-taking, and, consequently, how much and exactly what the client learns from the exercise. Typically, the therapist may seek to sit alongside the client as a dyad. The therapist–client dyad can then initiate dialogues with specific modes. Furthermore, the therapist can model Healthy Adult responses to various modes within the client's case conceptualisation and help prompt and coach responses from the client. Such a seating arrangement can help with enhancing the 'team therapy' aspect of the interplay.

'Empty Chair' When Directly Confronting or Challenging

A primary objective of using chairwork is to help the client distance their perspective from that of maladaptive modes. Were the therapist to challenge or confront modes and schemas by talking directly to the client (e.g., 'You seem to be avoiding my question'), the client might fuse further with the mode (i.e., the client experiences the therapist as making no distinction between the client's mode and the client's self). Moreover, the client may become defensive and resolute. However, the therapist can emphatically confront an empty chair (typically with the client sitting alongside them). As a result, the therapist can efficiently address therapy-interfering issues, while the client sees the challenge as being directed more towards a circumscribed way of behaving than towards themselves as a whole person.

Chairwork Technique in the Various Phases of Treatment

Chairwork is suitable for each phase of treatment. However, the exact method of working with chairs will change throughout the phases of therapy. Table 8.1 presents an overview of how mode work can be enhanced via the use of chairs in various phases of treatment. The use of the chair technique will then be explicitly elaborated upon in each phase.

Table 8.1 Chairwork in different phases of treatment

Phase of treatment	Application
Case conceptualisation	• Chairs for diagnostics • Interview modes
Initial phase	• Chair technique 'from the sidelines' • 'Moding out' triggers • Negotiate with Protector • 'Contaminate' the chair of the Vulnerable Child • Manage and restrict the impact of critic modes • Limited reparenting to the empty child mode seat
Middle phase	• Coaching Healthy Adult in compassion • Practise the three steps of the Healthy Adult • Use of chairwork as a forum to discuss change/explore feelings (e.g., grief) ambivalence
Final phase	• Strengthen Healthy Adult: Therapist plays coping or parent mode; client responds • Client responds to Vulnerable Child in the empty chair

Case Conceptualisation Phase

Within the case conceptualisation phase, the main aim of chairwork is to increase schema or mode awareness. At this stage, interviewing and identifying the mode interplay is sufficient. In subsequent phases, chairwork is used to manage and/or reduce the activation of those modes: to limit the internalised Critic modes and bypass the Protector modes through 'understanding and negotiation' so that contact can be made with the emotional part(s) of the client for corrective experiences.

A mode conceptualisation of a triggering event or life pattern can be translated into a chairwork exercise. Here, the therapist can allocate chairs to modes and provide a cognitive understanding of the interplay of modes in the client's life and treatment. The therapist can explore a mode's function and experience relative to a specific 'anchor' via an interview. In Box 8.10, the therapist invites the client to sit in an adjacent seat and 'be the mode'.

Initial Phase

The two main objectives of the initial phase of therapy are: (a) to learn to become more aware of the modes; and (b) to gain corrective emotional experiences. Chairwork is an essential tool for meeting both objectives. Therapists can explore recent triggers or problematic situations described by the client via chairwork approaches.

'Moding Out' a Trigger. A case conceptualisation can be 'moded out' via the use of chairs. Here, the therapist anchors the conceptualisation to a specific trigger or life pattern (e.g., a mode interplay around substance misuse), associating particular modes with chairs and then asking the client to move between each location, noting each mode's perspective towards the triggering event (see Box 8.11).

Box 8.10 Case Example Using Chairwork to Complete a Mode Dialogue

A client speaks about feeling 'bad' the previous week and, as a result, cancelling the last appointment and withdrawing.

THERAPIST: *[pointing to empty adjacent chair]* In this chair, I would like you to be that withdrawn side of yourself. Be that withdrawn person when you *[gesturing at the adjacent chair]* felt so bad. How do you help her *[gesturing at the other chair]* by withdrawing like that? What would have happened to her *[gesturing at the other chair]* if you weren't there or hadn't intervened?

After this active mode has been explored, the therapist asks the client to return to the initial chair. In this way, the client can distance themselves from that mood and reflect upon it.

Box 8.11 Moding Out a Trigger

THERAPIST: OK, sounds like a part of you wanted to have the drink on the weekend, another part was really angry at you for drinking, and another side felt overwhelmed. Would it be OK if we tried a chairwork exercise?

CLIENT: Sure.

THERAPIST: OK, here's three seats. One seat here is the part of you that is sad, alone, hopeless: your Vulnerable Child side. *[Getting a second chair]* Here is the Self-Soother side of you, the drinker part of you. This side is the part that relapsed on the weekend. *[Getting the third chair]* The last chair is the Punisher mode, the Critic that is activated for relapsing. Can you sit in this chair that wants to drink? Be that side. What does that side say about drinking?

CLIENT: *[Now sitting in the Self-Soother seat]* 'Drinking is inevitable. You won't feel as bad if you drink; it's easy to just forget.'

THERAPIST: Yes, this makes sense. It helps ease the pain and loneliness. OK, how about moving into the Punisher chair now, be this side. How does this react to your relapse? What does that say to your vulnerable side?

CLIENT: *[In the Punisher mode seat]* 'You messed up again. It's because of you. You're weak, and you have hurt the people you love. You keep making stupid decisions'.

THERAPIST: OK, I now want you to leave the Punisher in the chair and move to the Little Nikki seat. How does it feel hearing this from the Punisher?

CLIENT: 'I just feel alone *[tearful]*. Hopeless. What's wrong with me!'.

THERAPIST: It's hard. Giving up drinking is tough stuff. I'm guessing when you feel this way, the Self-Soother side of you *[gestures to the chair]* is wanting to drink more. Am I right?

Negotiating with Coping Modes. Unlike the conceptualisation and assessment phase, the initial phase of therapy aims to generate new, corrective emotional experiences. The client should now be aware of their mode conceptualisation. The therapist must reason with and negotiate with coping modes to bypass this protective state and help the client experience underlying feelings. Once the client's schema-driven emotions and associated beliefs are identified, the therapist can provide experiences of emotions and beliefs that counteract the schema.

'Watching From the Sidelines'. Some clients have trouble doing these emotionally oriented exercises. The related resistance can cause them to not want to switch chairs. In those situations, chairwork can also be applied 'from the sidelines'. The client remains seated in their original chair, but the therapist shapes the situation and related feelings using chairs placed in the space. As a result, the therapist 'works around' the client's reluctance. The approach allows the client to examine the various modes and their mutual interaction from the sidelines. The therapist uses chairs to sketch the mode model as they could do on a whiteboard.

The therapist can use chairwork to explore the pros and cons of a coping mode. For example, a 'protective chair' can be viewed as a gatekeeper guarding the entrance to the client's emotional inner world. Excessive pressure will not make a gatekeeper allow passage. Using a great deal of understanding, acknowledgement, and reassurance, and giving control, the therapist must offer sufficient security for this coping mode to be willing to share more of the client's underlying feelings. A typical case example for the use of chairwork to engage with a Protector mode is given in Box 8.12.

Box 8.12 Case Example of Working with the Protector Mode

THERAPIST: OK, so you protect her *[gesturing to the empty chair where the client first sat]* by just keeping all those feelings away, concentrating on other things and certainly not talking too much about the feelings ... I can imagine that you try to keep those feelings away if they bother you so much. I also have a protective side that tries to keep sadness or fears away. But what happens to her emotions when you do that? Does pushing them away solve them?

CLIENT: No ... No, well, at that moment, yes, but I could feel the same way again later.

THERAPIST: OK, so you can protect her from that sadness very well at the moment, but this doesn't solve the feelings. It just pushes them away temporarily. I think we can do more. I think I can actually help her to feel better. How does that sound to you?

CLIENT: Well ... Great, but I can't really imagine it.

THERAPIST: I understand. It might not sound believable. I would like to have the opportunity to prove that it's possible. But I do need your cooperation: if you give me a chance, I'd like to get in touch with her and let her know that there are more options than just pushing away sadness and fear. Could you give me this chance? You can always intervene if you want to stop. You're in control!

CLIENT: Alright.

[Therapist asks the client to switch chairs.]

THERAPIST: OK, I'm now going to ask you to get up from this chair and sit on the chair next to me. But do bear in mind that when you get up from that chair, the Protector stays there. Leave her superglued there while you come and sit here next to me.
[Now to the client in the chair next to the therapist, who says in a softer voice]: So there *[gesturing to the protector's chair]* is that Protector who is trying to help you by pushing away all your sadness and fears. see above does that by thinking about it as little as possible,

by staying focused on work. But in the meantime, you feel sad, and you have felt anxious in the past week. Can you tell me what made you so sad and anxious in the past week?

CLIENT: *[becoming tearful]* 'It's hard coming here.'

THERAPIST: When I listen to you, I don't find it strange at all that you felt sad and anxious. I think everyone in this situation *[gesturing to a place near the client]* would feel a bit uncomfortable: it would be a tricky situation for anyone. Of course, you also feel sad and anxious. But when I think of your history, I also realise that you often experienced these kinds of situations in your life. It is the umpteenth time that you are alone, and you feel threatened. Of course, you are completely out of sorts at that moment because, after all, it is an old pain that plays a part.

How does it feel when you hear me say that it makes sense, the way you felt? How does it feel to be understood in this? Is it a nice feeling to be understood *[the therapist holds his thumb up]* or not so nice *[moving thumb down]*.

CLIENT: *[gives thumbs-up gesture.]*

Attention is placed on the positioning of the chairs: the therapist sits closer to the Vulnerable Child mode than the Protector mode. Furthermore, the therapist's tone of voice is modified based on which mode is being addressed in the exercise. Responses to the Vulnerable Child mode can have a softer, more emotional tone than the rational and 'adult' negotiation with the Coping mode.

Although offering compassion has a soothing effect, it is still essential to ensure the client is aware of this effect. Clients tend to mainly pay attention to the situation that made them feel rotten and the emotional pain caused as a result. Focusing attention on the effect of compassion can increase its impact. In some cases, the client does not yet wish to participate in this kind of chairwork; in those cases the therapist can invite an exercise where they will first play the 'vulnerable side' as a way of scaffolding the client's participation (see Box 8.13 for an example).

Chairwork and Child Modes. Nurturance and care may have been scarcely experienced in the life of the client. As a result, limited reparenting can be uncomfortable and awkward when applied face to face with the client. The therapist can use an empty chair and respond to the client's needs in an indirect way that the client tolerates. Moreover, by observing the therapist's care and nurturance towards the client's child modes, the client is better positioned to model appropriate forms of care and nurturance to the self. Chairwork can also help the client understand and manage anger emanating from the Angry Child mode. The therapist may use two back-to-back chairs to highlight the interplay between anger and more vulnerable feelings. For example, Chair A = Angry Child mode: 'This is ridiculous, what is this? . . . "Forget the client day" or something?!' Chair B = Vulnerable Child mode: 'This side feels like I don't matter. No one is there for me.' In addition, the Angry Child mode can be allocated to an empty chair, and the therapist can then validate, empathise, and ultimately contain the anger within this mode. Typically, this approach is conducted when the client has gained some distance from the Angry Child mode and is more reflective. For example, the therapist may say 'So, the angry "Fireball" side of you is in this [empty] chair in front of me. *[Addressing the empty chair]* It's not nice for the therapist to be late, I really want you to know that, but stomping around giving me the silent treatment limits me in understanding what's going on for you. We have to work out a way for you to communicate how you feel without doing it in this way.'

Box 8.13 'Contaminating the Chair'

Although mode work in chairs can be an effective way to bypass coping modes and contact the vulnerable part of the client, some clients don't feel any different when they sit in various chairs. This lack of response may be due to several factors. The coping mode might be too active: the client may have never learned to allow and experience vulnerable emotions. In this case, the therapist can use chairwork to 'infect' the chair with emotions. Here, the therapist can ask the client (who remains detached or unaware of feeling) to sit in the therapist's seat. The therapist then sits in the seat representing the Vulnerable Child mode and starts talking 'from this side' based on knowledge derived from the client's conceptualisation. The therapist imagines the client's Vulnerable Child mode and acts out and verbalises their probable feelings and needs.

THERAPIST: If I was to think about you as a child, and I connected and stepped inside and vocalised your Vulnerable Child mode, I would say ... why doesn't anyone like me? I wish people were kind to me; I just want someone to like me being around, to notice me. I feel really lonely sometimes.

The therapist asks the client to take their place in the Vulnerable Child chair (which has been 'infected' by emotion). The therapist can then encourage the client to express and build upon notions laid out by the therapist. In this case, the therapist names potential core feelings and sentiments linked to the case. Doing so provides the client with an opportunity to express such feelings that may be typically blocked or avoided.

Chairwork and the Management of Critic Modes. A central aim of schema therapy is to provide corrective emotional experiences. Chairwork can offer the therapist a method to generate experiences that combat old dysfunctional rules and internalised messages from the past. The client can experience someone standing up for them and disagreeing with noxious and demanding sentiments. As noted in Chapters 3 and 4, Critic modes are conceptualised and managed in varying ways. In chairwork exercises, the therapist needs to adapt their responses based on the type of mode.

a. Punitive Critic mode: The therapist aims to defend and stand up for the client in chairwork. When confronting Punitive modes in chairwork, the therapist's tone is generally defiant, stating that the punitive and blaming notions and rules are wrong. For example, Therapist: *[to the empty Punitive Critic chair]* 'I don't agree with you, I don't care what you say; it's wrong, you're not good for her, and I've had enough of it.' Box 8.14 provides a case example of the use of chairwork with a Punitive Critic mode

b) Demanding Critic mode: The therapist does not generally take an adversarial stance in interactions with this mode via chair work. In contrast, the therapist appeals to and reasons with the mode that is pressuring and demanding. For example, Therapist: *[to the empty Demanding Critic chair]* 'Look, I know you have good intentions, but if she keeps listening to you, she will always be unhappy, is that what you want?'

c) Guilt-Inducing Critic mode: The therapist aims to be a strong advocate for the client's needs. The therapist appeals for the client's needs and rights, taking an unwavering stance. Therapist: *[to the empty Guilt-Inducing Critic chair]* 'Nikki is allowed to have some time to herself. It's normal for her to have an opinion. You put all this responsibility on her – it's too much! I want you to back off and give her some space.'

Box 8.14 Case Example: Chairwork with a Punitive Critic Mode

THERAPIST: Listening to you, it sounds like you're looking at yourself *[gesturing to a place diagonally from the client]* not with compassion, but with anger and criticism. Is that true?

CLIENT: But it's true, I mess everything up!

THERAPIST: Exactly, that's what I notice. It's like you're looking at yourself being completely convinced that you're a loser. If that punitive side is so active, let's literally give it a place in this room and hear what it has to say.

Come over here and sit in this chair *[Therapist pulls up a chair]*. Now be that critical voice, that punitive side. And I want you to look at *[clients's name and pointing to the original chair]* from this experience and tell me what you have to say about him.

It can be useful for the therapist to look at the original, empty chair too, not to draw the clients's attention to the interaction with the therapist but to focus more on the dynamic of self-criticism. Many clients do not find it difficult to come up with a list of criticisms of themselves. The therapist then wants to know what the substantive criticism is so they can provide substantive counter-arguments. It is, however, not advisable for the client to berate themselves with critiques. After several pieces of criticism, the therapist stops the client and asks them to return to the original chair.

THERAPIST: OK, OK, I'm going to interrupt you. You're doing fine, but I'd like to ask you to come and sit beside me. But do bear in mind that when you get up from that chair, I'd like you to leave behind the angry, critical voice. This *[gesturing at the chair of the punitive side]* is where you can express all that criticism, but when you get up, you leave the punitive voice superglued to that chair.

THERAPIST: *[Leaning towards the client and talking in a soft tone, gesturing to that other, empty chair]* When I hear the criticism from that corner, it's pretty harsh. It's not just the words but the tone in which they are said. It sounds a bit like dad speaking to you. When I hear this criticism, in that tone, I wonder how you feel when this is being said?

CLIENT: I don't know . . . rotten . . . I think sad.

THERAPIST: I don't agree with that punishing voice, but I know it's normal for you to speak to yourself that way. I know how much criticism you had growing up, and when I imagine you as a child with your dad speaking to you harshly, it makes me angry. I feel a strong urge to say *[facing the empty punitive chair and speaking in a determined and uncompromising tone]* 'Stop! Stop talking to *[name of the client]* like that. Stop it. What you're saying doesn't make any sense, and you're wrong.'

THERAPIST: *[softly to the client next to him]* How do you feel when you hear me say this, that there's nothing wrong with you *[pointing to the critic side]*, that you're not the problem here, but he is?

Clients regularly answer that they agree with the punitive side. This response is understandable because they're so used to hearing and believing punitive messages. However, it is important to note that the therapist didn't ask if the client believed the punitive messages, but how it felt to have someone stand up for them.

CLIENT: Well, it's nice of you, but let's face it, I'm a loser.

THERAPIST: OK, but now I hear you say that you believe and agree with that punitive voice. But to be honest, that's not what I was asking you. I was asking how it felt when I stood up for you. What was it like?

CLIENT: Well, it was nice to hear, of course.

THERAPIST: That's good to hear! And how does he *[gesturing to the punitive side]* respond to what I'm saying? Is he behaving?

CLIENT: That punitive side? No, he really wouldn't let you speak to me like that and would just get angry at you.

In some cases, the critic mode can be strong and dominant. However, the therapist seeks to win the exchange and provide a corrective experience: one of reattribution and someone standing up to the critical sentiment. In such cases, the therapist can then move to take away the chair and dramatically reposition it from the exchange.

THERAPIST: Oh, he's getting angrier? Then he should get out of here! *[The therapist stands up, diagonally in front of the client, facing the empty chair of the punitive side. He stands here briefly and once again addresses the punitive side in a strong, uncompromising tone.]* 'I've had it up to here with you. I won't stand by and watch how you talk to [name of the client] like that! She's not the problem. You are!' [Turns to the client and says softly] You're not the problem, they are [pointing at the punitive side]. [Now again facing the punitive side, in a strict voice] 'I want you to leave now' [points to the door, picks up the chair, opens the door, removes the chair and closes the door. Sits back down beside the client].* This is a safe place for you, where there is care and support, not those old punitive messages that don't make any sense. How do you feel now that the punitive side is gone?

What if ...?
What if the client keeps emphasising that the Punitive Critic cannot be dismissed?
On some occasions, the client can be very 'fused' with the critic mode. Linking these punitive or demanding messages to historical figures can assist the client in gaining more insight into the origins of such rules and messages. Naming the Critic as the historical figure that initiated the message can be helpful. For example, 'Your Father, together with those bullies from primary school, are sitting in the chair, and they're saying all those bad things about you again.'

Middle Phase

In the initial phase of treatment, the therapist provides a model of the Healthy Adult mode. In later stages of treatment, the therapist takes a receding role in mode work with chairs. Instead, the client is encouraged to access their own Healthy Adult mode and manage their problematic modes. Box 8.15 outlines a five-step chairwork exercise for strengthening the Healthy Adult mode.

Chairwork in the Final Phases

The final phase aims to further strengthen the Healthy Adult part of the client (see Table 8.2). In the final stage of chairwork, the therapist acts out the client's problematic modes (e.g., Protector, Critic modes). The client practices their Healthy Adult responses in direct dialogues with the therapist, increasing the challenge for the client and building their confidence to face their modes alone once therapy is concluded.

The therapist can also help coach the client to refute sentiments as in Box 8.16. Several tips for overcoming common roadbloacks to chairwork are outlined in Box 8.17.

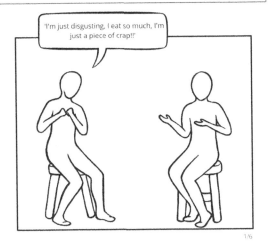

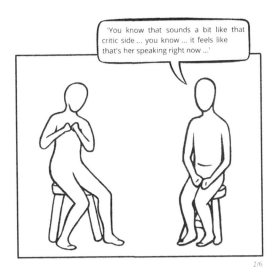

Cartoon 8.2 Chairwork with the Punitive Critic

Other Experiential and Emotion-Focused Techniques

Historical Role-Play

Therapists can use role-play to come to new interpretations and insights. In a role-play session, meaningful situations from the past or present are re-enacted. When situations

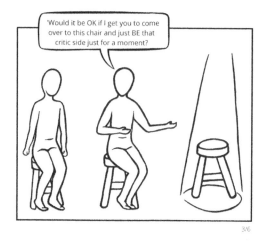

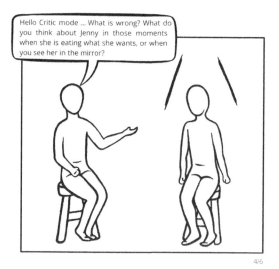

Cartoon 8.2 (cont.)

from the past are re-enacted, this is referred to as a *historical role-play*. Re-enacting an historically significant situation can have various objectives:

- To identify relevant schemas and their historical roots
- To gain greater insight into the interaction patterns between the client and attachment figures
- To provide an opportunity to try out new behaviour

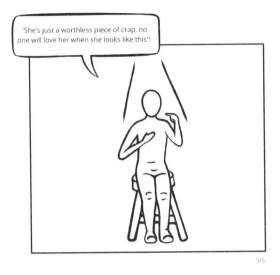

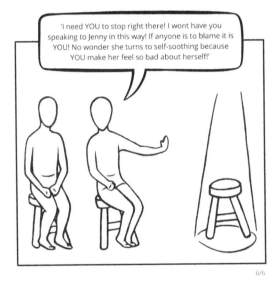

Cartoon 8.2 (cont.)

In several respects, historical role-play resembles imagery rescripting. In both techniques, meaningful situations from the past are brought to life and, in doing so, offer insight into the meaning of those events. In addition, both techniques also offer an opportunity to rewrite these events and thereby generate corrective emotional experiences in the process.

Box 8.15 'A Five-Step Chairwork Exercise' for Strengthening the Healthy Adult Mode

The following exercise can assist the client to strengthen their Healthy Adult mode. It involves rehearsing facilitative statements in three key domains when facing events that would usually trigger Critic, child, and maladaptive coping modes:

1. Compassion to self and others: explicitly acknowledging, understanding, and accepting emotions evoked from problematic situations and adopting an attitude of willingness to alleviate them.
2. Cognitive restructuring: correcting old beliefs from the protector and critical modes and realistically approaching the challenging situation.
3. Behaviour modification: rather than reverting to old coping-mode-induced behavioural patterns, the Healthy Adult mode tries to handle the problematic situation and maintain awareness of the self's basic needs.

This chairwork exercise can help the client internalise the three components of responding to schema and mode triggers. Instead of each chair representing a separate mode, a chair now represents a particular step in the Healthy Adult response to triggers.

Step 1: Exploration of the Problematic Situation

The therapist and client identify a problematic situation that recently occurred or look ahead towards a potentially challenging situation in the future. The therapist can help identify emotional experiences, critical or demanding mode cognitions, and schema/mode-driven behavioural responses (that either did occur [for past events] or might occur [in future events]).

Step 2: Place Three Chairs Opposite the client

The therapist explains that this situation is used to practise the three steps of the Healthy Adult. The three chairs are placed and named as the three steps of the Healthy Adult.

Step 3: Allocate a Chair for Compassion

In this chair, the client is initially asked to embody their Healthy Adult side. A short imagery exercise can assist them in accessing compassionate sentiments whereby the client visualises their Healthy Adult mode. The therapist can then coach the client in expressing explicit compassion and understanding towards the chair where the client was initially seated.

The therapist coaches the client to express out loud their understanding of the client's difficulties and challenges and their compassion towards the client.

THERAPIST: So, now be that Healthy Adult and look back on that situation you were just talking about (gesturing to the original empty chair, naming the client). I think we can easily understand why he felt so sad and alone in that situation, right? Could you express that out loud: 'Of course you feel so alone and sad because . . .'

Step 4: Allocate Chair for Cognitive Restructuring

In this chair, the critical or coping mode is identified. The therapist and client discuss how to counter distorted and unhelpful assumptions. Following this, the therapist coaches the client to contradict the punishing or coping mode. The therapist may encourage the client to repeat statements with a firmer tone or support them by adopting more assertive postures or gestures.

CLIENT: 'Well, I really did my best, and I don't know how to better prepare myself for that situation.'

THERAPIST: So, what do you think about the accusation that you should not have made mistakes?

CLIENT: It's actually not true.

THERAPIST: Can you say that directly to that punitive side? That you disagree with him?

CLIENT: *[turns to the imaginary punitive side]* 'Well, what you're saying is not true.'

THERAPIST: Say it louder, 20 per cent louder.

CLIENT: 'What you're saying is not true!'

THERAPIST: Great! How does it feel to say that?

CLIENT: Yeah, good. Powerful, better.

Step 5: Allocate a Chair for Behaviour Modification

In this chair, the therapist and the client discuss a healthy way of responding to the problematic situation. The best solution is the one that best meets the relevant core emotional needs of the client. At the same time, the therapist cautions that, in finding a solution, compromises will always need to be made, and situations can never be ideal.

THERAPIST: If there's one thing that's important for you to keep an eye on, what is it?

CLIENT: *[Seated in the Behaviour Modification chair, embodying the Healthy Adult's response]* Well . . . I'm allowed to feel OK about myself, and I don't have to immediately withdraw when I start feeling nauseous.

THERAPIST: Exactly! So, what's the best way of dealing with this situation without having to withdraw when you feel nauseous? Can you say that to him: 'What you have to do now is . . .' What would you advise him to do?

Step 6: Return to the Initial Chair Switching Perspective

As a final step, the client may return to the original chair (where they started the exercise), after which the therapist can summarise and reflect on the previous sentiments from the three?! elements of the Healthy Adult. As a result, the client can receive messages instead of expressing them, intensifying the experience.

Table 8.2 Chairwork to develop Healthy Adult in various treatment phases

Initial phase
- Stand up with the client and look at the chairs together

Middle phase
- Have the client sit in the therapist's chair and coach in expressing compassion
- Arrange a separate chair for the Healthy Adult side of the client with a chair for the Vulnerable Child between the client and the therapist
- Use three separate chairs to practise the three components of the Healthy Adult side

Final phase
- The therapist sits in the chair of the Protector or Critic mode and the client responds to the sentiments of the problematic modes

---

Box 8.16 Example of Therapist Coaching Client to Refute Critic mode Messages

THERAPIST: We have another ten sessions left. I suggest that we use the final sessions to prepare you more for the difficult moments you're bound to encounter in the future.

CLIENT: Yes, alright.

THERAPIST: Let's use the chairs again but in a slightly different way.

CLIENT: Oh . . . ?

THERAPIST: Yes, now I realise that there will be many situations in which your Protector will take over, and that means that at that moment, you may believe that it's better to withdraw. Let's prepare for those situations, in which I will now play your Protector mode.

CLIENT: Oh?

THERAPIST: I would like you to contradict my arguments from the chair of the Healthy Adult. But don't worry – if it's tricky I'll help you. You don't have to do it all on your own yet. We're just practising how to do it in the future.

Box 8.17 Chairwork Tips

What Chair Goes Where?

Chairwork is a rich methodology, and therapists can apply it in many different ways. There are no exact rules for using this technique, only the guiding principle to make it an emotionally oriented approach. Each chair represents a different side of the client, almost as if there were multiple people in the room.

There are various options as to who is being addressed in the original chair. Some therapists opt to approach this chair as the Healthy Adult, the client who came to therapy, with reflections being made towards the other modes from this location. Other therapists choose to address the more emotional part of the client in the original chair.

What If the Client Doesn't Want to Move?

If the client doesn't want to move or is hesitant, you can still proceed with mode work and bypass the client's resistance. Put the part that 'doesn't want to move' (typically a Coping mode or Angry Child mode) into a chair. Here, the therapist can respond to the mode within the empty chair without the client moving.

I'm Not Sure If My Client Will 'Buy Into' Chairwork

Clients can be cynical or pessimistic about doing chairwork. Typically, this is a way to avoid doing the exercise and throw the therapist off track. However, clients typically seek and respect a therapist who is confident in their skills and suggestions: if a client isn't buying a chairwork technique, back yourself and your suggestions.

THERAPIST: Yes, I know, I'm talking to a chair, you can laugh at me, but I'm serious. This technique can be really helpful. I would prefer to do something helpful than just to avoid it because it might look silly to you.

What Can I Do If the Client Flips Modes During a Chair Work Exercise?

If a client flips to a new mode, you can do several things. First, you can acknowledge the mode activation and use hand gesturing. For example, 'It sounds like the Critic is showing up [pointing to the corner of the room]. She can stay out of this exchange. Come back to that side of you that is hurting.' Alternatively, the therapist may want to allocate another chair to represent the new mode and continue with a dialogue with this mode.

How Many Chairs Do I Need? I Have a Small Office!

Keep things simple. Many therapists typically work with one mode at a time. In this case, you will only need one chair to base your mode work.

Box 8.18 Example of a Situation Suitable for Historical Role-Play

Sandra felt rejected by her friend when she told them about her relationship problems and they didn't respond to what she said. Sandra felt sad and alone, didn't say much more and left as soon as possible. The therapist recognises that this behaviour is emblematic of the pattern of avoidance which the therapy has previously focused on, and therefore suggests that another situation be examined more closely.

The physical interaction with another person in a historical role-play can increase the vividness and authenticity of the experience.

The re-enactment of meaningful events makes historical role-play inappropriate for situations in which the basic need of safety was missing. Memories involving verbal, physical, or sexual violence are therefore not suitable for this technique. However, historical role-play lends itself particularly well to all other situations.

The specific impetus in the session for considering historical role-play could be that the client talks about a strong emotional or behavioural response which is an illustration of the patterns that the therapy focuses on. For example, the client could talk about a situation in which avoidance, surrender, and/or overcompensation are at play. Or, the client may talk about a recent situation in which they felt ignored, attacked, or excluded (see Box 8.18).

If the therapist and the client agree that this situation is worth examining, a significant situation from the past is identified that may be related to this recent event. When the therapy is still in its initial phase, a diagnostic imagery exercise can be conducted to gain insight into this historical experience (see Box 8.19). When there is already greater insight into the historical roots of the patterns, the therapist and client can discuss together which of these historical events will be explored in more depth.

Now that a historical event has been selected, this situation can then be re-enacted. The re-enactment of this event takes place in a different part of the room than the chairs where the conversation has taken place so far. A clear distinction between the area in which the past is staged and another spot in the room in which that situation is reflected on contributes to the vividness and authenticity of the historical event.

Box 8.19 Example of Imaginal Assessment Linking Recent Situation to Historical Event

The therapist asks whether the client has any idea as to how this withdrawal behaviour as a reaction came about in her life. The therapy is still in its early stages and the client doesn't have a clue how this pattern evolved. At this point, the therapist asks if the client would like to close her eyes and allow an image of the situation with the friend to form in her mind.

THERAPIST: If you think back to the situation with that friend, and then in particular, the moment that you felt genuinely affected by it, what can you see now?

CLIENT: That moment when she looks away a bit bored.

THERAPIST: Describe what you can literally see now.

CLIENT: I've just told her that Tom [my boyfriend] and I have been having a lot of arguments lately and she doesn't say anything and she looks away.

THERAPIST: How do you feel right now when you see this now?

CLIENT: As if I'm a burden to her ... Sad ...

THERAPIST: Concentrate briefly on that feeling, that sadness, believing that you are a burden to the other person ... Hold on to that feeling but allow the image to fade away ... Is this a familiar feeling for you?

[Client nods.]

THERAPIST: Then concentrate on this feeling and just allow images to emerge from your past, images of situations which, in one way or the other, affect this feeling of being a burden to the other person ... what can you see now?

CLIENT: ... My mother ... In the kitchen and I am just coming in from school ... I want to tell her about my day but she is tired, and she waves me away ...

Historical role-play has three phases:
1. The original event is re-enacted as realistically as possible and the client plays herself as a child (see Box 8.20).
2. Historical role-play featuring role reversals where the client now plays the role of the other person and the therapist interprets the role of the client as a child (see Box 8.21).
3. Trying out new behaviour in a last role-play wherein the client tries out new, schema-breaking behaviour (see Box 8.22).

Therapeutic Letter Writing

Therapeutic letter writing and journaling can be used as a powerful way to develop compassion, empower, motivate, grieve, and assign responsibility [22]. In schema therapy, the therapist may encourage the client to write an unsent letter to caregivers involved in the development of EMS. Typically, the therapist encourages the client to write from their Healthy Adult mode on behalf of their child self. In contrast, the client may also write to various modes that are a part of the conceptualisation. For example, the client may write a letter from their Healthy Adult mode to their Vulnerable Child mode expressing care and compassion, or from their Healthy Adult mode to a coping mode highlighting the lack of future reliance on this mode. The therapist can then ask the client to read aloud the passage in session, enhancing the experiential aspects of the task. The therapist can enhance healthy emotional responses via

---

Box 8.20 Example of Historical Role-Play – Step 1: Re-Enactment of Original Event

THERAPIST: Good, this has evidently been a significant event for you. In order to gain a good understanding of what exactly you have learned there, I want to suggest re-enacting this situation as if it is taking place again. I also want to ask you to play yourself as a young girl and then I'll play your mother. Can you explain to me once more what exactly she is saying in that situation, as well as how she is saying it?

[The client describes her mother's behaviour as specifically and realistically as possible so that the therapist knows how to interpret this role.]

THERAPIST: We are going to re-enact this situation in a moment. So, I would ask you to try to put yourself in the shoes of the girl you were in this situation as best as you can. How old are you?

CLIENT: . . . I don't know . . . Eight years old, maybe?

THERAPIST: Otherwise just close your eyes for a moment . . . And just imagine that girl in this situation . . . Can you see her?

CLIENT: Yes . . . I believe I can . . .

THERAPIST: Could you describe her to me, so that I can see her too?

CLIENT: She's little, she's wearing a dress and has her hair hanging in two pigtails on each side of her head . . . She is standing close to her mother but her mother is busy doing the dishes . . .

THERAPIST: Now just be that little girl, put yourself in her shoes . . . You are now standing next to your mother and she is busy washing dishes . . . When you're ready, open your eyes . . .

[Client opens her eyes and the role-play begins.]

Debriefing. The first question asked about the role-play is whether this situation resembled how the client remembers it. The role-play may have taken a different form than the client remembers and may need to be re-enacted in a slightly revised manner. Afterwards, the meaningful learning experiences related to the self-image and the image of the others are identified and scored on a credibility scale.

Box 8.21 Example of Historical role-play – Step 2: Role Reversals

THERAPIST: Let's re-enact this situation again to make sure that we have a good overview of everything. But I want to suggest that I play the role of you as a child and you therefore play the role of your mother. So, put yourself in your mother's shoes as best you can. What did her life look like back then?

CLIENT: Well . . . she was a housewife, and her husband, my father, was often absent because he worked so hard. I believe my father was experiencing problems at work during that period – the threat of redundancy or something like that . . . So, I think they were worrying about that . . .

THERAPIST: Can you close your eyes for a moment? Now try to picture your mother, as you see her standing in front of you in that situation . . . Just be her, put yourself in her shoes . . . You are married, a housewife, your husband works hard, there are worries about his work . . . When you're ready, you can open your eyes and we will begin . . .

[The client opens her eyes and the situation is re-enacted again.]

Debriefing: During the debriefing, the therapist gives feedback from the role as a child as to how the mother's behaviour came across. The fact that the therapist also experiences being ignored due to the mother's behaviour can help the client reattribute responsibility for their feelings of being neglected away from their own defectiveness and towards the mother's actions. The role reversal can prompt a shift in perspective that can lead to new insights. For example, the client may discover that the father was mainly preoccupied with his own problems and not necessarily judging the client in a negative way. Alternatively, the client may come to the realisation that the behaviour of the mother is more likely to stem from a sense of powerlessness than any intentional criticism of the client. On the other hand, a change in perception may not occur at all. For example, it can happen that, after the second role-play, the client has become even more convinced of the original assumption about the other person. Indeed, an often-seen change is that the client comes to the realisation that the problem did not so much lie with the client as with the other person, whether that was intentional or not.

Box 8.22 Historical role-play – Step 3: Trying out Schema-Breaking Behaviour

This last part of the technique is analogous to the rescripting phase of imagery rescripting. The aim of this phase is to generate a corrective emotional experience. The client can experience what it is like to express his or her opinion, to set a boundary, or to demand respect. Just as is the case with imagination exercises, this experience is not expected to lead directly to a change in behaviour in their present-day life. And, just like imagery exercises, nor is it the aim to change the antagonist, but mainly to stand up for your own basic needs.

THERAPIST: So, we now have a better understanding of how that feeling of 'not mattering' has come about in your life. These situations that we are now re-enacting have contributed to this. At the same time, we have also come to understand more clearly that it is not so much you that is the problem in this but that your mother was not in a position to offer you the time and attention that you needed. In that situation, you had no choice but to withdraw because, after all, you were still only a child. As a child, that was how you had to survive and I am pleased that you were able to. But now you are no longer a child, and you have learned a lot over the years, just like in the therapy sessions with me. If you now look back at that situation with all the knowledge you now have and imagine that you could then go back to that time, knowing everything you know now, what would you want to say to your mother?

CLIENT: . . . Well . . . Simply that she's my mother and that she should just give her child a bit of attention.

THERAPIST: That sounds very good! Once again, as a child you were unable to say that, but as an adult you can . . . Shall we re-enact the situation again, but now you stand up for what you need, tell her what you would like to say? Just so you can experience what it's like to stand up for your own needs?

The situation is then re-enacted, but the client now includes the adult insights and resolutions in the role-play. At that moment when the client stands up for her needs, the therapist will have to decide how the mother would respond in this new situation. In some cases, it is conceivable and credible that the mother would respond in a healthy way and the therapist can play this. In many other situations, however, it is really not plausible that the parent would be able to respond in a healthy manner. The therapist can then choose to briefly interrupt the role-play, explaining that they don't properly understand how the parent would have responded but that they are able to show how they, as a parent, would respond in such a situation. This is how the therapist models a response that is considered good enough from a loved one.

[The client just said to her mother that she finds it unacceptable that she is not paying any attention to her child. She has made that known in a powerful and clear manner.]

THERAPIST: Ok, I just want to stop here for a moment because I honestly don't know how your mother would respond to what you are saying now. So, I am not able to play her properly in this new situation. But I can tell you how I as a parent would respond if you were to say something like that to me. As a father I would say: 'There, there kiddo, it's great that you're telling me this! I'm so happy you told me because the last thing I would want is for you to feel ignored! I'm really happy to hear that you've had a good day.' And then I'd make a cup of tea and sit down to hear all about what you've done today. How does that feel when you hear that?

Debriefing. In the debriefing, the experience of this schema-breaking behaviour is given careful consideration: How did it feel for the client to express their opinion? Where in particular do they feel that in their body? What did they like most about it? This explicit attention to the corrective emotional experience helps with the internalisation of it. The implications of this experience for current situations in the client's life can also be considered: What would it be like to speak up for her own needs more often in present-day situations?

blending the technique with a chairwork technique. For example, the therapist may encourage the client to imagine the caregiver linked to adverse childhood experiences in an empty chair, with the client reading out the written material to the empty chair.

Concluding Remarks

Experiential techniques are essential methods for effecting change in schema therapy. The approaches allow for new, healing, corrective experiences to occur for the client. Furthermore, the client can receive modelling from the therapist on how to understand and meet core emotional needs. Often, emotional techniques are avoided by therapists learning the schema therapy model, typically because they lack confidence in using the interventions and fear making things 'worse'. It is essential for the schema therapist to learn how to use emotion-focused exercises in ways that are helpful and tolerable for the client. Such techniques can result in powerful therapeutic changes for the client and synergs with the other important aspects of treatment (e.g., cognitive, behavioural, limited reparenting).

References

1. Patterson C, Alexander F, French T. Psychoanalytic therapy. *Journal of Social Psychology.* 1948;**28**(1):179.

2. Lang P. Imagery in therapy: An information processing analysis of fear. *Behavior Therapy.* 1977;**8**(5):862–86.

3. Epstein S. *Cognitive-experiential theory: An integrative theory of personality.* Oxford University Press; 2014.

4. Teasdale J. Clinically relevant theory: Integrating clinical insight with cognitive science. In Salkovskis P, ed. *Frontiers of cognitive therapy.* The Guilford Press; 1996. pp. 26–47.

5. Aafjes-van Doorn K, Barber JP. Systematic review of in-session affect experience in cognitive behavioral therapy for depression. *Cognitive Therapy and Research.* 2017;**41**(6):807–28.

6. Young J. *Cognitive therapy for personality disorders: A schema focused approach.* Professional Resource Press; 1999.

7. Simpson S, Arntz A. Core principles of imagery. In: Heath G, Startup H, eds. *Creative methods in schema therapy.* Routledge; 2020. pp. 93–107.

8. Utay J, Miller M. Guided imagery as an effective therapeutic technique: A brief review of its history and efficacy research. *Journal of Instructional Psychology.* 2006;**33**(1):40–43.

9. Najavits L. *Seeking safety: A treatment manual for PTSD and substance abuse.* Guilford Press; 2002

10. Young J, Klosko J, Weishaar M. *Schema therapy: A practitioner's guide.* Guilford Press; 2003.

11. Weertman A, Arntz A. Effectiveness of treatment of childhood memories in cognitive therapy for personality disorders: A controlled study contrasting methods focusing on the present and methods focusing on childhood memories. Behaviour Research and Therapy. 2007;**45**(9):2133–43.

12. De Haan K, Lee C, Fassbinder E, et al. Imagery rescripting and eye movement desensitisation and reprocessing as treatment for adults with post-traumatic stress disorder from childhood trauma: A

randomised clinical trial. *The British Journal of Psychiatry.* 2020;**217**(5):609–15.

13. Louis J, Wood A, Lockwood G. Psychometric validation of the Young Parenting Inventory-Revised (YPI-R2): Replication and extension of a commonly used parenting scale in Schema Therapy (ST) research and practice. *PloS One.* 2018;**13**(11):e0205605.

14. De Jongh A, ten Broeke E, Meijer S. Two method approach: A case conceptualization model in the context of EMDR. *Journal of EMDR Practice and Research.* 2010;**4**(1):12.

15. Arntz A. Imagery rescripting as a therapeutic technique: Review of clinical trials, basic studies, and research agenda. *Journal of Experimental Psychopathology.* 2012;**3**(2):189–208.

16. Farrell J, Reiss N, Shaw I. *The schema therapy clinician's guide: A complete resource for building and delivering individual, group and integrated schema mode treatment programs.* John Wiley & Sons; 2014.

17. Dibbets P, Arntz A. Imagery rescripting: Is incorporation of the most aversive scenes necessary? *Memory.* 2016;**24**(5):683–95.

18. Polster E, Polster M. *Gestalt therapy integrated.* Brunner; 1974.

19. Kellogg S. *Transformational chairwork: Using psychotherapeutic dialogues in clinical practice.* Rowman & Littlefield; 2014.

20. Pugh M. *Cognitive behavioural chairwork: Distinctive features.* Routledge; 2019.

21. Roediger E, Stevens BA, Brockman R. *Contextual schema therapy: An integrative approach to personality disorders, emotional dysregulation, and interpersonal functioning.* New Harbinger Publications; 2018.

22. Pennebaker J, Evans J. *Expressive writing: Words that heal.* Idyll Arbor. Inc, Enumclaw; 2014.

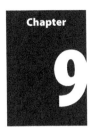

Intervention Strategies for Schema Healing 4
Behavioural Pattern-Breaking Techniques

Introduction

Behavioural pattern-breaking is arguably the most important phase of schema therapy. Whilst some behavioural changes may take place spontaneously alongside positive shifts in cognition and emotion, the last phase of therapy is dedicated to addressing the schema-driven behaviours that contribute to the perpetuation of presenting issues, and which often serve to block the client's capacity to get their needs met in healthy ways. In this chapter, we discuss how schema therapists' attention to client behaviours shifts across the course of treatment, how they prioritise which behaviours to address and which to leave, and how they employ schema therapy interventions to address clients' behaviour at different stages of treatment.

Behaviour Changes During Early Phase of Therapy

In the early stages of therapy, the schema therapist emphasises forming an attuned thera-peutic connection with the client to establish trust and rapport. Often, schema therapists are more tolerant of minor transgressions or therapy-interfering behaviours during this stage, whilst the client becomes accustomed to the therapeutic process. This is especially the case when working with clients with BPD traits as they are expected to have a reduced capacity to understand the boundaries of a healthy relationship and to manage their impulses and coping behaviours at the start of treatment.

Behaviour Change Interventions to Address Therapy-Interfering Behaviours

Although the focus on behavioural pattern-breaking largely takes place during the second half of therapy, it is often necessary to start to incorporate some specific behaviour changes during the earlier phases. Early in therapy, behaviour pattern-breaking may be required to reduce avoidant coping that either blocks attendance or prevents the client from engaging fully in sessions. During this phase, empathic confrontation may also be used to confront other overcompensatory therapy-interfering behaviours. The limited reparenting relation-ship, formed at the beginning of therapy, is then used to leverage and push for behaviour change throughout the subsequent phases. Many therapists wait too long before confront-ing therapy-interfering behaviours, such that these become the established norm, making it increasingly difficult to raise them as problems. This can lead to ruptures in the therapy relationship due to unexpressed resentment on the therapist's part. In the following sections, we discuss several common therapy-interfering issues that might come up in the early phases of treatment that would likely require an initial focus in terms of behaviour change.

1. Maintaining Regular Session Attendance. Behavioural change interventions that may need to take place in the earlier phases of therapy may address issues such as late cancellations and non-attendance of sessions, use of addictive substances that affect the client's engagement in therapy sessions, and other compulsive or avoidant behaviours that might lead to decreased efficacy of the session (e.g., co-rumination). Therapy-interfering behaviours often mirror the kind of problems clients experience in daily life, and thus become a useful initial target in therapy. To adequately address the entrenched schema-driven patterns characteristic of personality disorders and other severe acute psychological difficulties, schema therapy sessions must take place regularly – and ideally, in the initial phases, at least weekly. For those attending both group and individual sessions this can be managed relatively easily. For clients with an Abandonment schema, sessions that are too infrequent or spaced out will lead to ongoing activation of the Abandoned and Angry Child modes, with associated acting out or detached coping behaviours. For those with avoidant personality traits, an infrequent session schedule is likely to reinforce avoidance associated with the Defectiveness, Emotional Deprivation, and Social Isolation schemas, in which the client keeps the therapist at a distance, thereby reducing the opportunity to challenge fears that vulnerability and interpersonal connection will lead to rejection.

2. Maintaining Boundaries Linked to Entitled or Demanding Behaviours. Clients with narcissistic or overcompensatory traits may also benefit from early challenges to therapy-interfering behaviours such as not paying for sessions or acting entitled to the therapist's time (e.g., demanding additional time when they are late for an appointment), acting in a domineering or aggressive manner, or other aggrandising behaviours which prevent them from engaging in experiential therapeutic work. The fee-for-service arrangement that characterises much of our therapy work can trigger issues to do with basic respect and boundaries that may reflect the client's wider problems. Everyday financial transactions can often activate a kind of 'master–slave' expectation from the client that needs addressing early. If you work in a setting that is not fee-for-service, self-aggrandising may manifest more as a devaluing of your time – for example, an attitude of 'it's free anyway, isn't it?'

Box 9.1 provides an example of narcissistic behaviours presenting early in therapy. In this vignette, Fern's behaviour was primarily linked to an Entitlement/Grandiosity schema. She had learned that she came from a family with special status and privileges and that she should not have to follow the same rules as others. Furthermore, she struggled to take responsibility for the effects of her behaviour on others, instead perceiving herself to be the victim of their lack of understanding of her plight. The origins and unmet needs linked to this therapy-interfering behaviour were a lack of limit setting in childhood, whereby she did not have an opportunity to learn the basic principles of reciprocity. These grandiose-entitled behaviours were further modelled and normalised by her narcissistic mother. Consequently, she also developed an Emotional Deprivation schema through consistent emotional neglect and invalidation. She had learned to hide her vulnerability and presented in therapy either in a Self-Aggrandiser or Victim/Self-Pity mode. Unbeknownst to her, these entitled coping behaviours actively sabotaged her relationships outside of therapy, causing others to keep her at a distance and ultimately preventing her from getting her needs for genuine connection and support met. At this early stage of therapy, it was important for the therapist to

Box 9.1 Example of Narcissistic Behaviours Early in Therapy

Fern was a 42-year-old woman with a history of interpersonal difficulties. Her husband was threatening divorce because of her highly critical and demanding interpersonal style. However, during the first sessions she complained that he was unsupportive and inadequate as a partner. She was also on poor terms with her two adult children, but she viewed this as mostly due to their lack of cooperation and attentiveness to her stress levels. Behavioural patterns characteristic of narcissistic traits emerged relatively early in the therapy. She would commit to paying for sessions, then 'forget' to bring her credit card or default on paying and fail to reply to messages about payment after each session. Although she was given the benefit of the doubt on the first couple of occasions, this behaviour continued intermittently. When questioned about this, she protested that her husband was withholding funds, whilst indicating that she expected the fees to be waived, claiming that others (such as her GP) had taken pity on her and recognised her 'special' circumstances. She then began to take phone calls during sessions, on each occasion stating 'This is very important, I have to take this'. These conversations would continue for several minutes, and, on one occasion, even beyond the finishing time for her session.

Self_Aggrandiser_Mode ⋮   **Illustration 9.1** Self-Aggrandiser mode

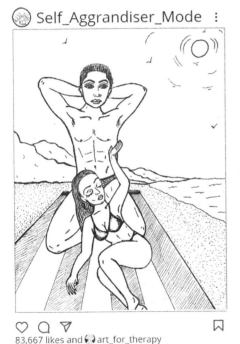

♡ ◯ ▽   🔖
83,667 likes and 🔊 art_for_therapy
Self_Aggrandiser_Mode "Everyday life"
#highsociety #lifestyle #vip #goat #perfection
#billionairesclub #beautifulpeople #famous #$$$

Box 9.2 Example of Empathic Confrontation of Narcissistic Therapy-Interfering Behaviours Early in Therapy

THERAPIST: Fern, I know you are going through a really tough time at the moment and that finances are really tight, and I can see how stressful that must be. I realise as well that this is a source of friction between you and your husband. However, as we are intending to work together, it's really important that we can be really upfront and honest with each other. You probably don't realise it, but when you promise to pay for our sessions but then drop off the radar without following through, it has the effect of making me feel like you don't respect me or the time that we have spent working together in therapy. The therapist part of me understands that of course there are a lot of difficult circumstances that are contributing to this happening, but there is also a part of me that feels slightly irritated about not being paid. Although it might not seem significant to you, I want our time together to be focused on your needs, and so although on the one hand it's no big deal, there is a bigger issue of us respecting each other. I don't want anything to get in the way of us working together, so that is why I am being so upfront with you. It's also important to talk about because if you do this with others, including your friends, then they might not be so understanding and may distance themselves from you. This sort of thing gets in the way of others getting close to you and giving you the care and understanding that you deserve. That's why it's important for me to raise this. Can I check in with you now . . . what did you hear me say?

---

empathically confront this behaviour and encourage her to be respectful of the needs of others. As this was the early stages of therapy, the therapist placed strong emphasis on the empathic aspect of this interaction to ensure that rapport was not unduly affected. The therapist started by empathically confronting the behaviour that interfered most with therapeutic rapport and phrasing the confrontation in a way that helped the client link the behaviour to their own unmet needs (see Box 9.2).

3. Empathically Confront Inconsistent Attendance. If a client consistently misses or cancels sessions at the last minute, this should be empathically confronted. Once we have begun to introduce the modes, we can also use chairwork to facilitate these dialogues (see Box 9.3).

Identifying Other Relevant Therapy-Interfering Behaviours

In the early phase of therapy, the schema therapist works consistently to uncover behavioural patterns which perpetuate the client's schemas. A detailed list of problematic behaviours should be constructed and linked to common triggers described by the client. This, of course, will inform the therapist's conceptualisation of the predominant modes that are responsible for the behaviour. Whereas some of these patterns may become apparent within the therapy room, it is also essential to differentiate the client's narrative of interpersonal interactions from the schema-lens through which they are perceived, and which is potentially distorted. It is essential that the schema therapist asks questions to gain a less biased perspective on the specific behaviours (i.e., as they actually took place). Box 9.4 provides an example of this type of interviewing.

Box 9.3 Empathically Confronting Non-Attendance Through Chair Dialogues

THERAPIST: Trevor, there is a part of me that feels awkward about bringing this up, as the last thing I want to make you feel is uncomfortable, but there is also another part of me that is determined to help you to get your needs met through our work together. So, I need to let you know that when you miss sessions we have planned, it makes me worry about what's going on with you. Does that surprise you at all? Do you remember that we discussed the idea that we all have different 'parts'? I wonder, could it be that the same Avoidant Protector part that stops you going to work sometimes, and other events that you have been invited to, also stops you from coming to therapy sometimes? I wonder if we could put that part in the chair, so I can understand what that side is afraid will happen on those times that it persuades you to avoid? . . . . Trevor's Protector, I know that you have helped Trevor to survive by keeping a low profile when he was a little boy. You helped him back then, but I wonder what you are afraid might happen on those days that you get him to skip therapy sessions?

TREVOR: *[in Protector chair]* 'By keeping him at home, I stop him feeling hopeless. Nothing will ever feel better. It's better just to hide away, that way you won't be disappointed.'

THERAPIST: *[speaking to empty Protector chair]* Protector, I can see you are working hard to stop Trevor from feeling disappointed, but at the same time I worry that if he doesn't come here, he will end up feeling even more hopeless, because we can't work together and make changes. I know that in the past things were different, and this might have been the best way to protect him. You learned to protect him by keeping him out of his parents' way so that they wouldn't criticise him. But now it's different; I am here and I want to help him learn healthier ways of coping. So, it's important that you don't hold him back, otherwise, you'll end up having the opposite effect to your intention: instead of protecting him, your avoidance will make it harder for him to have a better life. I wonder if you could let go a little bit, and test out what it might be like to come to all of our sessions, and allow Trevor to tell me if he is feeling afraid or hopeless, instead of avoiding?

THERAPIST: *[speaking to Trevor in the Vulnerable Child chair]* I know this is scary, but it's not like it was back then, you can count on me to be here to support you. I want to hear about how you feel.

Unpacking the exact details of the interaction gives the therapist a more accurate understanding of how their schemas increase the client's sensitivity to specific interpersonal triggers, and an opportunity to observe how clients' coping behaviours perpetuate their difficulties, preventing them from getting their needs met. From the vignette in Box 9.4, Mary's Mistrust/Abuse schema developed during childhood as a consequence of parents and other family members taking advantage of her and lying to her. Her father was emotionally and sexually inappropriate and reacted aggressively if she tried to protect her privacy. He behaved as if she were his 'property'. She learned to be suspicious of others' behaviours and wary of their hidden agendas. Mary had recently moved into a property and hadn't checked the deeds in sufficient detail to know that her neighbours rightfully had access to the woodshed. When she saw them approaching, she automatically assumed the worst: that they were intruding on her property and taking advantage of her. Her

Box 9.4 Clinical Example of Schema-Perpetuating Problematic Interpersonal
Behaviour

Mary attended the session complaining that her neighbours were rude to her. She described an incident whereby a neighbour had come to collect wood from their woodpile alongside her house, and she had become angry with him for intruding on her property. The therapist asked a series of questions to uncover the way in which this interaction had unfolded:

MARY: My neighbour was so rude, I can't believe this sort of thing always happens to me. People just have no respect!

THERAPIST: Mary, I'm really curious, can you think back to how the argument started?

MARY: Just like I told you, my neighbour came down and started taking wood from the pile.

THERAPIST: Okay, and what exactly did you say? What were your exact words? And what was your tone?

MARY: What does it matter, I am telling you what happened, can't you just take my word for it? He was rude, and I just had to put him in his place.

THERAPIST: Of course, I can see it's frustrating to go through it all again, but it's really crucial for us to understand this in detail. How did you 'put him in his place'? Can you replay it for me in the exact words and tone?

MARY: I told him . . . 'Back off, what do you think you're doing?! How dare you come down here. You're invading my privacy!'

THERAPIST: What were you feeling at that point?

MARY: Annoyed! How dare he just barge in like that!

THERAPIST: How did he reply? What did he say?

MARY: He told me that the wood pile is on his property, and it's his right to access it.

THERAPIST: What do you think he was feeling? . . .. What happened next?

accusatory tone is also likely to have increased the probability of some kind of retaliation or counter-response, thereby reinforcing her perspective that they were 'not nice people'. Ultimately, this schema-driven behaviour is likely to have resulted in her neighbours keeping their distance from her, thereby removing future opportunities for neighbourly connection and support.

Where feasible, the therapist should also consult with significant others in the client's life to gather details of behaviours that may create interpersonal difficulties (and thereby perpetuate the underlying schemas). Difficulties are especially likely to arise when clients exhibit overcompensatory coping behaviours. Significant others should be asked to provide detailed examples of how coping modes play out in interpersonal situations. This will enable the therapist to identify which EMS are repeatedly being triggered within the client's relationships. Again, the therapist should ask specific questions to find out the exact details of what the client said and how they behaved in specific situations. Speaking with significant others may also reveal discrepancies between the client's account of events and others' perspectives, thereby highlighting the schemas that may be influential on both sides.

Schema inventories can provide a useful mechanism for identifying behaviours that cause difficulties in the client's relationships. The Young Schema Questionnaire is useful for identifying behaviours in clients who are surrendering to their schemas (i.e., where high scores indicate that the client is aware of their EMS, and believes their cognitive content is true). However, other questionnaires are likely to be more useful in identifying overcompensatory or avoidant coping behaviours: the Young-Rygh Avoidance Inventory [1], the Young Compensatory Inventory [2], and the Schema Coping Inventory [3].

The Importance of Understanding Therapist Schemas when Pushing for Change

To provide an attuned reparenting response when clients are faced with making difficult behavioural changes, schema therapists must maintain a parallel awareness of both the schemas and unmet needs of their clients, alongside their own schemas and needs. In the case of Mary (in Box 9.4), if the therapist had a Subjugation schema, they might avoid exploring this scenario in sufficient detail due to a fear of conflict and being faced with the client's Angry Protector mode. If the therapist had an Abandonment schema, they might be fearful that if they empathically confronted the client, the client would leave. Or, if the therapist had an Unrelenting Standards schema, they might push the client too much, prioritising their own urge to strive for achievement over the client's needs. In each scenario, the therapist's lack of awareness of their own schemas has the potential to prevent them from ensuring that the client's needs are met. This demonstrates the importance of therapists maintaining an ongoing awareness of their own schema-driven coping responses, especially when they block capacity to meet their clients' needs. Box 9.5 presents an example of a self-reflection exercise for therapists.

Box 9.5 Therapist Self-Reflection Exercise

Identify a situation in which you feel triggered by a client's behaviour in session that is linked to your own schemas. For example, are you fearful that the client will become angry if you push for change (due to a Subjugation schema)? Are you fearful that the client will leave therapy if you challenge their schema-driven behaviour (Abandonment, Defectiveness schemas)? Are you pushing the client too hard (Unrelenting Standards schema)? Are you overidentifying with client's schemas and not providing sufficient encouragement and empathic confrontation to motivate change?

Notice which of your behaviours may be activating or clashing with the client's schemas.

What are the client's underlying needs, and how can you work with them in a direct way to meet these?

What are the limited reparenting messages that they need to hear from you that they didn't get when they were growing up, to support them in making behavioural changes?

For example:

- I believe in you, you can do this! (Failure)
- I am here for you, I'm not going anywhere (Abandonment)
- It's going to be okay, you're safe now (Vulnerability to Harm)
- You are so much more capable than you know. I really value your ideas, and I can see that you have what it takes to do this! (Dependence)

As the therapist, what do you need in this situation? What does your little side need from you? What will you do to meet that need?

More detailed information about therapist schemas, and the role of self-reflection for the schema therapist, are discussed in Chapter 18: Schema Therapy for the Schema Therapist.

Middle Phase of Therapy: Breaking Patterns of Life-Interfering Schema-Driven Behaviour

Once the client has entered the middle stage of therapy, there will be a strong emphasis on experiential, interpersonal, and cognitive change work, which represents a lot of the 'healing work' in schema therapy. Once the client can: (1) understand the childhood origins of their schemas and modes; (2) recognise and label them when triggered; and (3) engage in schema dialogues, the schema therapist starts to prompt the client to transition into taking on the Healthy Adult role, whilst learning coping mechanisms which are more aligned with their values and getting their needs met. When the client has begun to demonstrate a capacity to protect and nurture themselves within imagery rescripting and chairwork exercises, this will indicate a readiness to start behavioural pattern-breaking.

The first behavioural pattern-breaking target midway through therapy is for clients to try out small behaviour adjustments without prematurely resorting to major life changes that they may later regret (such as leaving a marriage or a job). When clients report a sudden unexplained improvement, the therapist should be alert to the possibility that this may be a manifestation of an avoidant or overcompensatory coping mode, masquerading as Healthy Adult mode. If the client expresses a desire to embark on a significant change, the therapist should investigate this thoroughly with the client through evaluating the pros and cons of taking an 'act-now' versus 'wait-and-see' approach. The schema therapist provides guidance in making healthy choices and taking manageable steps (and discourages impulsive decisions that may lead to regret). The client is encouraged to make incremental changes within their current circumstances and relationships to see whether these can transform their circumstances sufficiently to allow them to get their emotional needs met. For example, in a poor relationship that the client has been considering leaving, the therapist might first assist the client to attempt to address some of the specific sources of dissatisfaction (e.g., lack of intimacy), before considering more permanent solutions (e.g., divorce). For significant life decisions, in the first instance the client is coached to manage difficult aspects of these situations before making decisions about leaving (except in situations involving abuse). Although it may appear that the other person is solely the problem, the client must learn how to overcome their own schemas, to connect with their vulnerability and express their emotional needs more directly, before reaching any decisions about ending a relationship. Furthermore, clients will need help to prepare in advance of any significant changes, such as through learning to regulate emotions, endure discomfort, and manage practical and/or unexpected difficulties.

There are two key things that characterise a schema therapy approach to behaviour change. The first is that we scaffold everything. Schema therapists are patient; the client can make as much change as they like, so long as they are supported to make such changes incrementally. We often use the term 'slicing it thin'. This makes the change process less overwhelming (and risky) for the client, as the impact of changes can be analysed and understood over time. Second, in schema therapy, behavioural pattern-breaking is thought to be most powerful when it is done in the service of a client's needs. Any proposed behaviour change should be explicitly linked to the client's stated needs in a situation. Behavioural pattern-breaking tasks are not undertaken to achieve habituation or 'exposure', as may be done in traditional CBT, but are designed to connect the client with their stated needs and evaluated on the extent to which this occurs. This helps to optimise client motivation for change.

Box 9.6 provides the case example of Fern again, illustrating problematic behavioural patterns that occur both inside and outside therapy sessions. The therapist's observations of

---

Box 9.6 Clinical Example: Problematic Behavioural Patterns Inside and Outside the Session

Fern attended therapy complaining that her husband was insensitive to her needs, describing him as an 'emotional dolt'. She and her husband had lived together as a married couple for more than twenty years and had three grown-up children together. She was on the verge of leaving him, having concluded that he would never be able to meet her needs, and that he had never really understood her or supported her in the way she wanted. She described a recent incident as evidence that he was the problem. In this situation, she was adamant that she had told him how she had felt, had shown her vulnerability, but he had not been supportive of her in any way. When asked about the words and tone that she used to communicate her vulnerability, it turned out that she believed that because she felt hurt and upset, he should be able to recognise this and provide the support she craved. However, it became apparent when she repeated what she had said that her tone had been angry and accusatory, making it almost impossible for anyone to detect her vulnerability or to ascertain what she needed in that moment. Although she felt that her needs should have been blatantly clear to her husband, in reality her overcompensatory coping mode manifested as defensive and passively angry, making it difficult for him to hear her plea for support or sense her underlying need for connection.

The therapist's understanding of this dynamic was also informed by Fern's schema-driven behaviours in therapy sessions. When asked how she was feeling, she rarely, if ever, used emotional labels to describe her inner experience, instead relying on lengthy, intellectual descriptions of her state of mind. She repeatedly stated that the therapist should come up with 'solutions' to her problems, but insisted that the therapeutic model did not really resonate for her and that the experiential techniques were not relevant to her difficulties. In the countertransference, the therapist sensed that whatever she did and however much she strived to meet Fern's emotional needs, it would never feel enough – and that Fern would remain dissatisfied and misunderstood.

Fern's behaviour within sessions and her exploration of countertransference reactions enabled her to begin to conceptualise the relationship dynamics between Fern and her husband. It became clear that it was important to address overcompensatory behavioural patterns in therapy by encouraging Fern to learn to express her vulnerability more explicitly before she would be able to make a clear decision as to whether she should stay in the relationship or end it. In the sessions ahead, the therapist began to gently and empathically confront Fern. By the middle phase of therapy, the therapist was more insistent that these changes would be essential to enable Fern to overcome her longstanding pattern of not getting her needs met. Chairwork was used to encourage Fern to dialogue with her overcompensatory mode and learn about the unmet needs underlying this way of coping. As she learned to take risks and express her vulnerability more often in sessions, she was encouraged to practise the same at home with her husband, keeping a detailed diary of how these dialogues unfolded and her own emotional and behavioural reactions. As Fern learned to communicate more openly with her husband, she discovered a new side to her relationship, as well as the possibility of getting her needs met. She was surprised to find that there was a side to her that was unfamiliar and uncomfortable with getting her needs met and the newfound intimacy that ensued from this. It was at this point that she made the decision to commit to working on her relationship further rather than leave. Therapy then shifted focus to helping Fern to build skills for dealing with conflicts and relationship blocks in the future, and especially for maintaining openness and vulnerability in times of stress and during moments of schema activation.

Box 9.7 presents recommended steps in the development of targets for behavioural pattern-breaking.

Box 9.7 Steps in Developing Targets for Behavioural Pattern-Breaking

1. Collaboratively develop a list of behavioural targets based on the client's common triggers and coping mode patterns.
2. Prioritise behaviours based on the client's primary presenting problems – the ones that will impact on their capacity to get their emotional needs met in relationships.
3. Explain that behaviours will be targeted one-at-a-time, rather than focusing on the entire schema-driven pattern all at once.
4. Start by assisting the client to identify one behaviour to change. Choose the most problematic behaviour, with the highest impact on emotional well-being and both personal and work functioning.
5. If client feels unable to tackle the highest-priority behaviour, identify the behavioural target highest on the list that they can manageably address.
6. After establishing the first target behaviour, use motivational strategies to stimulate change.

   a. Clarify the link between the target behaviour and childhood experiences and unmet needs to increase self-understanding and the capacity to relinquish attachment to this coping mechanism in the here and now.
   b. Link behaviour to previous experiential and cognitive work that has been carried out in therapy.
   c. List pros and cons of coping behaviour, with a focus on capacity to reach life goals and find emotional well-being.

7. If the client feels the current behavioural goal is too overwhelming, break it into smaller more manageable steps.
8. If the client still feels too overwhelmed to address changes related to the main presenting issue, switch to another presenting problem, and then return later to re-target the original behavioural patterns linked to the primary problem.
9. Client and therapist write a detailed plan of a behavioural homework task, based on a comprehensive list of tangible steps. The client is encouraged to complete the homework, using the flashcard as support, and to record the outcome, including thoughts, feelings, and reactions of others.
10. The therapist prioritises enquiry about homework at the start of the following session, and provides praise and reinforcement for progress, and support and encouragement in the face of failure.
11. Therapist and client work together to adjust the behaviour plan (e.g., break task down into smaller steps, change incentives) to facilitate progress.
12. Develop awareness of blocks, then challenge schemas and modes creating the block.
13. Develop flashcards to address blocks.

Therapist Tip: This process can be aided by use of the pattern-breaking forms, as seen in Figures 9.1 and 9.2

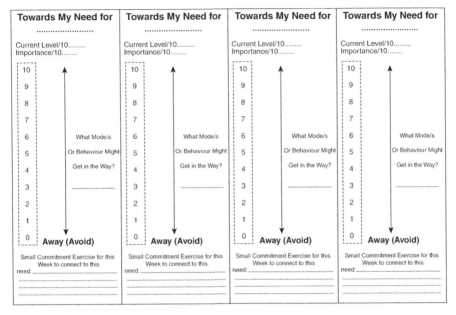

Figure 9.1 Blank pattern-breaking form

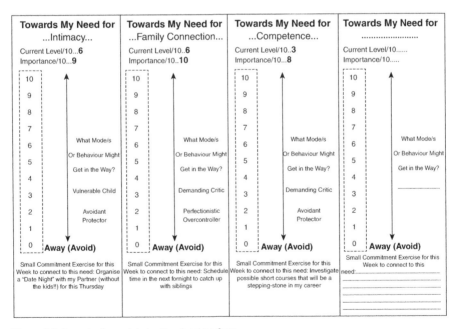

Figure 9.2 Example of completed pattern-breaking form

Identifying Schema-Driven Behaviours That Cause Problems and Impede Goals: Linking Behaviours to Childhood Unmet Needs, Schemas, and Modes

To structure the behavioural pattern-breaking work, therapists can make a list of all of the behaviours that the client recognises are self-sabotaging, behaviours that are reported as problematic by significant others, and any remaining therapy-interfering behaviours. Before working on actually changing behaviour, the next step is to conceptualise the relationship between each behaviour and its underlying schemas (and modes) and explore how the behaviour was learned during early experiences in the client's life. For example, a client with an Emotional Deprivation schema may be emotionally avoidant, use humour to avoid showing their vulnerability, and ask for their emotional needs to be met in direct ways. Alternatively, they might actively engage in self-sacrificing behaviour (Compliant Surrenderer mode) as a means of trying to show others what they need or exert a sense of obligation on others to meet their needs, whilst avoiding expressing their needs directly. A client with a Defectiveness schema might cope via overcompensation, by finding subtle ways of putting the therapist down or giving the impression that the therapist is taking up his valuable time. Box 9.8 presents a case example (Mario) demonstrating the role of schemas and modes in influencing coping behaviours that arise in therapy.

In the case presented in Box 9.8, the therapist works alongside the client to explore the ways in which their behaviour can be made sense of within the context of their childhood experiences, schemas, and modes. This can open a discussion of the role of schema-perpetuating behaviours, including distorted thinking patterns that exaggerate information that is consistent with schemas, whilst minimising other information that is inconsistent. The therapist and client can then explore ways in which these behaviours prevent the person from getting their emotional needs met, such as through distancing or alienating others. This would lead to a clear plan for incremental behaviour change, to be set via homework.

Box 9.8 Case Example: Addressing Schemas and Modes Influencing Client Coping Behaviours in Session

Mario grew up in a rural environment and his parents were farmers. His father had missed out on opportunities to achieve his full potential due to poverty. He therefore expected Mario to be achieving at all times, either by helping on the farm or carrying out his schoolwork to perfectionistic standards. Mario was expected to use every hour of the day in a productive manner. Mario's father was highly authoritarian, setting strict rules that Mario and his siblings were expected to follow without question. He would often become angry or use guilt-inducing statements to ensure Mario's compliance. Mario's mother was caring, but passively compliant, and focused on serving her husband and managing the domestic aspects of farm life to her husband's high standards. Mario's primary schemas were Emotional Deprivation, Unrelenting Standards, Emotional Inhibition, and Subjugation.

Mario repeatedly turned up late for therapy sessions from approximately session 12 onwards. Up until this point, Mario had attended promptly and had been highly compliant with the therapeutic process. Although he was outwardly compliant, the therapist began to notice some passive resistance to his suggestions. Homework was completed intermittently, and whenever he gently questioned Mario about this, he noticed that Mario reacted in a defensive and irritated manner. The therapist began to suspect that a transference reaction was taking place, whereby his therapeutic requests were activating Mario's Subjugation schema and a behavioural coping pattern characterised by passive resistance, just as he had done with his father. In the following dialogue, the therapist starts by making tentative links to help Mario to make sense of his own behaviour. He then works with the client to identify other situations which trigger this behaviour and discusses tentative steps towards learning healthier ways of expressing the underlying needs.

THERAPIST: Mario, I have noticed that in recent times you have been late for many of our sessions. I know that you have a lot on your plate, and there are practical reasons that make it tricky for you to fit everything in. But you know me . . . as your therapist I can't help but wonder about the role of your schemas and modes, and how they might be impacting on you. One of the aspects of your childhood that appears to have made a big impact on you was your father's controlling parenting style. You have told me about his demanding standards and many rules, leaving not much space for you to have any autonomy or freedom over your own life. His high expectations were attached to almost everything you did, and as a result you learned to subjugate to avoid him getting angry with you. It's not uncommon that if we subjugate our own needs, the Angry Child side simmers away under the surface, feeling annoyed that he has lost his freedom. Sometimes this angry side might try to regain his freedom in small ways, such as by breaking rules or rebelling against others' demands, often without the person even being consciously aware of it. This mode has learned to go underground for fear of being crushed or punished. I wonder, could it be that this [Angry Child] freedom-fighter side of you comes to the surface when I tell you that our session starts at a particular time . . . almost like in that moment this side perceives that I am just like dad?'

MARIO: Maybe . . . I don't really think about it that way. All I know is that you set the time of the sessions, and here I am, late again.

THERAPIST: When I set the time of our sessions, does it feel like you don't have a say in it, that you are not allowed to have a voice? Could you possibly close your eyes and notice what feelings come up for you? Where those feelings arise in your body?

MARIO: In my throat and chest . . . a tension. It's a feeling that I often get, I don't know why . . .

THERAPIST: Throughout your childhood, you didn't have enough opportunities to get your needs for control and autonomy met. You were punished and made to feel guilty for speaking out, for asking for what you needed. As a result, you have learned to disown this part of you that has the power to voice what you want and what you need. I would very much like to see more of that part. It's not like it was when you grew up; I want to see this freedom-fighter part of you. And although there might not be much scope to change the time of our sessions, I wonder if there are other aspects of our time together where you could take more control and be more assertive . . . how would that feel . . . to practise getting those needs met?

I also wonder if you might consider noticing when this feeling comes up in your day-to-day life, and seeing if you can figure out what you really want or need in those moments . . . just notice the times when that Angry Child part inside feels frustrated and digs his heels in because his needs have been overlooked in some way? Would that be useful to you?

Behaviour Change Targets for Pattern-Breaking

Whereas the earlier phase of therapy might focus on behaviours within the therapeutic relationship, towards the latter end of the middle phase of therapy behavioural pattern-breaking focuses on behaviours that interfere with the client's capacity to get their needs met in their daily life. A behavioural hierarchy can be generated collaboratively by therapist and client, based on common triggers and coping mode patterns. Traditionally in schema therapy, this kind of real-life behaviour change is often reserved for the middle to later stages of therapy when the client has a severe disorder (e.g., a personality disorder), but in practice, with less complex clients or clients with a capacity for early change, this can be brought forward to achieve some early success. Behaviour patterns to change can then be prioritised according to their current impact on the client's life, especially on interpersonal relationships. The first step is to choose the highest-priority target on the hierarchy that the client can realistically manage. The aim of starting with high-impact behaviours is to increase the probability that the client will experience a positive change in their life as soon as possible. Motivation for addressing behavioural patterns can be enhanced through revisiting the origins of this behaviour as a survival mechanism linked to coping with unmet needs during childhood. This linking can enhance the client's capacity for self-empathy; it reminds them that this coping behaviour emerged in the context of having limited options during their early years. Furthermore, revisiting the pros and cons of the behaviour in the present can highlight potential advantages of change and bolster motivation to invest in the effort required to make changes. The general strategy at this stage is for the therapist to remain focused on prompting new behavioural patterns whilst addressing interfering modes as they arise. Box 9.9 illustrates how behaviour change targets might be selected by the client and therapist together.

Box 9.9 Clinical Example of Setting Behavioural Pattern-Breaking Goals

Fern's overeating behaviours were linked to her Abandonment and Defectiveness schemas. During early childhood, her mother repeatedly told her that she was 'too much' and a burden. She frequently left the family home, announcing that she was sick of Fern and would not be coming back. In the absence of a consistent nurturing relationship, Fern learned to rely on food as a form of self-soothing, and to escape feelings of fear and shame linked to rejection and abandonment. Behavioural change work started with reminding her of these links and the work that had already been carried out in therapy to address these schemas. Her first behavioural goal, decided in collaboration, included two key steps: (1) to express her vulnerability and emotional needs with trusted friends (2) to reduce her pattern of turning to her overeating (Detached Self-Soother mode) as a way of tuning out her emotions.

With the help of her therapist, she explored the pros and cons of coping through overeating. Advantages of this coping behaviour listed by Fern included having a reliable and dependable source of comfort, an opportunity to indulge in tasty foods, reduced risk of rejection, a feeling of euphoria, escape from difficult feelings, an excuse to avoid social interactions, and that it 'gives a reason for why I don't see my friends'. The cons were 'I eat so fast that I don't get to experience the pleasure of food', 'I am gaining weight and losing fitness', 'I have lots of health problems', 'my clothes no longer fit me', 'I feel sluggish and lacking in energy', and 'I feel worse about myself'. By reflecting on this list, Fern was able to recognise that most of her pros were linked to short-term avoidance and relief, whereas the cons were linked to ongoing perpetuation of her difficulties and loneliness. This was followed by the development of an audio flashcard in her own Healthy Adult voice, which provided an additional source of motivation that she could tap into in the context of changing her behaviours.

In order to ensure that her expectations were realistic and to reduce the likelihood of giving up, Fern was warned that it is very common to encounter some initial discomfort, 'withdrawal effects', and awkwardness throughout the adjustment period associated with changing entrenched behaviours. Behaviours with an addictive quality can be particularly difficult to address due to the fact that they tend to be highly compulsive, habit-driven, and provide more intense and immediate reinforcement. As such, Fern was encouraged to write a detailed plan describing concrete steps needed to fulfil her homework task, including contingency management steps that would increase motivation and the likelihood of success. She decided that the first step that she would take in breaking this pattern was to reduce overeating through introducing three regular meals, and two snacks, each with a distinct start and end point. The only change that was introduced at this point was the time of eating; to avoid overwhelm, the quantity and content of food was not addressed. Fern believed that focusing on avoiding a negative consequence would provide more motivation than generating a reward for limiting her overeating. She therefore decided that she would look at a picture of the effects of diabetes (something her doctor had cautioned her about) for fifteen minutes for each day that she did not stick to the mealtimes. Furthermore, she decided to reward herself with her favourite coffee only on the days that she was able to meet her goal. In the following weeks, she went on to address further aspects of this pattern, through gradually introducing 'forbidden' foods into her mealtimes whilst adhering to her new meal structure. Naturally, this process was not straightforward and involved numerous setbacks, which provided an opportunity for problem solving and finding solutions that met her needs. Fern was then encouraged to work on the second aspect of her behavioural pattern, which was associated with her longstanding avoidance of seeking support and directly expressing her vulnerability and needs with others. Both aspects of this pattern (the overeating and the interpersonal contact) were equally important and required multiple steps to accomplish, with opportunities for troubleshooting in the face of setbacks.

These kinds of tasks are set as realistic and collaborative homework tasks. It is common for clients to come back to therapy sessions after setting pattern-breaking tasks having struggled to complete them in some way. In schema therapy, this is an opportunity to work on the 'blocks to change' within the session (see Box 9.10).

Fine Tuning the Case Conceptualisation Through the Pattern-Breaking Process over Time

Exploring behavioural coping mechanisms at this stage provides additional information that allows the therapist to fine-tune the case conceptualisation. In turn, the case conceptualisation provides a roadmap that enables the therapist to carry out behavioural pattern-breaking in an attuned way. For example, many clients have not experienced sufficient guidance or direction and will not be capable of generating Healthy Adult alternative courses of action on their own. A client with a Self-Sacrifice schema who was always given the message that her needs were secondary to everyone else's will benefit from a direct message from the therapist that gives permission for them to focus on their own needs: 'You are allowed to have your own job, and to take time for yourself

---

Box 9.10 Addressing Blocks in Behavioural Change Work

Investigate 'stuck points' that prevented the client from completing the behavioural home-work task [4].

a. Is the client aware of the reasons for their lack of progress?
b. If not, explore the reasons:

    i.   Did new impediments arise when the client tried to make changes?

    ii. Does the client fear the repercussions of change? (Vulnerable Child).

    iii. Is the client angry that they need to work so hard to bring about change? (Angry Child).

    iv. Is the client struggling to manage the discomfort and persistence required to bring about change? (Undisciplined Child).

    v. Is the client feeling hopeless about the possibility of change? Or fearful of trying and facing the disappointment of failing? (Vulnerable Child; Hopeless Resigned coping mode).

2. If the block is still elusive, use imagery to take the client through the behavioural change step by step, to identify the point at which they become stuck.

3. Set up a mode dialogue (chairwork or imagery, empathic confrontation) between the stuck side and the Healthy Adult side to work through the block.

4. Develop a flashcard to manage the block through challenging maladaptive schemas and coping modes, including information from the pros and cons exercise, and skills for managing difficult moments.

5. Fine-tune contingencies whereby the client rewards themselves for progress as part of the homework task.

6. Client re-attempts behavioural change for homework.

7. If the client continues to incur difficulties, consider breaking the task into smaller steps and re-attempting for homework.

8. If the client continues to be unable to manage homework, refocus on a different behavioural pattern for a period of time, before returning to the original behaviour.

9. Use empathic confrontation to push for behavioural changes and emphasise the importance of breaking patterns in the context of client's long-term goals.

In highly resistant cases: Following a lengthy period wherein the client is unable to make any changes, suggest a provisional break in therapy, making it clear that the therapist is ready and willing to recommence sessions when the client is able to proceed with the behavioural change work. Life circumstances may need to change for the client to reach a point where the cons outweigh the pros of the coping behaviours.

---

apart from your family ... this is healthy, and something that everyone needs.' A client with a Failure schema who has never received sufficient encouragement and praise is likely to benefit from the therapist providing these unmet needs in a direct way: 'I know that your schema is telling you something different, but I really believe in you. I know you are smart and capable. I've seen this in our work together. You can do this!' It is essential that these messages are expressed with gusto, with the therapist in the position of cheerleader, just as we would when parenting our own child or supporting a good friend. Emotional authenticity is key; we want the client to really feel that the message stems from an experiential connection, rather than simply being a rational response. Furthermore, the therapist must also take into account the client's fears associated with behaviour change and ensure that these are incorporated into the preparatory planning. For example, a client with a Subjugation schema may fear that if they are assertive and ask for what they need, others will become angry and reject or abandon them. A client with an Unrelenting Standards schema may fear making mistakes, performing at less than 100%, or being criticised by peers. A client with an Abandonment schema may fear that if they stop clinging, others will leave and they will be left all alone. A client with a Grandiosity schema may fear that if they give up striving for status, others will judge them as mediocre or 'nothing'.

In the example in Box 9.11, Mario and the therapist agreed to use imagery rescripting to work with his Subjugation schema, whilst encouraging him to be more assertive about his needs and to take more control of other aspects of the therapy process.

Box 9.11 Clinical Example of Chairwork to Address Therapy-Interfering Behaviour (Non-Attendance)

THERAPIST: Mario, I'm really curious about the side that is blocking you from coming on time . . . could we get to know that part a bit better to find out what is making it difficult for it to come along? I know that, from what you have told me, this side also affects your work attendance, so it might help us both to understand what is happening a bit better if we do some detective work together and give this side a voice. Would you be okay with that?

MARIO: Ok, it seems a bit strange.

THERAPIST: Yes, it can seem that way at first, but using the chairs can help us to understand more easily what is happening under the surface . . . So, can you sit on that empty chair, and really embody that side of you that slows things down before you come to our sessions. Really try to get into the head and body space of that side. What is it saying?

MARIO: [long pause] . . . There's really no point. It's hopeless . . . I'll just mess it up anyway. I'll fail.

THERAPIST: If I understand correctly, it sounds like there are two parts coming up . . . one part is the part that feels hopeless and downhearted, and another part that is telling you that you will fail. Am I getting that right? So, this side of you would be the child part, that holds the emotions and feelings.

MARIO: I guess so.

THERAPIST: [introducing an extra empty chair] Can you now move to the chair of the critical side, that is telling Little Mario that he will fail? What does he say?

MARIO: [moves to chair] 'You will fail at this just like you do with everything. Face the facts, you are a loser. Why you even bother to go to therapy, I don't know. It will come to nothing, just like everything that you attempt.'

THERAPIST: Ok, Mario can you please move back to Little Mario's chair, so that I can talk to that critical chair? What does it feel like to hear that message?

MARIO: It feels normal . . . hopeless, like nothing will ever be possible. It makes me feel like giving up. And ashamed of myself.

THERAPIST: *[therapist shifts to a stronger tone of voice]* Critical side, it's not okay that you treat Mario this way. It's too much. It's over the top. You are the one who is sabotaging his progress when you treat him in this mean way. How do you expect him to feel motivated, when you are dragging him down? You are from the past, but you are still interfering too in his life. This has to stop. I won't allow you to hold him back in this way! *[Therapist re-directs attention to Mario in 'Little Mario' chair.]* Mario, you have been working so hard, and I want you to know that I believe in you. I see that you are capable of doing this work. I really mean it . . . you can do it! I will be right by your side. To set limits on that Critic that is stuck in the past, and to remind you that change is possible, that you don't always have to feel this way . . . that what you learned as a child was wrong. You are capable of so much more than you know . . . what is it like to hear me say that?

MARIO: It feels good . . . its always felt this way, I've never believed in myself. But your words felt different . . . it touched me somehow.

THERAPIST: We will be doing more of this work, to change the old messages in your head. And to strengthen your healthy side so that you can give your little side the encouragement that he missed out on in the past. Could you move over here to stand behind the Healthy Chair for a moment. Is there anything you would like to say to your little side from this part? This is the part of you that sticks up for justice. The compassionate, strong part. What do you want to say?

MARIO: *[softly]* 'You can do this.'

THERAPIST: Can you say it 10% louder? Can you show him you mean it?

MARIO: *[louder]* 'You can do this!'

THERAPIST: Excellent. And we will be working together to help this part of you to grow stronger and to help you to get more of the things you need. Shall we make an audio flashcard together to help you to connect with your health voice and to set limits on the Critic to use before our sessions?

A flashcard was generated to help him to access his Healthy Adult mode when his Subjugation pattern was triggered, and he was encouraged to use the flashcard before sessions. Mario promised to work on coming to sessions on time and agreed that this topic would be re-visited in future sessions. However, after five further sessions, the same pattern re-emerged and Mario felt unable to find an explanation. In order to investigate further, the therapist invited 'the part that is blocking you from attending sessions on time' to sit in an empty chair.

Final Phase of Therapy

In the final phase of therapy, behavioural pattern-breaking increases, with a strong emphasis on working through the hierarchy of behaviours that affect their daily functioning outside of therapy. Most schema-driven behaviours are highly entrenched and, although they cause distress, they provide familiarity, a sense of coherence in the client's world. Giving them up can feel frightening and disorienting. We warn the client that schemas 'fight for their own survival' and will try to convince the client to continue their familiar schema-perpetuating behaviours. When blocks are encountered, the therapist helps the client to identify which schemas and modes are involved, and to work through these therapeutically and make continued attempts to change the pattern.

The specific patterns addressed in the behavioural change phase must be driven by the client's case conceptualisation. A list of general behavioural targets linked to common modes is presented in Table 9.1.

The Use of Future Pattern-Breaking Imagery and Chair Dialogues to Support Behaviour Change

Future pattern-breaking imagery is, in a sense, the opposite of imagery rescripting. Rather than rescript childhood and other painful memories of the past, future pattern-breaking imagery connects the client to images of problematic or avoided scenarios, usually represented on the client's behaviour change hierarchy. This kind of imagery becomes a useful experiential technique especially in the later phases of treatment as the therapist pushes the client for concrete change. The aim is to be able to help the client experientially process and rehearse new, more adaptive patterns of behaviour that have been identified for behaviour change. This allows clients – with the help of the therapist – to become aware of, work through, and ultimately anticipate problematic schema-based reactions to support behaviour change. Generally, if the client is not able to carry out behaviour change in imagination (or through other methods such as chair dialogues), their chances of doing so in the real-life situation change are significantly reduced. However, to the degree that clients can participate assertively and adopt a Healthy Adult perspective in the imagery, they are better prepared to make changes in their daily lives. It should be noted that the dialogues can also often be processed similarly using chairs (e.g., having an assertive conversation with a parent). The basic steps for the implementation of pattern-breaking imagery are given in Box 9.12 [5]. You will notice that they basically describe the process of imagery rescripting, but in reverse, applied to future scenarios.

Concluding Remarks

Behavioural pattern-breaking is arguably the most important phase of schema therapy. Although some degree of behavioural pattern-breaking occurs throughout the therapeutic process, the most significant changes occur primarily in the middle and final phases of therapy. Empathic confrontation is used to gently push for changes to take place in the early phases of therapy, to address therapy-interfering behaviours, and to set limits on behaviours which may lead to danger for clients and/or others. As therapy proceeds, the therapist becomes more insistent about the need for behavioural changes, such that old habitual schema-driven coping mechanisms must be overcome to ensure that the client can get their needs met in healthy ways. If coping modes continue to dominate, schemas will be perpetuated and lasting progress will not be possible. It is therefore crucial that the therapist work to address both their own schemas and the client's schemas that block change, to enable them to overcome presenting issues and to facilitate authentic emotional vulnerability and interpersonal connection.

Table 9.1 Common behaviour change targets for common modes

Coping Modes		Behavioural Targets
Surrender	Compliant Surrenderer	• Set limits and boundaries on other's demands and intrusive behaviours
		• Reduce urge to 'rescue' others
		• Find balance between own needs and those of others
		• Practise asking for needs to be met, rather than 'acting out' or trying to 'earn' the right to get needs met by self-sacrificing
		• Learn to express healthy anger and assertiveness
	Helpless Surrenderer	• Practise taking responsibility for own emotional needs
		• Practise asking others to meet needs in direct ways
		• Maintain awareness to ensure relationships are based on reciprocity rather than dependency
		• Develop balance between own and others needs
Avoidant	Detached Protector	• Practise mindful awareness of interoceptive and proprioceptive experience
		• Allow underlying Vulnerable Child to express emotional needs when appropriate
		• Practise *choosing* to adjust the switch of detachment/numbness in daily life
	Detached Self-Soother	• Notice tendency to rely on compulsive behaviours (drugs, alcohol, eating, work, gambling, sex, etc.) as a means of numbing self
		• Recognise needs and emotions underlying compulsive behaviours, and work to actively get these needs met
		• Learn to seek connection (rather than relying on substances to disconnect)
Overcompensatory	Self-Aggrandiser	• Reduce grandiose behaviours, boasting, put-downs, scathing remarks
		• Reduce tendency to 'use' others, or to treat relationships as transactions
		• Learn to respect the rules and to pay your way
		• Practise reciprocity in relationships
		• Practise showing vulnerability to trustworthy others and asking for emotional needs to be met
		• Reduce focus on appearances, status, materialism, and nurture values that are focused more on connection with others and nature
		• Learn to be respectful of others' needs and to provide nurturing for significant others

Perfectionistic Overcontroller	• Introduce play and fun into daily life
	• Allow self to make mistakes and perform less than perfectly
	• Resist urge to describe experiences in overly detailed way
	• Tune into bodily experience (interoception)
	• Develop somatic awareness/mindfulness skills
	• Tune into emotions of Vulnerable Child
	• Learn to communicate about vulnerability
	• Resist urge to intellectualise or 'fix' problems
	• Resist urge to objectify self and others, and to reduce relationships to transactions
	• Increase capacity to connect to vulnerability and to nurture self and others
Child Modes	
Vulnerable Child	• Allow closeness with others who are *trustworthy* and *capable* of meeting your needs
	• Practise asking directly for needs to be met
	• Allow healthy interdependency
Angry Child	• Validate underlying unmet needs
	• Learn to ask for needs to be met in direct ways
	• Reduce tendency to avoid anger through suppression, somatisation, or acting out/discharge of anger
	• Process unresolved childhood anger and rage through Imagery Rescripting
	• Express healthy anger in the present and set healthy boundaries
	• Find constructive focus for expression of anger
Impulsive Child	• Practise setting healthy limits on behaviours
	• Set healthy incentives and rewards that reinforce healthy behaviours
	• Get needs (e.g., for freedom and self-expression) met in overt ways so that Impulsive Child is not forced to 'grab and run'
	• Identify fears associated with giving up impulsive behaviours, and address directly to meet the needs

Table 9.1 (cont.)

Coping Modes		Behavioural Targets
	Undisciplined Child	• Practise setting realistic goals
		• Break goals into small steps
		• Use flashcards as mechanism for staying connected to short-term and long-term life goals
		• Explore pros and cons of setting limits on undisciplined child
		• Gradually build up self-control 'muscle' by practising every day
		• Reward self for meeting mini-goals and more significant goals
Inner Critic [Parent] Modes	Punitive Critic	• Set limits/challenge Inner Critic in daily life
		• Make a list of all of the aspects of life that are avoided due to feeling 'undeserving' – arrange in a hierarchy (most to least difficult)
		• Gradually work through behavioural hierarchy
		• Be actively rebellious against Inner Critic – use anger in constructive manner to fight back
		• Challenge Critic through flashcards and chairwork
	Demanding Critic	• see above as for the punitive critic
	Guilt-Inducing Critic	•

PUNITIVE INNER CRITIC

Illustration 9.2 Punitive Critic mode

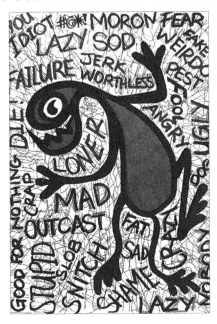

Box 9.12 Future Pattern-Breaking Imagery: Step by Step

Step 1: Provide a Rationale and Negotiate a Future Image Target

It is important to provide a rationale for applying future pattern-breaking imagery. By the time the client has made it towards the ending phases of treatment, they are generally socialised to the use of imagery techniques. The rationale (as with Imagery Rescripting) should emphasise both the advantages of experiential learning and the opportunity to practise. Processing future challenges in imagery provides the client with an opportunity to anticipate and rehearse overcoming any obstacles, with the benefit of the therapist's support. Once the client agrees to participate, the therapist works with the client to agree on an imagery target that is representative of their future chosen pattern-breaking scenario (e.g., having an assertive conversation with dad). It is useful at this stage to also help clients to anticipate and discuss any obstacles they might experience in the image.

Step 2: Visualising Healthy Adult (Optional)

This step is a more recent addition to the protocol and, as such, can be considered optional. The idea is to activate and prime the client's Healthy Adult mode in a brief imagery exercise as preparation for sending the client, in the next step, in to confront their agreed future pattern-breaking image. A full protocol for visualising the Healthy Adult mode is outlined in Chapter 10: Building Connection to Healthy Modes: The Healthy Adult and Happy Child Modes as a stand-alone technique. When visualising the Healthy Adult mode in this context, it may be useful to use a positive image that is thematically related to the schema/s and needs activated in the future image (e.g., autonomy and healthy boundaries).

Step 3: Activate an Image of a Future Pattern-Breaking Scenario

THERAPIST: Can I get you to close your eyes now and get an image of your upcoming meeting with your father. Really take the time to paint the picture of this scene. Where is your dad? What is happening in the scene? What do you see in the image? What do you hear? What do you feel?

Step 4: Bring in the Healthy Adult Part to Implement Healthy Behaviour (Pattern-Breaking)

THERAPIST: Now I want you to imagine your healthy side . . . big, strong Jenny . . . the side of you that knows you need to set a boundary with dad. Can you do that? Can you imagine big Jenny 'tapping in' in this scenario?

CLIENT: Yes.

THERAPIST: Great. Now just sit upright . . . adjust your posture . . . you are in charge now. Now, what do you need to say to your father? *[Encourage the client to implement the new behaviour.]*

Step 5: Coaching in Self-compassion, Cognitive Restructuring, Behavioural Change

Allow the client to complete the dialogue. The goal is to give the client an experience of mastery over the future situation. If the client is at some risk of failing to master the image, the therapist can play a coaching role, feeding healthy messages and cognitions.

THERAPIST: . . . I want you to tell him that it is ok for him to share his opinion, but it is also OK for you to disagree, and have your own thoughts on the matter . . .

If the client struggles to master the image with this coaching, then the therapist can enter the scene and take charge, modelling what might be needed (from a Healthy Adult) in the scenario, as is done in imagery rescripting of past images.

Step 6: Reflection and Homework

Once the scene is complete, have the client open their eyes, and spend some time reflecting on the imagery exercise. What were the key takeaways from this experience? What did they learn? Would this change anything about how they approach the situation in vivo? What barriers to change remain? What does all of this mean for our behaviour change hierarchy? Are you ready to work on one of the steps this week?

Once the client has been able to imagine being successful at changing the pattern, collaborate with the client to attempt some pattern-breaking 'for real' as part of homework.

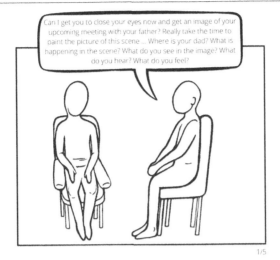

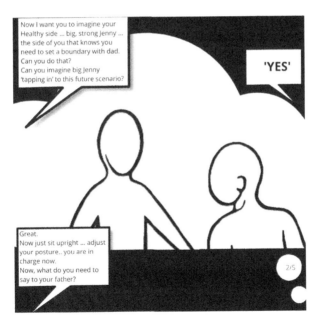

Cartoon 9.1   Future Pattern-Breaking Imagery

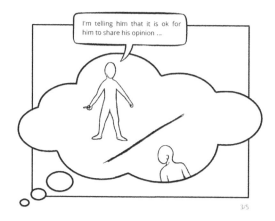

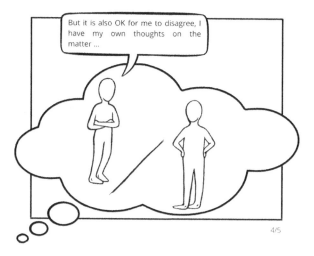

Cartoon 9.1 (cont.)

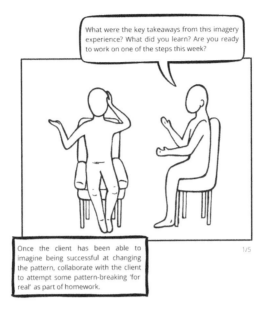

Cartoon 9.1 (cont.)

References

1. Young JE, Rygh J. *Young-Rygh Avoidance Inventory (YRAI)*. Cognitive Therapy Centre; 2003.

2. Young JE. *Young Compensatory Inventory (YCI)*. Cognitive Therapy Centre; 1995.

3. Rijkeboer MM, Lobbestael J, Arntz A, van Genderen H. (2010). *Schema coping inventory*. University of Utrecht Press.

4. Young J, Klosko J, Weishaar M. *Schema therapy: A practitioner's guide*. Guilford Press. 2003.

5. Van der Winjgaart R. *Imagery rescripting: Theory and practice*. Pavilion Publishing & Media; 2021.

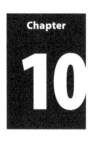

Building Connection to Healthy Modes
The Healthy Adult and Happy Child Modes

Introduction

Although schema therapy is often characterised by its focus on healing painful and mal-adaptive aspects of a client's presentation, it is equally important to nurture and grow psychological health and resilience.

Jeff Young, in his seminal book, outlined the importance of two positive modes that often require development during schema therapy: the Healthy Adult mode and the Happy Child mode [1]. In this chapter, we elaborate on the nature and function of healthy modes, and present when and how schema therapists seek to develop these capacities in clients throughout treatment.

Conceptualising the Healthy Adult Mode

The Healthy Adult mode is primarily responsible for healthy self-regulation. As maladaptive modes become more readily identified and appropriately addressed in therapy, it becomes important to also focus on strengthening the healthy aspects of the self. A central aim of schema therapy is to strengthen the Healthy Adult mode of clients well enough that they can take care of their own core emotional needs outside of therapy. In the early phases of schema therapy, the therapist acts as a role model for this Healthy Adult side. For the most complex clients, the therapist may present the first healthy role model and limited reparenting provider they have encountered. It is hoped that the healthy, adaptive attitudes (cognitions) and responses (behaviour) of the therapist will be internalised and serve as building blocks for the development of the client's own Healthy Adult repertoire. During the middle to ending phases of schema therapy, the client must also learn to be able to invoke the Healthy Adult by forming a mental image of this mode and imagining how they would deal with common problematic situations in daily life. It is useful to think about the Healthy Adult mode as both a trait and a state; schema therapy aims to build both a healthy general pattern of responding (Healthy Adult as a trait), but also help the client to be able to access or invoke this mode to effectively regulate emotion and behaviour in the face of life's challenges (Healthy Adult as a state).

Functions of the Healthy Adult Mode

Young and colleagues [1] described several functions of the Healthy Adult mode. The Healthy Adult mode is characterised by:

1. Higher functioning and healthy schemas of capability and strength.
2. Adaptive behaviours and cognitions that are required for undertaking appropriate adult functions, such as taking responsibility, working, parenting, commitment, etc.

3. Positive or adaptive schemas.
4. Being motivated by the satisfaction of core emotional needs. This mode is primarily concerned with helping meet needs in a stable and enduring way.
5. Its role as a nurturer to the Vulnerable Child.

In Chapter 1 we provided a broad description of the Healthy Adult mode:

> The Healthy Adult recognises, protects, and nurtures the inner Vulnerable Child and their needs, and demonstrates compassion for self and others. This mode demonstrates flexibility, seeking to balance prioritising the needs of self and others, and can manage adult responsibilities (sustaining a job, self-care, managing finances, caring for others). The Healthy Adult strives for a flexible balance between pleasant adult activities (intellectual/cultural/physical) and maintaining commitments. This mode experiences the body and mind as integrated aspects of the self, can give and receive nurturance and care, and gains meaning from authentic self-expression and connection with others and the world. This mode, when activated, can step back with awareness from one's automatic schema-based reactions and choose adaptive reactions with respect to one's longer-term needs. (P10)

Recently, authors have built and expanded upon the original definition, describing the Healthy Adult mode as involving two key processes or abilities [2]:

1. Healthy self-processing characterised by self-awareness, mindfulness, and distancing (or defusion) from schema or mode activation (e.g., 'I notice that a part of me is afraid that you will leave if I ask for my needs to be met').
2. Accessing healthy beliefs about the self and the world (positive/adaptive schemas) and related functional patterns of behaviour (e.g., 'It will be OK . . . it's normal to ask for my needs to be met. Other people expect that relationships should be a two-way street and if they don't then that is *their* problem').

Strengthening and Connecting with the Healthy Adult Mode

In Young, Klosko, and Weishaar [1]), the process of strengthening the Healthy Adult mode was described mostly as an implicit process, derived through observing the therapist and via interventions largely focused on healing maladaptive schemas and modes. Considerable attention has been paid in recent years to methods of explicitly building the Healthy Adult mode as a separate therapy objective. A plethora of cognitive, experiential, and behavioural treatment strategies have been proposed to explicitly strengthen the healthy side of the client [2, 3, 4]. However, this range of methods can be narrowed down to four core skills necessary for healthy self-regulation: (1) healthy self-awareness; (2) self-compassion; (3) cognitive restructuring and accessing healthy perspectives; (4) behaviour change. These can be considered the building blocks of the Healthy Adult, and key targets for positive schema therapy. These abilities both build the Healthy Adult 'trait' over time and can be used to induce or 'connect with' the Healthy Adult 'state' within treatment sessions or during daily life (e.g., for mode management). These four skills are presented here as a series of steps. Before beginning skills development, schema therapists will gauge the strength of the client's Healthy Adult mode by assessing the client's existing strength in these four areas. If the client has difficulties in any specific areas, these can be used to prioritise relevant positive interventions.

Four Aspects of Healthy Adult Functioning

Step 1: Healthy Self-Awareness (Mindfulness)

In the early phases of schema therapy, clients typically present as overwhelmed or dominated by the activation of maladaptive modes (e.g., critics, Vulnerable Child, Detached Protector). Consequently, they have very poor self-awareness: they do not understand their feelings, where they come from, what their needs might be, or how to adaptively respond to challenging situations. Such clients are often stuck in automatic and engrained patterns of mode-responding, which allow them to survive but ultimately disconnect them from satisfaction of their core emotional needs. To the degree that clients are not aware of these automatic, schema-driven patterns of responding, they remain destined to repeat them. Thus, it is important in the early phases of treatment for schema therapists to help clients to identify their schemas and modes and understand which childhood memories, emotions, bodily sensations, cognitions, and coping responses are associated with them. The goal is for clients to understand how to notice and label these experiences (as schemas or modes) as they arise in the here and now, while recognising any links to developmental origins and their experience of their current problems. It is hoped that by doing so, clients learn to be able to 'step back' and notice their automatic schema- or mode-driven reactions when their schemas and modes are activated, providing them crucial time to be able to formulate healthy or adaptive responses. An important part of this process is that clients also become aware of their needs and values in the situation. Schema activation will often indicate that one's needs and values are threatened in some way. Knowing which needs and values seem threatened is necessary to select an adaptive behavioural response.

Building schema and mode awareness traditionally occurs via the education and conceptualisation process at the beginning of therapy, through the use of schema/mode monitoring forms, and via attunement within the therapy relationship (see Chapter 6: Intervention Strategies for Schema Healing 1: Limited Reparenting). In recent times, authors have recognised the potential applicability of mindfulness practices and other 'third wave therapy' approaches (e.g., values clarification exercises) to explicitly build or induce healthy self-awareness (see [2] for a more thorough overview). For example, highly ruminative clients (high in Over-Analyser coping) might be encouraged to start treatment sessions with a brief mindfulness practice as a way of connecting them to the present moment and, in turn, to their Healthy Adult mode at the start of a treatment session.

Step 2: Self-Compassion

Many clients report being subjected to heavy doses of demanding, critical, or punitive messages during their childhood, and did not receive adequate levels of care, compassion, or kindness. These kinds of negative messages were delivered either verbally, were modelled, or were interpreted as such after traumatic or difficult life events. Having not received much of it, these clients have difficulty experiencing kindness and difficulty showing kindness to themselves. Instead, they may have an overdeveloped 'Critic' voice.

It is generally accepted that experiencing compassion stimulates systems in the brain that calm a person down [5, 6]. Therefore, as the therapy starts to reduce the dominance of the Critic mode(s), it is also important to help the client experience more compassionate thoughts and feelings. In practice, once a client has become aware of their own schema-driven reactions, and then made initial contact with their Healthy Adult side, the next step is to induce some calming within the self by responding to emotions with compassion.

Self-Compassion Involves the Following Four Processes:

a. Recognising and naming the emotions evoked: 'I feel sad/scared/angry . . .'
b. Explicitly expressing why situational circumstances make this reaction understandable: 'of course I feel sad, because this is a difficult situation . . .'
c. Explicitly expressing that old pain from past events makes these emotional reactions understandable: 'of course I feel so sad, because after all I've been through, this really is a difficult situation . . .'
d. Paying attention to the soothing and calming felt sense that self-compassion evokes.

Schema Therapy Intervention Approach to Building Healthy Self-Compassion:

1. *Mode/Schema Awareness.* Clients low in self-compassion tend also to be dominated by critic modes and associated schemas (e.g., Punitiveness, Unrelenting Standards). Initially, through the case conceptualisation, education, and process of self-monitoring, clients need to be made aware of the negative influence of their Critic mode on their problems, and their ability to regulate emotion with self-compassion. The hope is to create some initial distance or defusion from the Critic and start to make this voice more ego-dystonic (and less ego-syntonic). It is also useful for clients to gain awareness of the historical antecedents that have led to these Critic messages; this starts the process of understanding and having compassion for these (vulnerable) experiences.

2. *Limited Reparenting.* As clients start to become aware of this, the therapist uses the therapy relationship to directly meet their needs for acceptance, validation, compassion, and care. The therapist meets the client's needs directly and models how to be caring.

3. *Cognitive Techniques.* Cognitive techniques in this context have three aims: (i) to build a willingness in the client to let go of Critic messages and commit to the notion of self-compassion as an alternative (healthy) path to self-regulation (pros and cons technique can be useful here); (ii) challenge the adaptiveness of schemas that block self-compassion (e.g., standard cognitive techniques for Punitiveness or Unrelenting Standards); and (iii) help the client establish new, desired adaptive schemas (e.g., healthy self-care.) All three of these aims are important, but we have found the first aim to be the foundation, and the one that is often neglected in treatments that target compassion.

4. *Experiential Techniques.* Standard experiential techniques to build self-compassion tend to revolve around chair and imagery dialogues that (i) challenge any Critic activation or messages, and then (ii) convey care and compassion to the child (see Box 10.1 for a clinical example). For some clients, giving and receiving care and compassion can be overwhelming; thus, experiential techniques aiming to increase self-compassion should be applied according to the client's window of tolerance. One exercise that evokes relatively low emotional arousal is the *Little Boy or Girl on the Street Dialogue* [2]. It is worth noting that many experiential techniques exist within the Compassion-Focused Therapy tradition that have been designed specifically with these goals in mind [7] and can quite readily be integrated into schema therapy.

5. *Behavioural Techniques.* As the client starts to heal and develop some capacity to experience self-compassion, it is also important for them to change their behaviour. This often involves a reversal of some form of maladaptive coping, but should also include a commitment towards compassionate, kind, and caring behaviour towards oneself (e.g., committing time for relaxation). The client should start to adopt healthy and adaptive behaviours that reflect the attitude 'I am worth it; I'm worthy of self-care and kindness.' As clients develop more capacity to experience self-compassion, their capacity to turn this outward and show others compassion is also enhanced and can be threaded into Healthy Adult pattern-breaking (some clients in particular struggle with this).

Box 10.1 Clinical Example of Self-Compassion Using Chair Dialogue with the Vulnerable Child Mode (Experiential Technique)

In response to an argument that took place over the past week, a chair technique was introduced. A chair is placed between the therapist and the client, symbolising the little girl that the client once was. To intensify this image, a photo of the client as a little girl has been placed on the chair. Since the conceptualisation of the case and the first phase of treatment, it's been known that this girl has often been the victim of verbal and physical abuse by her father. The therapist now coaches the client in dealing with this emotional pain in a healthy manner.

THERAPIST: I think we understand very clearly why she is so scared and sad, don't we?

CLIENT: Yes . . .

THERAPIST: Can you say that out loud, that you do understand? Please finish this sentence: *[therapist turns towards the small child's chair]* 'Of course you feel so sad because . . .' *[therapist turns back towards the client again]* Please express why is it actually perfectly logical that she feels so sad in this situation?

CLIENT: . . . Well, there was that argument, of course . . .

THERAPIST: Exactly, can you express loudly that understanding you felt, the understanding that this situation was also very sad to her?

CLIENT: *[turns towards the small child's chair]* Well . . . Of course, you feel sad, because an argument is never fun. Anyone would feel anxious and sad in that situation . . .

THERAPIST: Excellent! You're doing great! But I think that an argument is very difficult for her in particular, don't you think? What with everything she's been through . . .? Can you also say something about that?

CLIENT: . . . Yes . . . You've already experienced so many arguments; you've been shouted at so often . . . even as a child, growing up. Of course, it makes complete sense that this frightens you and also that it makes you sad . . . I get that . . .

THERAPIST: You did great! . . . How do you feel when you voice that understanding of the situation so loudly? Do you feel worse than before? Just as bad? Or a little better?

CLIENT: I do feel calmer, yes . . .

[Note: for some clients this part can trigger the critic mode, as a barrier to the experience of healthy compassion. The critic mode would then become a target for intervention within this session.]

HEALTHY ADULT (NURTURER) MODE

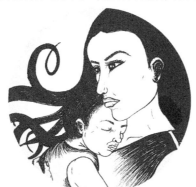

Illustration 10.1 Healthy Adult (Nurturer) mode

Step 3: Cognitive Restructuring and Accessing Healthy Cognitions

The calming effect of self-compassion is a prerequisite for being able to reflect realistically on the situation, the emotions evoked, and how to deal with them in an adaptive way. Negative self-evaluations from internalised Critic modes need to be contradicted and reflexive methods of self-protection stemming from coping modes need to be adjusted. Cognitive restructuring of these old assumptions is a key step in strengthening the Healthy Adult part of the client. In the beginning phases of therapy, the therapist presented the cognitive arguments needed to contradict the Critic mode messages and to make the client more aware of not just the advantages, but also the disadvantages of the old coping modes. In this middle phase, the client should increasingly make the cognitive arguments (that contradict old assumptions) on their own by voicing them and repeating them frequently.

In this phase focused on the Healthy Adult, the goal is for the client to access healthier and more functional thoughts and attitudes (healthy self-talk) that reflect positive or adaptive schemas [8]. We have found that an important theme here is the notion of basic hope and optimism. Clients will often 'borrow' from our hope for them through the reparenting messages, but in the later phases of treatment they will need to be able to access this hope for themselves to effectively regulate their schema-based reactions (e.g., 'It's going to be OK, even this will pass'). See Box 10.2 for an elaboration of the previous clinical example.

Step 4: Behaviour Change

The fourth and final step in strengthening the healthy side of the client is to learn to *respond* to problems and emotions in a healthy way. However, each situation requires a different kind of behavioural instruction as the specific factors of each situation tend to vary. In addition, there may also be a range of other basic needs, motivations, and values surrounding problematic situations. The Healthy Adult mode is ultimately concerned with long-term need satisfaction [2]. Connecting the clients with their needs will tend to connect them to their Healthy Adult mode. When the client is triggered in session and reflects on some urge

---

Box 10.2 Clinical Example of Cognitive Restructuring for Developing Healthy Cognitions

After the client has been coached in expressing self-compassion, the negative self-evaluations that were triggered by the argument with her boyfriend are addressed.

THERAPIST: When I hear what was going on in your head during and after the argument – that it was all your fault and that you always ruin everything – who do we hear saying this? What side of you?

CLIENT: My Punitive side!

THERAPIST: That definitely sounds like it . . . However, you have now made contact with that Healthy Adult side of yourself, that captain of your own ship. In the meantime, you have calmed down a bit by first observing your reactions with a sense of compassion and understanding, instead of criticising them as this 'Punisher' tends to do. Now let's think about why what the Punisher is saying isn't true. Why it isn't true that it is all your fault and that you ruin everything?

CLIENT: . . . But that's what I think.

THERAPIST: Who thinks that – you or that Punisher?

CLIENT: I think I . . . hmm . . . I don't know . . .

THERAPIST: That's why we really need to take some time now to think about that, not coming from reflexes, but really coming from your Healthy Adult side. You know how the saying goes: Where two people argue or fight . . . it takes two to . . .?

CLIENT: Tango?

THERAPIST: Exactly . . . What do you think about that? Could that be the case?

CLIENT: Yes, that seems about right . . . I guess it can't be ALL my fault.

THERAPIST: But if that is true for others, then why shouldn't it be true for you now – and are you really the only one who is to blame for all of this? Or is that just what the Punisher would have you believe? Does that make any sense?

CLIENT: I guess so, if you look at it that way.

THERAPIST: So, this is an important point, one to remember and bear in mind. Can you say that literally to the Punisher, that in an argument, there is never only one party at fault? Like it takes two to tango!

CLIENT: *[speaking softly]* . . . Well, where there are two people arguing, both are responsible . . . so it's not just my fault . . . There are two sides to the story.

THERAPIST: Very good, say it again but now 20 per cent louder.

CLIENT: *[slightly louder]* Where two people are arguing, both have to take some responsibility, so it's not all my fault, because he was being really mean to me!

---

to cope reflexively, ask them 'what do you think you need in that situation?' Consequently, in learning to regulate with the Healthy Adult mode, the client must learn to first ask themselves what they need in problematic situations, and how that need can be validated or met in that specific situation. The complexity of different problematic situations and the presence of other people who may have different needs than them make it almost impossible to reach an ideal outcome in all situations. Dealing with problematic situations is therefore a constant balancing act. A metaphor that can be used to convey this to the client is the Healthy Adult who, as captain of a ship, tries to stay on course even though that course sometimes faces strong currents, storms, and as such, is never sailing in a perfectly straight line. Initially the client starts to speculate, through their self-monitoring, on how to bring their needs into play in various situations. The therapist will then guide the client to elaborate and add to their initial observations.

Connecting with the Healthy Adult Mode Using the 'Healthy Adult Connection Form'. The Healthy Adult Connection Form (see Figure 10.1) can be used to help guide clients through the process of connecting with their Healthy Adult mode and build Healthy Adult capacities over time. Clients are often more able to complete the initial (basic) aspects of this form early in treatment. The form provides a structured method to build mode awareness: clients learn to become aware of aspects of a triggering situation, their own reactions, and their needs, and recognise their own mode activation. The monitoring form kind of 'force feeds' the Healthy Adult mode. Encouraging the client to step back and reflect on Healthy Adult questions induces the Healthy Adult. Over time, clients become better able to complete the form right through to the end, including forming a plan to respond in a healthy way. Don't expect clients to achieve a healthy response independently, early on in treatment; the ability to plan a healthy response follows a developmental process. By a later stage of treatment, the form can also be used to facilitate mode management; clients can use the form in difficult situations to help access their Healthy Adult mode. Such a form, if used for homework, will provide a helpful focus for the sessions and priceless data on where the client struggles to regulate, and will suggest potential intervention targets.

Connecting to the Healthy Adult Through Imagery. The client can learn to form a mental image of their Healthy Adult side. We have found it helpful for the client to practise accessing this healthy side in imagery, to feel vividly and realistically what might otherwise only be an abstract concept.

1. Rationale. The therapist overviews the later phase of therapy in which the client must learn to handle any problematic situations and emotions in a healthy way. The Healthy Adult side is described as a mode, a side of the client, and, as was the case with other modes, attention is focused on the recognisable signals of this state of mind.

2. The Therapist Gives a Personal Example of Their Own Healthy Adult Mode. The therapist also gives personal examples of what their own healthy side looks like in various situations. An example is given of a challenging, difficult situation from the therapist's everyday life where old patterns were activated but the therapist managed to handle these patterns and the situation itself, in a healthy way. The therapist might choose an example where they had to balance meeting their own needs with meeting the needs or demands of others. There are various reasons why the therapist gives a personal example. First, it illustrates that being a Healthy Adult does not ostensibly mean that everything is easy and problem free. The therapist has already made it clear that everyone, including the therapist, has schemas. It has also been explained that it is not the presence of these schemas that determines whether or not you are a Healthy Adult, but rather how you deal with these schemas and problematic situations. Nevertheless, experience has shown that clients still have unrealistic

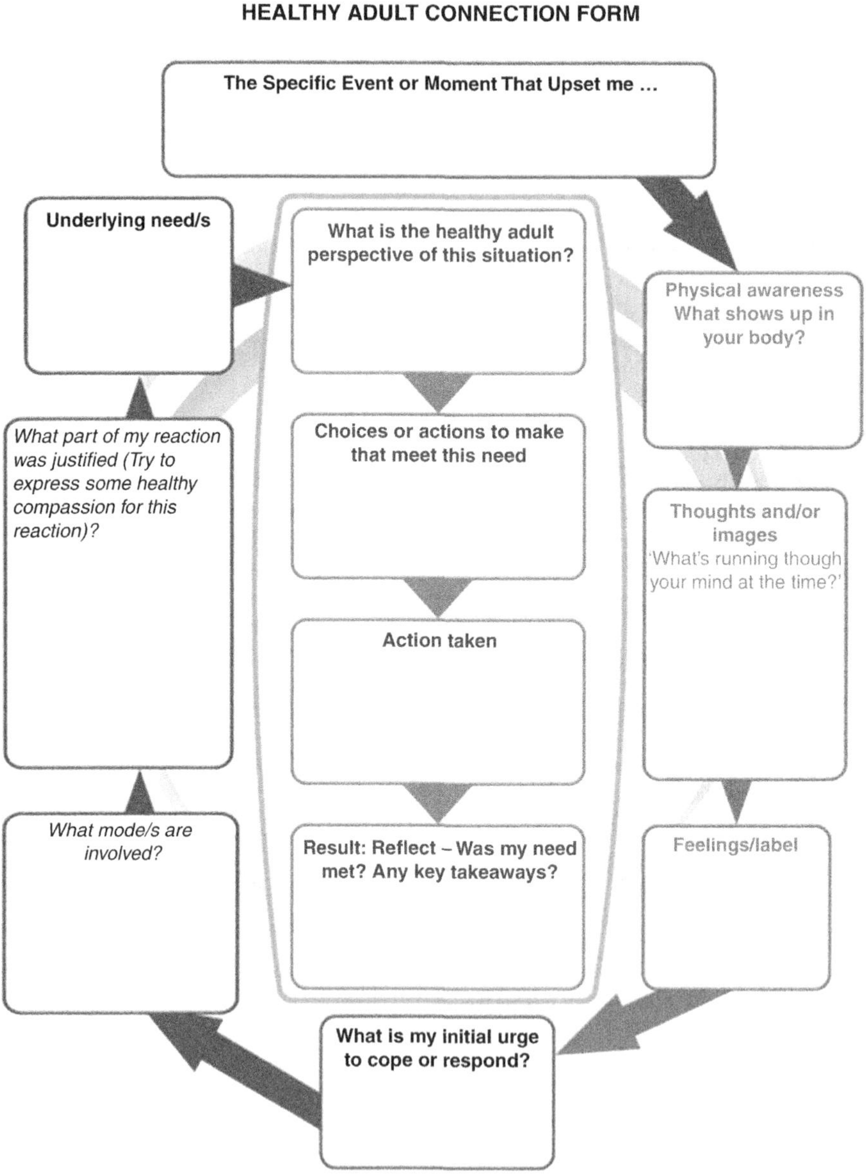

HEALTHY ADULT CONNECTION FORM

The Specific Event or Moment That Upset me …

Underlying need/s

What is the healthy adult perspective of this situation?

Physical awareness
What shows up in your body?

What part of my reaction was justified (Try to express some healthy compassion for this reaction)?

Choices or actions to make that meet this need

Thoughts and/or images
'What's running though your mind at the time?'

Action taken

What mode/s are involved?

Result: Reflect – Was my need met? Any key takeaways?

Feelings/label

What is my initial urge to cope or respond?

Figure 10.1 Healthy Adult connection form

expectations when it comes to what it means to be a Healthy Adult. Citing a personal example reinforces an important message – namely, that therapy goals should be realistic goals.

Box 10.3 Step-by-Step Plan for Learning to Visualise (Invoke) the Healthy Adult Mode

1 Explain the rationale behind the imagery exercise.
2 The therapist gives a personal example of their Healthy Adult.
3 The client visualises their own Healthy Adult mode.
4 Identifying the embodiment of Healthy Adult mode.
5 Evaluation and homework.

A second reason for citing a personal example is to provide the client with the opportunity to experience contact on a more equal footing. In preparation for the end part of therapy, the client needs to develop more autonomy and self-confidence, which will be undermined if the therapist remains on a pedestal as someone who can effortlessly handle all problems and is never plagued by concerns and feelings of fear, sadness, or anger. The middle phase of therapy can be likened to the puberty phase of children. In this phase, adolescents have to learn that their parents are not able to do everything in the way in which they had experienced as small children and are people with their own limitations and shortcomings. This process of 'coming down from a pedestal' offers room for autonomy to grow.

3. Client Visualises Their Own Healthy Adult Mode. The therapist invites the client to recall a visual image of their healthy side. The client is asked to think back to a situation that they found difficult but that was ultimately handled well, and that the client looks back on with a sense of satisfaction or pride. In this imagining, the client is asked first to focus on the difficult part of the memory and to become aware of the emotions that are being evoked. Next, the client is asked to concentrate on the part of the memory where they handle these emotions and the situation well. The therapist explicitly labels these acts of competent emotional and situational management as the operation of the client's Healthy Adult.

4. Identifying the Embodiment of the Healthy Adult Mode. The therapist asks the client to become aware of the physical, sensory qualities of the Healthy Adult state of mind (associated with the memory identified in step 3). What feelings are associated with this part of the memory? Where does the client experience these feelings in their own body? Which posture best suits this feeling? Can the client assume that posture now? What urges to act does the client experience? The client is also asked to take a mental photograph of themselves in this state of mind. **Therapist Tip**: The client can also be encouraged to make a basic artwork or drawing representing this 'photograph'.

5. Evaluation and Homework. In the follow-up discussion, both the memory itself (from step 3) and the embodied qualities are named as potential gateways to this Healthy Adult state of mind. The client can then consciously choose to use these cues to access their healthy side in future situations – for example, by assuming the same posture, recalling the image of themselves in that state, or focusing the attention on the part of their body where they felt that specific feeling. Homework involves the client practising this imagery exercise. A recording can be made during a session to guide the homework practice, if desired.

Developing and Expressing the Happy Child Mode

In addition to the Healthy Adult mode, schema therapy recognises the Happy Child mode as a second functional mode to nurture. Theoretically, the Happy Child mode is intrinsic (like the Vulnerable Child or Angry Child modes). As humans, we all have a Happy Child mode: the capacity to be light-hearted, to experience fun and enjoyment. This mode can act in a dyad with the Healthy Adult mode to maximise well-being; the Healthy Adult allows for the activation of the Happy Child mode and helps meet its core needs of spontaneity and play when it is appropriate.

The Happy Child mode is evident when the client describes a sense of joy, fun and playfulness. The Happy Child mode is thought to represent the first kind of developmentally appropriate healthy mode for children. Much of what is learned about the world in childhood comes through this playful state. In Happy Child mode the client engages in more light-hearted behaviours and takes a less serious and more playful view of events around them. They engage in fun behaviours and interact with the world with an attitude of curiosity and enjoyment. It is important to note that the Happy Child mode does not function as a coping mode. For example, although the Self-Aggrandiser mode may use humour to jeer or tease others with the guise of being 'playful', its function is to gain superiority or take a position of power. Within Happy Child mode, the function of humour and play is not to avoid, hide, or mask emotional states but to experience positive affect (e.g., joy, happiness, curiosity).

The suppression of the Happy Child mode typically occurs in developmental environments where play, spontaneity, and fun are restricted, discouraged, or not valued. As a result, the child's experience of positive affect (e.g., happiness, joy, spontaneity, curiosity) is thwarted. For example, clients may have excessively structured routines, they may have had excessive pressure to achieve, and caregivers may have viewed fun and play as not being a priority compared to 'accomplishments'. Adult clients whose Happy Child mode was neglected might struggle to describe childhood memories where caregivers played and had fun with them. In addition, in some caregiving environments, any display of emotion – positive or negative – was inhibited and the caregiver presented as being self-conscious or overly controlled in their emotional expression. Where emotional expression is inhibited, the experience of play for the child is restricted. Adults with a limited capacity to express their Happy Child mode may present as overly inhibited in their experience of positive emotions and related behavioural repertoires (e.g., play). Chronic disconnection from positive affect experiences represents a vulnerability factor for psychopathology such as depression. The Happy Child mode can also be conceptualised as a healthy regulator of positive affect. Positive affect can buffer against more acute, grave, and aversive emotional states (negative affect).

In cases where the Happy Child mode is undeveloped and linked to clinical problems, the therapist may need to incorporate the Happy Child mode into case conceptualisations with a view to strengthening the mode and the dyad with the Healthy Adult mode. The client's Healthy Adult mode allows for playfulness, permitting the client to 'lighten up' and go 'off duty'. Clients experiencing high levels of the Unrelenting Standards schema may benefit from developing and building the Happy Child mode. In such cases, the schema's excessive focus on achievement or the compulsion to 'get things right' comes at the expense of engagement in fun or enjoyable activities. Such adult clients may feel guilty or stressed when engaging in Happy Child mode pursuits and require intervention. Alternatively, individuals with high Emotional Inhibition schemas may feel uncomfortable engaging in or displaying any positive emotions. They may present as being emotionally 'uptight' and unable to feel positive emotional experiences. If the Happy Child mode is conceptualised as 'underdeveloped' and linked to clinical problems (e.g., depression), then the development of the Happy Child mode would be a target for intervention.

Methods to Strengthen the Happy Child Mode

Intervention approaches that aim to develop and express the Happy Child mode involve some flexible and creative combination of all four classes of intervention characteristic of schema therapy: limited reparenting and cognitive, experiential, and behavioural strategies.

Limited Reparenting. The therapist models the use of the Happy Child mode to the client, demonstrating being 'real' and at times modelling a light-hearted approach. The therapist directly meets the need for spontaneity and play by affirming to the client that it is 'ok to have fun and feel light-hearted' and framing the sessions more within this playful stance.

Cognitive Techniques. The therapist encourages the client to challenge the belief that fun, playfulness, and spontaneity are redundant and unnecessary. Here, psychoeducation regarding play in childhood development can be helpful to validate the core emotional needs that underpin the mode. It is also likely that EMS (e.g., Unrelenting Standards, Punitiveness, Emotional Inhibition) or modes (Demanding Critic, Avoidant Protector) that directly thwart the expression of the Happy Child mode will need to be directly addressed. The therapist may also construct flashcard recordings for the client to listen to as homework when they feel uncomfortable engaging in healthy, 'Happy Child' behaviours (see Box 10.4).

Experiential Techniques. In imagery rescripting exercises, clients may access childhood images where the need for play was evident. The therapist can enter the image and play with the child and validate the need for playful interaction. It will often be necessary to first address any caregivers in imagery that are actively inhibiting the expression of positive emotions. For example, the therapist may challenge the parent's message that 'play always comes second, what is important is to work hard'. The exercise can end with the therapist encouraging, supporting – and perhaps participating – in playful activities and experiences in the imagery (see Box 10.5).

Box 10.4 Example Excerpt of Flashcard Recording for Connecting with Happy Child mode

'Right now, you may be feeling uncomfortable, tense. This is the right time to start engaging in something fun, something you like to do, and would like to be able to enjoy. This is your Happy Child mode. You may be thinking that this is not a priority, that you should be doing something more 'productive'. Your Happy Child mode is underdeveloped because your parents discouraged normal fun and enjoyment over their financial goals and 'hard work'. This has resulted in you now feeling stressed and "pressured" by your Demanding Critic whenever you try to have fun. So even though you want to go back to work or do something "productive", it's important to allow yourself to lighten the load and have some fun. It's OK . . . you deserve this . . . it's OK to just "have fun".'

> **Box 10.5** Example of Playful Imagery to Foster Happy Child Mode
>
> THERAPIST: Now that things are a bit more relaxed here, what does Little Johnny want to do with all this free time?
>
> CLIENT: Play on the swing.
>
> THERAPIST: Let's do that then ... Can you imagine that ... we are at the park, and I am pushing you on the swing ... How does that feel?

Mode Work with the Happy Child mode. The therapist can 'mode out' (i.e., conceptualise) the prospect of engaging in Happy Child mode. This allows the therapist to understand the interplay of other modes that may stifle spontaneous behaviour. Mode chair dialogues can be used to help challenge sentiments from the Demanding Critic mode or reason with the Perfectionistic Overcontroller mode. The therapist also aims to strengthen the dyad between the Happy Child and Healthy Adult modes. Late in treatment, the client's Healthy Adult can take the lead on chairwork exercises and advocate for the importance of the Happy Child mode. A plethora of Happy Child imagery exercises have been developed to directly encourage its expression, including 'Ice-Cream Imagery' [9] and 'Toy Store Imagery' [2].

Behavioural Techniques. The therapist encourages the client to engage in behaviours that represent 'lightening up' and enjoyment. Therapists may construct a list of behaviours that might function to strengthen the Happy Child mode. For example, the therapist may encourage the client to bring something funny to share to session (e.g., a funny comedy sketch on YouTube), often as a way of starting sessions on a playful note. We have found that children tend to be a great conduit of the Happy Child mode. If the client is a parent, they may be encouraged to set aside time to play, engage, and follow the lead with their child to develop 'playfulness'.

Concluding Remarks

When faced with the long problem lists, pervasive interpersonal difficulties, and frequent distress of chronic and severe clients, it is easy for therapists to become preoccupied with the negative qualities of the client's life. Furthermore, psychological health is not simply the absence of painful emotions; most of our clients have well-developed coping modes that minimise their painful emotions but do not enhance their quality of life. Growing the client's Healthy Adult mode is the ultimate aim of schema therapy, and cultivating their Happy Child mode is a critical component of that developmental process. All children are born with a capacity for joy, curiosity, and exploration, a basic need which western neoliberal economies arguably pay scant attention to. Schema therapy offers continual opportunities and numerous methods to counterbalance early child-rearing and wider socialisation forces, to promote the importance of play and self-compassion for a more authentic, enriched model of psychological health.

References

1. Young J, Klosko J, Weishaar M. *Schema therapy: A practitioner's guide.* Guilford Press. 2003.

2. Roediger E, Stevens B, Brockman R. *Contextual schema therapy: An integrative approach to personality disorders, emotional dysregulation, and interpersonal functioning.* New Harbinger Publications; 2018.

3. Claassen A, Broersen J. *Handleiding module schematherapie en de Gezonde volwassene.* 1st ed. Springer; 2019.

4. Claassen A, Hulsbergen M. *Schematherapie en de Gezonde Volwassene: Positievetechnieken uit de praktijk.* 1st ed. Springer; 2015.

5. Gilbert P, Tirch D. Emotional memory, mindfulness and compassion. In Zinn J. *Clinical handbook of mindfulness.* Springer; 2009. pp. 99–110.

6. Neff K. The role of self-compassion in development: A healthier way to relate to oneself. *Human Development.* 2009;**52** (4):211–14.

7. Kolts R. *CFT made simple: A clinician's guide to practicing compassion-focused therapy.* New Harbinger Publications; 2016.

8. Louis JP, Wood AM, Lockwood G, Ho MH, Ferguson E. Positive clinical psychology and Schema Therapy (ST): The development of the Young Positive Schema Questionnaire (YPSQ) to complement the Young Schema Questionnaire 3 Short Form (YSQ-S3). *Psychological Assessment.* 2018; **30** (9):1199.

9. Farrell J, Reiss N, Shaw I. *The schema therapy clinician's guide: A complete resource for building and delivering individual, group and integrated schema mode treatment programs.* John Wiley & Sons; 2014.

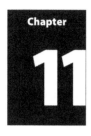

Bypassing Maladaptive Coping Modes to Support Change

Introduction

Coping modes embody the client's most successful survival strategies from their most adverse earlier experiences. However, to the extent that their adult life no longer resembles the context in which their coping modes developed, these modes often become *schema maintaining*. To effectively deal with coping modes, the therapist must deeply understand the roles those modes have served, the vulnerability they protect the client from, and the ways in which they now interfere with needs satisfaction. In this chapter, we describe how schema therapists negotiate with clients to lower their guard and allow the therapist to help them achieve deeper healing and growth, rather than continuing to settle for 'coping'.

The Function of Coping Modes

Coping modes represent the 'survival' parts of the self that are currently active for an individual, which would have developed as a means of coping with unmet needs during childhood or adolescence. Coping modes function to avoid or escape schema activation and can be categorised within three overarching styles: avoidance, overcompensation (inversion), and surrender (resignation). In individuals with chronic interpersonal or psychological difficulties, coping modes are not under adequate voluntary control. Maladaptive coping modes are often either rigidly maintained regardless of how well they work to meet the person's needs in a situation (such as in Cluster C presentations, wherein the person becomes rigidly 'stuck' in one or more coping modes) or flip chaotically between alternative coping modes with minimal stimulation (such as in Cluster B presentations). Coping modes may also become dissociated. The degree of dissociation operates along a spectrum, at the highest end of which is dissociative identity disorder (DID), wherein the modes operate as multiple independent 'selves' with minimal awareness of each other. By contrast, in a healthy person there is natural and flexible control of coping modes as the individual maintains a consistent self-awareness across the ebb and flow of different modes assuming momentary prominence. The Healthy Adult mode encapsulates a stable sense of self as the 'conductor' of the 'internal orchestra'. As a person becomes healthier, they become more consciously aware of the presence of their coping modes, have more control over their intensity (can 'dial' them up and down), and are less reliant on using them in extreme ways.

Schema therapy is based on the premise that differentiation is integrative; it is by recognising the different aspects of self that we become aware of them and begin the process of bringing them together into a coherent sense of self. Schema therapy interventions in the initial phase of therapy are aimed at differentiating the coping modes, labelling them, noting their character and felt sense, and acknowledging their functional intention. The goal is to help clients recognise that their coping modes make sense because they were adaptive in the childhood context in which they emerged. Later in therapy, the focus gradually shifts to exploring how problematic coping behaviours are no longer serving the client and often prevent them from getting their needs met or cause interpersonal problems. It is important to recognise that, in many cases, the coping modes are the closest that clients have to a Healthy Adult side. These states of mind helped the person to survive their childhood, to protect their Vulnerable Child self, to manage unmet needs, and to 'make sense' of an otherwise confusing or chaotic environment. They have provided inner coherence and, in some cases, a 'surrogate identity'. Often, the coping modes have developed an 'addictive' quality because the associated behaviour provides an experience that mimics partial need fulfilment, and dysfunctional behaviour has been reinforced by the pleasure or relief from frustration it provides. Thus, our goal is not to 'remove' or eliminate the coping modes, but to help the client gain more flexible, context-dependent control over them. We teach clients to acknowledge and respect the mode-system in place, whilst negotiating for more access to the Vulnerable Child part, to enable healing to occur.

In this chapter, several strategies for bypassing coping modes will be described in detail: labelling, interviewing coping modes, chairwork to bypass coping modes, and empathic confrontation. However, these dialogues between therapist and coping mode could equally well be carried via imagery work, whereby the client closes their eyes and is asked to 'play the voice of the side that doesn't want to do imagery rescripting'. In some cases, just asking the client to close their eyes and allow an image of their 'little self' to arise will automatically bypass coping modes, thereby eliminating any need for direct dialogue with the coping mode. In the example in Box 11.1, the therapist discovered the context in which Frank's coping mode emerged. This information provided the foundation for the therapist to show a deep level of understanding when dialoguing with the coping mode through chairwork or empathic confrontation.

Box 11.1 Clinical Example of Coping Mode and Its Development

Frank described a childhood characterised by loneliness, disconnection, and lack of belonging. His parents worked long hours, and Frank's needs often went 'under the radar', with minimal opportunities for family connection or expression of emotional needs (Emotional Deprivation, Emotional Inhibition schemas). His parents relied heavily on alcohol on weeknights as a means of unwinding from work. Frank recalled frequent parties on weekends, where the house would be full of adults intoxicated with alcohol. He never quite felt that he belonged, either within his family or within his peer group in his rural hometown (Social Isolation schema). Most of the boys in his peer group played football, and this was the focus for all community activities and most conversations. Frank, on the other hand, was a sensitive child. He had no interest in sport but was creative and aspired to become an artist or interior designer. He described feeling a lack of acceptance, value, and belonging, and craved approval and recognition for his achievements (Approval Seeking schema).

Frank coped with his loneliness through distraction; he escaped into books, online gaming, and comfort eating (Detached Self-Soother/Self-Stimulator mode). Once he reached early adolescence, his gaming time gradually increased to the point where he often stayed up all night and spent entire weekends playing, barely leaving the house except to attend school. Frank became increasingly competitive, seeking the thrill of winning a game and enjoying the sense of achievement and admiration from peers. By the time he attended therapy in his mid-twenties, he described a longstanding 'addiction' to gaming. He experienced relationships and life outside of the gaming world to be unsatisfying and 'boring'. Further, he had become increasingly isolated from his 'real-world' peers, leading to social anxiety and loneliness when not gaming. Frank described feeling ambivalent about working on his addiction; it had become his sole source of connection with the world, and his only means of accessing recognition and acceptance. Frank's Detached Self-Soother also blocked his capacity to attend therapy sessions regularly, and he frequently cancelled at the last minute due to feeling exhausted following all-night gaming sessions.

In the example in Box 11.1, Frank's Detached Self-Soother/Stimulator mode had become a source of both comfort and escape from his lonely childhood, and partially compensated for unmet needs of belonging and approval. Over time, it became an entrenched coping mode that was strongly reinforced by recognition from peers for his gaming prowess. Furthermore, the emotional 'high' of intermittently winning compensated for the lack of feelings of warmth and joy associated with unmet needs for connection, warmth, and care. The pleasure and relief offered by this form of detached self-stimulation became increasingly intertwined and led to Frank relying on gambling as a safe means to access company while avoiding anxiety about being rejected or seen as 'different' in a real-life setting.

Labelling, Bypassing, and Interviewing Coping Modes via Chairwork

During the early phase of schema therapy, coping modes often present as the 'default' mode in sessions, presenting a façade that largely keeps the child modes at a distance. It is easy to be blindsided by coping modes that mimic the Healthy Adult mode, such as by giving the appearance of being highly rational, logical, independent, and even successful. However, further investigation will reveal that if the client is inhabiting a coping mode, they do not access and share their more vulnerable thoughts and feelings, or show themselves compassion, as they would if they were inhabiting their Healthy Adult mode. It is the therapist's job to recognise and negotiate with the 'front stage' coping modes to bypass them and to reach the Vulnerable Child mode which has been relegated to 'back stage' (i.e., outside of conscious awareness).

After roughly three to six sessions, once the therapeutic alliance is strengthening, the therapist can begin to draw clients' awareness to modes as they appear in session and invite the client to label them using their own vernacular. For example, labels such as 'the Security Guard', 'the Wall', or 'the Smokescreen' are common names the client might come up with for the Detached Protector mode. The 'Alcoholic Haze' or 'Binge Trance' are typical names for the Detached Self-Soother. Ideally, the function or the felt sense of the mode is captured in some way by the label. Next, key identifying features of the coping mode are explored, including its felt sense in the body, somatic signs, typical mental state, thoughts, feelings, and behavioural urges or action tendencies. These might be written on a whiteboard or handout. The client is invited to monitor their modes between sessions, such as through a schema-mode diary, self-monitoring circle, or mode-schema pie chart [1]. In session, the therapist can use a chair to represent the client's coping mode, to set up a dialogue with it. By

Detached Protector Mode

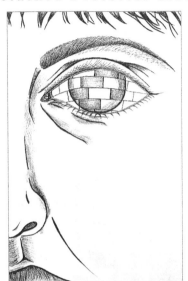

Illustration 11.1 Detached Protector mode

inviting the client to move back and forth between the Vulnerable Child and Coping Mode chair, they can begin the process of differentiating between these sides of self. Through inviting the client to physically move, we are making their implicit internal processes explicit. This enables them to begin to disidentify from the maladaptive messages of the coping mode, and to increasingly identify with their Vulnerable Child side. The case example in Box 11.2 provides an illustration of this process.

In the exercise illustrated in Box 11.2, the therapist negotiates with the coping mode and addresses its main concerns. If the main concern is that they will be flooded with emotions (in the case of a Detached Protector or Overcontroller mode driven by an Emotional Inhibition schema), the therapist can reassure the client that they can learn to experience emotions again gradually, whilst building new strategies for managing their intensity, such as safe/calm place imagery and positive imagery. Similarly, if the client fears that they will lose control of their behaviour (e.g., self-harm), then the therapist can reassure them that they will learn new healthier ways to contain the intensity of their emotions. If the client fears that the therapist will humiliate and shame them for showing their vulnerability (as in the case of a Paranoid Overcontroller mode driven by a Mistrust/Abuse schema), then the therapist must validate the existence of their concern (that it is understandable that they learned this from previous relationships) but also gently teach the client to question the validity of the fear in this situation. The therapist can ask the client whether they have noticed any indications that the therapist will humiliate or ridicule the client. The therapist must reassure the coping mode that they will not ever intentionally hurt the client, but also

---

Box 11.2 Clinical Example of Bypassing the Coping Mode via Chairwork

Over the course of her assessment, Marisa described several traumatic experiences through-out childhood, including emotional neglect, sexual abuse, and witnessing domestic violence between her parents, followed by being raped and a terminated pregnancy during adoles-cence. She described her current life as a 'rollercoaster', marked by chaotic and incontrollable changes in mood and episodes of impulsivity and parasuicidal behaviours. As she recalled these events during childhood, she appeared emotionally numb and unaffected by the traumatic events she described. Her tone of voice was flat, with no obvious sign of distress, almost as though she were talking about someone else's life. In session six, the therapist expanded on the concept of modes.

THERAPIST: Marisa, I'd like to share with you something that I notice as you are telling me about the troubles and emotional struggles that you have suffered. There seems to be a side of you that appears to be slightly detached from your feelings as you are talking . . . like this side is protecting you from feeling too much . . . almost as though its job is to carry on with 'business as usual', even in the face of highly distressing situations. I wonder if this is something you might have noticed at all?

MARISA: What do you mean? . . . This is me. This is who I am.

THERAPIST: Oh yes, it is you, but only one part of you. And just to reassure you, this is no criticism at all . . . you might not realise, but as humans we are not just one-dimensional creatures. We all have several different parts that make up who we are. These parts all come to the surface at different times, depending on what is needed. And in this situation, as you are telling me about difficult parts of your life, I am noticing one part of you.

For example, I have a confident outgoing part of me that I can access when I am teaching. And at other times, when I am with my partner or my family, I might be more in touch with my spontaneous, fun side. Or, if I have had some upsetting news, but then need to attend a meeting, I have a side that can 'carry on' and focus on what is important without getting too caught up in my emotions. Does that fit with your experience at all, where different parts are stronger at different times? *[Marisa nods.]* At the moment, as you are telling me about some really painful memories, it makes sense that the side of you that detaches from feelings might get stronger, to protect you. But it can feel a little bit like talking to you through an interpreter that doesn't want me to get too close. I wonder if we could try a chair exercise where we find out more about that side . . . would that be okay?

MARISA: I guess so, I don't really see the point but . . . I'll give it a go.

THERAPIST: *[smiling]* Ok, thank you for indulging me with this strange technique! So, over here we have a chair that is for your Detached side that doesn't really want to talk about or express feelings. If we gave that part a name, what would it be called? Like 'the Wall', or 'the Security Guard', or something else?

MARISA: Well . . . maybe the 'Snow-Storm'? It's like everything in my mind is in white-out, and I'm numb and don't have to think about anything.

THERAPIST: Perfect, that makes sense! Let's call it the Snow-Storm mode. Can we put that side on this chair here, and this other chair that you are on now will be the Vulnerable Child chair . . . to represent the side of you that has the feelings. This is 'Little Marisa'. Now, I am going to ask the empty Snow-Storm chair some questions: 'I know that you are here to protect Marisa, and I completely respect that. I would like to find out more about Marisa's feelings, so I can connect with her more and help her to learn some healthy ways of managing emotions. I wonder if you might tell me what you are afraid will happen if you allow her to tell me about her emotions?' *[Therapist turns to Marisa.]* Marisa, could you go over to that chair to reply, trying your best to be that side that doesn't want to think or talk about it . . . what would it say?'

MARISA: *[reluctantly moves]* I don't know . . . I guess that the problem is that it will be like a can of worms. Once I start feeling, it will all come flooding out. And I won't ever be able to stop. And when my feelings get strong, that is when trouble happens, like when I self-harm and end up in hospital.

THERAPIST: Ok, thank you, that makes sense. Can you move back to the Little Marisa chair now so that I can reply to this detached side? *[Marisa returns to Vulnerable Child chair, next to the therapist.]*

THERAPIST: *[addressing the empty chair]* Snow-storm, I can see you are working hard to protect Marisa, and you have been a big help throughout her life. You have helped her to survive all sorts of traumas. I respect that, and I want to reassure you that I am not trying to get rid of you. You have an important role in her life. But I can also see that it's a heavy job for you to be working so hard all the time, protecting her all on your own. And I can see that the painful feelings underneath are still there, as she has never had the chance to learn healthy ways of managing them. I wonder if it might be possible to allow me a little window of time with her, just a few minutes, so that I can start to help her with those painful emotions. Would that be possible?

[Therapist turns to Little Marisa's chair] What is it like for you to hear me talk to that protector side from your Little Marisa side?

MARISA: It feels kind of weird. And a little bit scary.

THERAPIST: That is totally understandable. You've rarely had the opportunity to talk about your feelings, and from what you've told me, when you were a young child, there was no one there to support you with your feelings. So, you created this detached Snow-Storm part to protect you by shutting down the emotions. But I want to get to know this side of you, and to find out more about what it was like for you to go through those experiences. There is a part of you that is suffering, and I am here by your side to help you with those feelings of sadness and hurt. We can just do it a tiny bit by bit, at your pace. And each session you can decide how much you want to say. Would that be okay?

MARISA: I guess I could try.

that they recognise that it will take time for the client to trust them. In short, the therapist must listen to and address the fears of the coping mode.

To understand the coping mode better and build trust, the therapist can also ask questions and ask the client to reply from the coping mode chair. A coping mode can also be interviewed, to learn about its function, both in the past and the present, and to begin the process of getting to know it as an 'old friend' which made sense in the context of their childhood circumstances (see Box 11.3).

It is important to make the links between coping mode avoidance and unmet childhood emotional needs explicit for clients. Our goal is to help them recognise that the role of coping modes is to prevent schema activation. For example, in the earlier example, Marisa's Detached Protector mode is protecting her from a fear of being overwhelmed and all alone

Chairwork with a Detached Protector

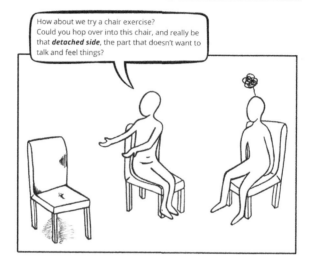

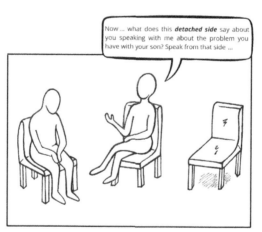

Cartoon 11.1 Chairwork with the Detached Protector

with her emotions. Our goal is to help Marisa understand that the reason her coping mode is working so hard to protect her from this fear is that her needs for nurturance, warmth, and attunement weren't met in childhood so she continues to expect this will be the case within current adult relationships, including with the therapist. Once the client understands this link, it opens up opportunities to explore ways in which – in spite of its good intentions – the coping mode is, in practice, blocking the client's capacity to get their needs met, thereby

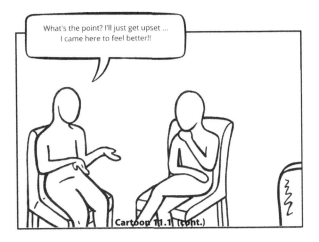

What's the point? I'll just get upset ... I came here to feel better!!

Cartoon 11.1 (cont.)

Cartoon 11.1 (cont.)

Box 11.3 Clinical Example of Interviewing the Coping Mode

THERAPIST: Frank, I wonder if we could get to know this side of you a little more? Let's bring in an extra chair, and on this chair *[therapist points to empty chair]* I can see the gaming side of you sitting there in my mind's eye. I'd like to ask that side some questions to get to know it a bit better, if that's okay with you? And if it's okay with you, you could either tell me what it's saying, or move over to the chair and reply from that side of you. Would that be okay?

- When did you come into Frank's life?
- How did you help him in the past?
- Can you tell me how you protected him in the past? What kinds of things did you do to provide protection?
- Did you help him to feel better about himself in any way?
- Was there anything difficult going on that you were trying to distract him from?
- What were you trying to give him that he needed and wasn't getting enough of back then?
- And what about now that he is older ... how are you helping him now?

---

perpetuating the schema. The therapist can then help the client to explore ways of meeting these needs more effectively in the here and now.

The therapist can also check in regularly with the client's coping modes to 'show respect' for the role the Protector parts play in the client's life. For example: 'I'd like to suggest that we do some imagery or chairwork today, and I want to check in with you as to whether you have a preference, and also whether your Protector parts would be on board with us doing that?' The coping modes often feel less threatened if they feel heard and respected. On the other hand, the therapist must balance the need to slow the pace of work sufficiently to allow the client to feel safe, while also pursuing the overarching goal of maximising access to the Vulnerable Child in therapy, to ensure healing exercises can occur. This 'checking in' process is an example of the highly collaborative nature of schema therapy, which in turn is a robust transtheoretical predictor of client outcomes in therapy [2].

Mode-bypassing exercises may need to be persistently repeated for many weeks or months until the therapist starts to build enough trust that the client can be more open and show their vulnerable side more willingly. Mode interviewing of the type described earlier can be carried out with any coping mode. Mode dialogues can also be conducted via imagery, whereby the client is asked to get an image of the side that doesn't want to do the imagery work. The therapist asks the client to 'be that side and tell me why that side thinks it's a bad idea to do the imagery'. The goal is not to have a long conversation with the coping mode, but to have the client access their emotional responses. Once the client is feeling emotion, the therapist can proceed with limited reparenting, via any of the experiential techniques.

Bypassing Coping Modes When the Client Believes They Don't Have a Vulnerable Side

In some cases, the coping modes are so effective at keeping the Vulnerable Child mode outside of the client's conscious awareness that the client can struggle to recognise the existence of this side of themselves. The client might talk about difficult circumstances or situations, but in a detached manner. The therapist can begin to introduce the vulnerable side through the 'Contamination of the Chair' exercise, illustrated in Box 11.4.

Box 11.4 Contamination of the Chair to Access Vulnerable Child Mode

THERAPIST: *[talks to client in Protector chair]* I understand that there is this side of you that is most comfortable being in the 'Protector' mode, but today I'd like to explore a way of helping you in a completely different way from just blocking the feelings. So, I have brought in an empty chair. What I would like you to do is to stand up and leave this 'Protector' chair and move over to this other chair. When you do, just notice if you can leave the Protector side behind and come over here to sit next to me. *[Client moves to Vulnerable Child chair.]*

THERAPIST: *[talks to client in Vulnerable Child chair, gesturing toward the Protector chair]* I understand that this side is just trying to protect you but I also hear it talking about feeling lonely and struggling. So over on this chair where you are now, I want to hear from the side that is feeling the loneliness and struggles.

MARISA: No, it feels the same to me.

THERAPIST: Can you maybe try to connect to the emotional side that feels lonely and upset? What were you feeling upset about?

MARISA: Nothing really, it doesn't feel different over in this chair.

THERAPIST: That's okay. I can hear that this Protector side is still here, so can you move back to the Protector chair that blocks the feelings? And I will sit in the Vulnerable chair *[therapist moves]*. In this chair, I will really try to keep connected to the five-year-old child that you showed me in the photographs. And that she is all alone and was often alone. When others paid attention to her, it was with anger. It makes me so sad to think of her. If I was that child, I would feel so lonely, like no one is there for me and the only ones who give me attention get angry with me. I feel sad in my stomach. I want people to be kind to me, warm to me.

Okay, now I will move back to my chair. And I wonder if you can move back to the Vulnerable chair and sit next to me again? When you come back to this chair, can you recall what I was talking about?

MARISA: Well, it was about when I was small. And not being treated very well.

THERAPIST: And when you focus on that time of your life, what comes up for you?

MARISA: Well, it was hard, I felt sad a lot.

THERAPIST: And can you remind me what was making you so sad?

MARISA: No one was around to look after me.

THERAPIST: Yes, that makes sense. And when I was on the chair, I also mentioned the sense that this child needed something different. Can you remember that?

MARISA: I wanted my family to take care of me.

THERAPIST: When you say that now, what feelings come up for you?

MARISA: Sadness.

THERAPIST: Where do you notice it in your body?

MARISA: Here [gestures toward heart].

THERAPIST: It makes sense that you would feel that. You are such a kind and sensitive person, Marisa. This is normal that you need others to be kind and warm for you. I want to be here for you. Together, you and I can be here together with these feelings, rather than you being on your own with them. How does that feel for you ... different from being over in that [Protector] chair?

Another version of chairwork that can be particularly useful when clients are unable to recognise the impact of their coping modes on their lives is when the therapist plays the role of the client's Vulnerable Child mode. In this exercise, the therapist's agenda is to express the emotional pain and longing that they sense is underneath the coping mode. The goal is for the client to begin to recognise and acknowledge that perhaps these 'back stage' emotions and needs linked to their Vulnerable Child mode do exist. The expression of these needs by the therapist once again makes the implicit *explicit* and reinforces their validity. Through this chairwork exercise, the therapist implicitly gives the client 'permission' to express needs and feelings which they previously denied. The therapist also aims to show the client's Vulnerable Child side that, despite them remaining hidden, they are seen and heard by the therapist. This method can also be a useful way of highlighting the impact of compulsive and/or addictive behaviours in covering emotional suffering and needs, as is illustrated in the example in Box 11.5 with Frank.

In the exercise in Box 11.5, the therapist draws on her knowledge (from earlier sessions) that Frank has been feeling lonely, depressed, and disconnected. Although Frank is currently unable to articulate or acknowledge this in therapy, the therapist recognises that the

---

Box 11.5 Clinical Example of Therapist Playing the Vulnerable Child Mode

THERAPIST: Frank, we talked last time about your plans to talk with your mum again. You mentioned that you were anxious that it was going to be a difficult conversation. I was wondering how you got on with that?

FRANK: It was fine. I don't really want to talk about it. I've barely had any sleep and I can't think straight. Maybe we could talk about something else today.

THERAPIST: Okay, I respect that, and we can easily do that, but before we do, I wonder if we can slow things down so that I can understand what is happening just now for you? When you say you didn't get much sleep, can you tell me more about that?

FRANK: Well, I had some all-night gaming sessions, and, if I'm honest, I was also binge eating quite a bit this week, and now it's hard for me to concentrate on anything.

THERAPIST: That sounds really difficult for you, Frank, and I can totally see why it feels too hard to talk about anything too triggering today. There is one side of me that just wants to let this go, but there is another side of me that cares a great deal about Little Frank . . . the side of you that really wanted to connect with your mum this week, and so I want to make sure that he still gets some airtime.

FRANK: No, honestly, I have been fine, apart from the lack of sleep.

THERAPIST: I'm not sure if I'm getting this right, but something that I noticed is that your gaming and bingeing compulsions sometimes get stronger when there are difficult feelings that have been triggered. It's almost as if they are working harder to keep the feelings underground. Can you relate to that?

FRANK: Not really.

THERAPIST: I wonder if we could try a brief chairwork exercise where we explore that a bit more – would that be okay with you? *[Frank nods reluctantly.]*

[NB: Chairs arranged as in Figure 11.1]

THERAPIST: Can I ask you to move to the coping mode chair and be that side that thinks the gaming and bingeing is a good idea? I want you to do the best you can at representing that side. I will move to sit in the Little Frank chair, and I will try to represent that side of you. Okay?

THERAPIST: *[as Little Frank]* When you don't let me talk about my feelings, I find it hard. I'm feeling really sad and lonely, but I have no one to talk to.

FRANK: *[a coping mode with therapist prompting]* Yeah whatever, it's not that bad. Just get over it.

THERAPIST: *[as Little Frank]* But when you keep gaming and bingeing, it makes me feel like you are pushing me away, like you don't care what I think. It makes me even more lonely.

FRANK: Oh, come on, it's no big deal. I enjoy gaming. Why shouldn't I have a good time? There's no harm in it.

THERAPIST: *[as Little Frank]* To me it is a big deal. And when you say that, I feel sad – like I'm not a big deal, like I don't matter. I want to talk about what happened this week. I want help to manage these feelings. I don't want to keep feeling like this. I don't want you to keep pushing me away, just like so many others have done in my life.

    [Therapist stands up to stand outside of the chair circle, and invites Frank to join her.]
Frank, just to step outside of this interaction for a minute, I'm just wondering what it's like for you to hear me speak from this little side of you?

FRANK: Well, this part of me doesn't really want to hear it. It just wants to keep blocking it out. But it does make sense. I can sort of see what you mean. There is a part of me that didn't feel great about this week.

THERAPIST: Ok, I know it's really hard to talk about it, but I also know that I don't want Little Frank having to cope on his own with these difficult feelings that come up when you talk to your mum. I wonder if you could move over to this [Little Frank] chair, so that this side of you could say a bit about what you've been feeling? Would that be okay? I'll be right here with you.

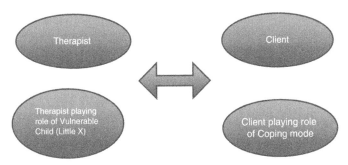

Figure 11.1 Chair arrangement for therapist playing the vulnerable child

first step toward recovery and reconnection is that Frank will need to acknowledge the existence and suffering of his vulnerable side. When the therapist takes on this role from a vulnerable yet persistent stance, it can provide validation to the voice of the client's 'little' side which has, until now, remained hidden.

Empathic Confrontation to Bypass Coping Modes

Empathic confrontation can be a powerful method to bypass extreme coping modes that drive therapy-interfering behaviours. Such behaviours include frequently missing or arriving late at therapy sessions, acting in contempt of the therapist's rights and boundaries (e.g., putting feet on the therapist's table, taking phone calls during sessions), being overly compliant to please the therapist at the expense of describing authentic feelings, and avoiding experiential therapeutic work.

Marisa's Angry Protector mode became activated when the therapist gently nudged her toward chairwork: 'I really don't see the point in this stupid exercise, or any of this work for that matter. You keep talking about the past . . . what's the point?! I've talked about it before and it doesn't help. And nor does this crazy talking to chairs business!' Typical fears that drive this type of hostile response include: fear of being rejected and/or abandoned; fear of being misunderstood; fear of revealing perceived weakness or flaws; fear of loss of control or becoming overwhelmed and being unable to function; fear of being unable to satisfactorily perform the exercise and therefore being a 'failure'; fear of triggering feelings of guilt or punitive responses from others as a result of breaking loyalties, casting parents in a negative light, or confessing secrets; fear of being controlled, coerced and compelled to subjugate; and fear of losing respect, 'one-up' status, or perceived specialness [3]. The therapist's role is to ask questions to identify the intention and function of the coping mode, as well as the current problems associated with staying in this mode. The more we can deepen our understanding, the more informed and prepared we will be to apply empathic confrontation as a method to reduce its negative impact.

The *implicit assumption technique*, developed by Behary [3], is based on the premise that the compulsion of the coping mode to detach from emotionally triggering experiences is based on implicit learning experiences early in life (see Box 11.6). The power of this technique draws on the therapist's capacity to make sense of these automatic coping mode reactions in the here and now, through 'making the implicit explicit'. By making sense of the various reactions of the mode under a range of activating circumstances, the client is helped to link the coping mode with early experiences which have become over-learned to the point of operating automatically, outside of conscious awareness. Once the client understands the implicit learning that drives their reactions, the pathway becomes clear for the therapist to offer reparenting messages that provide for healing of the

---

Box 11.6 Implicit Assumption Technique

THERAPIST: Something I am noticing, Marisa, is that while this 'Snow-Storm' side of you is front stage just now, I can't help but wonder whether Little Marisa is feeling afraid or under threat. I feel the force of the 'Storm' – which won't allow me to reach in to connect with Little Marisa, and also forbids her from coming out of her solitary confinement. I sense that Little Marisa must be very scared, as I can sense that security guard is fierce. And that makes sense, when I think about what you have told me about your background ... that allowing anyone else to see your vulnerable side and trying something new opens you up to being humiliated and put down ... just like when you were little and your dad and brothers would put you down or laugh at you when you showed any emotion or spontaneity. So, I can imagine that the uncertainty of a new exercise like this might make this Snow-Storm side feel you are in dangerous territory?

Marisa, I'd really like to speak to this Snow-Storm side that is putting so much energy into guarding you.

[Therapist speaks directly to the empty chair assigned to the Snow-Storm mode]: Snow-Storm, firstly, thank you for working so hard to protect Little Marisa. As a little girl, she was powerless and so you showed her how to keep quiet about her feelings and needs, so that she would feel safe from being humiliated by others. But many years have passed; it is such a burden for her to carry around these old messages into her adult life – such that she is still not permitted to express her needs and feelings, to express her thoughts, desires, wishes, nor to stick up for herself when others overstep the mark by hurting her feelings. I understand that she went through much suffering in the past, but I'm concerned that she no longer needs to be carrying around this burden. You might not realise it, but she is not powerless anymore, and she no longer has to tolerate her father or anyone humiliating her as a means of elevating his own sense of power. I am here now, and I want to be able to help her, but to do this I need to connect with her, because this way of protecting her is only making her feel more lonely, powerless, and frustrated. She deserves to be heard, to say what she feels, without fear of being shut down. She needs to have a voice, to say what's on her mind without having to worry about how others will react. She is perfect and lovable the way she is – and she is allowed to be authentically herself without having to deal with judgements and criticism. I am here to stand up for her – and she also has her own strong Healthy Adult side who is more powerful than she knows – and set limits on others when she needs to. I wonder ... could you consider taking a rest from carrying around this old burden for a short while so that Healthy Adult Marisa and I can connect with Little Marisa ... so that she doesn't need to feel so lonely?

underlying schemas, and build novel, healthy ways of relating to others, to maximise the possibility of getting their needs met [3].

The power of empathic confrontation depends on the authenticity and compassion of the therapist as they attempt to connect with the client's inner world. The therapist needs to be genuinely curious about how coping mode responses are the direct result of implicit learning during childhood and adolescence. The therapist should remember that when the client hears the therapist really understanding both what they went through in childhood and how that felt, the very experience of being heard and understood is itself healing and uplifting. When clients see that another human being can hear about their experiences and tell them that things ought to have been better for them and that others won't necessarily neglect their needs the way their early caregivers did, it gives the client hope that perhaps they can get their needs met in the future. In Marisa's case, negotiating with her Detached/Angry Protector mode was an entry point for her to let go of old patterns of self-protection which were keeping her locked in a world of loneliness and isolation, and her tendency to self-harm as a way of channelling her despair. By recognising, understanding, and bypassing her coping mode, she was able to begin actively working at a deeper level, nurturing her Vulnerable Child self, challenging her Inner Critic mode, and developing a Healthy Adult self-respect that involved trusting her inner signals and setting limits on others in assertive ways without hostility.

In the initial stages of therapy, the therapist takes on the role of the Healthy Adult within mode dialogue work, and the client gradually learns to take on this role over the course of therapy by learning to recognise and work with their own parts. If the therapist does not consistently recognise and bypass the coping modes, it is easy to become stuck in 'chatting' about the problems, rather than therapeutically working on the issues. This is more likely to occur if the therapist's own coping modes are present and the therapist's and client's coping modes (e.g., Detached Protector modes) collude to avoid working on emotions. Therapists must consistently check in with clients to ensure that they are connecting with their vulnerable side, by regularly enquiring about their current emotional state throughout sessions, especially during experiential exercises. If the client is in a coping mode, the potential benefits of techniques such as imagery rescripting and limited reparenting will be lost and the client will be unable to absorb the healing messages.

Concluding Remarks

It is often stated in schema therapy training workshops that 'a session in Detached Protector is a wasted session'. Although it is important to recognise that coping modes were needed as survival mechanisms earlier in the client's life, we also help the client recognise that these ways of coping are the result of outdated implicit learning, which now keeps them isolated and trapped in a self-perpetuating loop. In the present, coping modes block the client's capacity to emotionally connect with others and to achieve fulfilment of their needs. In schema therapy, experiential techniques are emphasised because information processing is enhanced in the presence of affect. All the methods and techniques described in this book rely on the schema therapist empathically bypassing any coping modes that block the client from experiencing their Vulnerable Child mode. Schema therapy relies on the client inhabiting Vulnerable Child mode to receive limited reparenting and corrective emotional experiences and messages that counteract outdated schema-driven messages. As this process unfolds in the therapy room, there is potential for the client to open up to new and unexpected ways of developing a revitalised capacity to connect with others in their own lives.

References

1. Farrell J, Shaw I. *Experiencing schema therapy from the inside out: A self-practice/self-reflection workbook for therapists.* Guilford Press; 2018.

2. Ardito R, Rabellino D. Therapeutic alliance and outcome of psychotherapy: Historical excursus, measurements, and prospects for research. *Frontiers in Psychology.* 2011;2:270.

3. Behary W. The art of empathic confrontation and limit-setting. In Heath G, Startup H, eds. *Creative methods in schema therapy: Advances and innovation in clinical practice.* Routledge; 2020. pp. 227–36.

Chapter 12

Preparing for Termination and the End Phase of Schema Therapy

Introduction

It is common that as the therapy approaches the ending phase, challenges emerge; as such, it can be easy for clients to fall back into their old schema-maintaining behavioural patterns. In these moments, clients may seem unable to continue independently without the support of therapy. This chapter discusses the way in which the end phase might be carried out, how the therapeutic stance of limited reparenting changes during this phase, and how the therapeutic strategies are implemented differently as compared to the earlier phases. Furthermore, we will review some common problems and challenging situations schema therapists might encounter in this end phase.

Introducing the Reality That Therapy Will End

As much as the schema therapist is an agent of limited reparenting, becoming a source of support for the client to help meet their needs, the reality is that the therapy will not last forever. The client will need to eventually learn to take care of their own needs and find healthy ways of connecting with their needs in 'real life'. The therapy plan created in the case conceptualisation phase clarifies to both therapist and client how important the ending phase is and when it might begin. Periodic evaluation or discussion of this plan is required, especially during the middle phase of treatment, so that the client remains aware of this reality. If no such timetable has been explicitly outlined, it is important that the therapist signals this ending phase well before the actual end of therapy occurs. The mention of the end of therapy can have a strong schema-activating effect, with the client feeling over-whelmed by feelings of fear, abandonment, and possibly anger. Timely reminders about the eventual end of therapy, and the ending phase, gives the client the opportunity to get used to this idea whilst there is still enough time in therapy to work through any issues or feelings that arise. In this way, the client learns that the therapist is there for them to help meet their needs, but this relationship exists in the service of change and building their autonomy, rather than to foster an unhealthy dependence.

The therapist will eventually have to make the reality of the ending of therapy definite, which will require answering many of the following questions:

1. How long will the therapy last before the final session takes place?
2. How many more sessions will be planned?
3. What issues and topics will be discussed in the time available?
4. What happens when we say goodbye? Will the client still be able to get in touch after the therapy has ended?

It is not necessary that all these questions be answered at once; rather, they are aspects of the final phase that will likely arise and require careful attention. We recommend that, as a rule, the therapist sticks to any agreements regarding timeframes and does not drop them too quickly because of an impulse to calm the client's activated schemas. After all, the goal of therapy is that the client must learn to handle their schemas in real life.

Objectives of the Final Phase

The objectives of the final phase often involve breaking through negative behavioural patterns (see Chapter 9) to strengthen the Healthy Adult mode (see Chapter 10) and to anticipate and overcome future problems and obstacles. Breaking out of patterns of behaviour means reducing old coping styles, such as avoidance, surrender, and overcompensation. Without an actual change in behaviour, the chance of relapsing into old patterns is very high. Strengthening the Healthy Adult mode means that the client becomes better at maintaining this mode in situations that inevitably activate schemas. Preparing for future problem situations is, in a sense, the formulation of a relapse prevention plan that is practised in advance with the help of imagery exercises and role-plays. These goals of the final phase of treatment have some implications for the therapeutic relationship, and the methods and techniques undergo a change in emphasis to meet these objectives.

Implications for the Therapeutic Approach

The role of the therapist in limited reparenting changes over the phases in the same way as the role of a parent changes as a child grows up and develops. In this comparison, the final phase of therapy is analogous to early adolescence. It is during adolescence that children need to be encouraged to apply what they have learned in childhood. In the final phase of treatment, the role of the therapist is more like a coach on the sidelines actively urging and 'pushing' for a change in behaviour whilst ultimately leaving responsibility for changes with the client. This change in attitude first requires an awareness of the need for it – an awareness that autonomy and competence in this phase are strengthened not by a therapist who takes over and determines what happens, but by one who is instead offering the client space to handle their own schemas or modes.

In concrete terms, this change in the therapist's attitude may manifest in them asking more open questions and respecting the client's answers. Respect, however, does not mean uncritically accepting the client's choices. Pushing for autonomy may mean that the therapist shows frustration or some mild irritation more openly when the client relapses into old patterns. Showing these emotions is a rather provocative tactic to encourage the client to fortify their efforts to change old maladaptive habits. This can again be likened to the frustration and irritation a parent might feel as the natural consequences of times such as when an adolescent drops his coat on the floor again when entering the house. They serve as a natural stimulus to encourage the child to do as they have been taught.

See Box 12.1 for an illustration of the therapist limited reparenting response as it may apply in the ending phase of treatment.

Implications When Using Methods and Techniques

In the final phase of therapy, the same cognitive, experiential, and behavioural techniques are applied as in the earlier phases of treatment. However, the aim of these interventions is now to strengthen the Healthy Adult part of the client and to break through behavioural

---

Box 12.1 Clinical Example of Therapist Limited Reparenting Response in Ending Phase of Schema Therapy

The client talks about the past week and how she has been feeling anxious and sad. She talks about feeling that this will never change and that she is not making any progress.

CLIENT: *[angry, frustrated in talking about herself]* I can't do it, I just can't! Whatever I do, I always fail, I'm really useless!

THERAPIST: Okay, okay ... who do I hear now?

CLIENT: I don't know!

THERAPIST: Well, I think you may have an idea who we hear when you talk about yourself like that ...?

CLIENT: I don't know! I really don't know! I don't know what you mean!

[In the early stages of therapy, the therapist would not have let the tension get to this point and would have certainly stepped in and indicated that they thought the Punitive Critic mode was active. But realising that this is the final phase of treatment, in combination with a felt frustration that the client again does not seem to recognise what has been discussed so many times before, the therapist chooses a more directive attitude.]

THERAPIST: I'm sorry, but I can't go along with that ... Who would I say is talking now ... which side of you? You know the answer to this ... you've heard me say that so many times, you know those words ...

CLIENT: That it is the Punitive side?

THERAPIST: Exactly! And why? How can you tell it's the Punitive side?

CLIENT: *[pauses, thinking]* ...

THERAPIST: That's alright, take your time, it's not an exam question but it is something to seriously think about .... and reflect on ...

---

patterns and teach new behaviour. The following sections present some examples of the way in which techniques are applied differently in the final phase.

Imagery Rescripting

In the final phase, imagery rescripting is used to prepare for future problem situations as discussed in Chapter 9. In an imagery exercise, future events can be 'previewed' in the same way that memories can be relived [1]. Future-oriented imagery can thereby lead to behavioural change [2]. Imagery rescripting (or, rather, in this context, future-confronting imagery) could therefore be an effective way of allowing clients to prepare themselves for future events and to have them practise a healthy way of reacting [3]. Future-oriented imagery rescripting can be used to support behaviour change in the following ways:

- to practise reconnecting to the Healthy Adult mode during schema activation
- to practise compassion when schemas are activated
- to learn to apply cognitive arguments against punitive self-evaluations or coping modes
- to practise new behaviour
- or a combination of these

The exercise works best if the therapist and the client discuss beforehand which new behaviour will be visualised because there are so many different possibilities. Also, if the client is clear about what they will visualise beforehand, there tends to be less need for the therapist to actively adjust or coach them during the exercise. See Box 12.2 for an illustration of future pattern-breaking imagery as it may apply in the ending phase of treatment.

Box 12.2 Clinical Example of Future Pattern-Breaking Imagery

Sandra regularly goes into her Detached Protector mode in her relationship with her boyfriend, which means she does not speak up about the things she does not like, such as the fact that he often goes out with friends without her. The therapist has discussed with her how she can try to contact her Healthy Adult in such moments and then say that she does not like it when he does not ask her to come out too.

THERAPIST: Good, now close your eyes and first get an image of that Healthy Adult, that captain on your ship. What do you see now?

CLIENT: Then I see myself back at work, when my boss asked me to do something that really wasn't my job and I said so.

THERAPIST: Fine, just see let it happen . . . just be that Big Sandra, the Sandra who says she doesn't want to do this job . . . how do you feel?

CLIENT: . . . Strong . . . confident . . .

THERAPIST: And where in your body is this feeling?

CLIENT: . . . Here . . . *[points to her chest]*.

THERAPIST: Lovely . . . let this feeling fill you, flow through you . . . and maybe you can adopt a posture that suits this strong, self-confident feeling . . .

CLIENT: *[sits up straight]*

THERAPIST: This is your Healthy Adult . . . Big Sandra . . . well, let this image fade away now . . . let it drift away and let the image of you and your boyfriend return . . . your boyfriend wanting to go out with his friends . . . it hasn't happened yet, but just let this film unfold as you expect it to . . . what do you see now?

CLIENT: I see him standing at the door, his jacket on and he says very casually that he will be away for the night . . .

THERAPIST: What do you feel when he says that?

CLIENT: . . . Sad . . . but also angry . . .

THERAPIST: Okay . . . and now I want to ask you to pause this image . . . at this moment . . . the moment your pleasing side takes over and you don't say what bothers you . . . I want you to bring in that Big Sandra now . . . be that Big Sandra, that Healthy Adult . . . good. Sit up straight . . . how do you feel?

CLIENT: . . . Yes, a little better . . . a little stronger . . .

THERAPIST: Good . . . so, what do you want to say?

CLIENT: . . . That I don't like him going out, without me . . .

THERAPIST: Say it to him.

CLIENT: . . . *[softly]* I don't really like it . . .

THERAPIST: How does this feel, does this feel like Big Sandra?

CLIENT: . . . No . . . *[with more force]* I don't like you going out without me!'

THERAPIST: Wow . . . how does this feel?

CLIENT: Yes, better . . .

Chairwork Dialogues

Chairwork can be used to strengthen the Healthy Adult during this phase. The therapist can take a seat in the chair of the coping mode or stand next to the chair of the parenting mode, which represent old messages. The client then confronts these messages from within their Healthy Adult and practices resisting the old beliefs of the coping or 'Critic' modes (see Box 12.3 for an illustration).

Box 12.3 Clinical Example of Chairwork to Strengthen Healthy Adult in Final Phase of Schema Therapy

THERAPIST: We have eight sessions to go and we have agreed to use this time mainly to prepare you for those situations in which your Protector threatens to take over. Isn't that right?

CLIENT: Yes, that is correct.

THERAPIST: And if you were to go back to the Pleasing side, what is your biggest concern, what could go wrong if you were to speak your mind?

CLIENT: Yes, I know him, then he will get moody and that will spoil the atmosphere and I don't want that.

THERAPIST: Like, if I give my opinion, he will get angry?

CLIENT: Yes . . .

THERAPIST: Good, then I want to work on that today, prepare you for those situations and practise now what you can do or say at those moments, okay?

CLIENT: Yes, that's fine . . .

THERAPIST: I want to do this again with the chair exercise we did earlier . . . *[takes a chair and places it opposite the client]* . . . but this time a little differently . . . This is the pleasing side *[points to the new chair]* and I will be sitting in this chair . . .

CLIENT: Oh?

THERAPIST: Yes, I will be the Pleaser and I would like to ask you to be the Healthy Adult, Big Sandra, to oppose me . . . *[sits down in the new chair]* . . . so here, I am the Pleaser; I find it very important to keep a peaceful atmosphere and I am willing to hold back my opinion *[points to the client's stomach]*. But you *[pointing to client's face]* are Big Sandra, that Healthy Adult. Maybe you can take a moment to step into that feeling . . . why not close your eyes for a moment . . .

Okay, and I, as your Pleasing Protector, say: 'All right, you don't like him going out with his friends again, but just let it go, otherwise he will be moody again and that is even more annoying.' Be that Big Sandra; why is holding back what you feel not the best thing to do?

CLIENT: . . . I don't know, I really hate it when he's moody, so I don't think it would help.

THERAPIST: *[laughing]* Now you're getting onto my chair! You can't do that, I'm there already. I could say what you said. Your job is to think about what Sandra really needs. Remember what she really needs?

CLIENT: . . . That she can be herself . . . and be heard and seen . . .

THERAPIST: Exactly, and is holding back her own opinion a good thing?

CLIENT: . . . No, I don't think so . . .

THERAPIST: Why not? Can you tell me directly: 'It's not good for Sandra because . . . .'

Cognitive Techniques

Compared to the initial and middle phases, cognitive techniques used in the final phase will increasingly resemble those used in regular cognitive therapy. Clients are required to fill in diary forms by themselves in which they investigate problem situations. In this phase, the responsibility for investigating and formulating more realistic thoughts is increasingly transferred to the client. The diary forms and the flashcards that are made can also begin to focus more on future problem situations.

Behavioural Techniques

Behaviour therapy is ideally designed to bring about behaviour change. Therefore, many methods and techniques from classical behaviour therapy can be applied in the final phase of schema therapy specifically aimed at behaviour change. Problem-solving strategies, role-playing, social skills training, self-control procedures, communication training, and applied relaxation exercises are some of the types of interventions that can be used in this phase of treatment. In contrast to regular cognitive-behavioural therapy, these exercises are linked to the modes from the case conceptualisation and are intended to strengthen the Healthy Adult in the ending phase of the treatment (see Box 12.4 for an illustration).

Box 12.4 Clinical Example of Behaviour Therapy Strategies Used in Final Phase of Schema Therapy

THERAPIST: In this last phase of the therapy, I would like to strengthen your captain as much as possible, so that in the future he will be able to handle all those crew members, that Punitive Critic, that Protector, and take good care of the needs of [name client]. After all, what is the most important thing in therapy – and also in life?

CLIENT: Basic needs.

THERAPIST: Exactly, basic needs, which you find with that emotional part, Little [name client]. And then what are the steps you need to take as captain of your ship?

CLIENT: First understanding, recognition, then standing up to that Punisher and Protector and then . . . uh . . . .

THERAPIST: Finally, you have to find your way in difficult practical situations. You really have to plan your course, and that is not always easy because you cannot always get what you need quickly. That is why it is called give and take . . . or compromising. In this process, it is important for you to know what you can say or do in situations with others. Because it is not easy to give your opinion when it is not exactly the same as that of others, is it?

CLIENT: . . . No . . .

THERAPIST: And that is why I want us to practise today how you actually do that, give your opinion when it clashes with that of others. Very practical; what do you say, how do you say it? Shall we practise this?

CLIENT: . . . Okay . . .

THERAPIST: Is there a situation that you know is coming up, in which this will happen in some way? That things will get so stressful that this Protector of yours might take over?

Saying Goodbye

The final phase concludes with saying an actual goodbye. Many clients do not have healthy experiences with saying goodbye – important attachment figures suddenly fell away, or contact was broken with a great deal of conflict or sadness and fear that was not attended to or cared for. Ending schema therapy therefore offers the opportunity to give the client a corrective emotional experience in which a goodbye is carefully planned and carried out. A healthy way of saying goodbye means looking back (reflecting) at the therapy process on the one hand, and looking forward to the future on the other.

Looking Back

We help clients reflect on the key question: What have you learned? Explicit attention is given to the changes that have been made. Allowing some space for clients to reflect together on what has been learned and experienced in therapy helps to consolidate their learning and hopefully leads to the client internalising this information within their Healthy Adult mode. Therapists should therefore take the time, possibly across several sessions, to consolidate all the information learned in therapy. To aid this process, the client can be given various homework assignments, such as to write down what they have learned, to check this list regularly, and add to it.

Looking Ahead

How can clients remember what they have learned and take it with them into the future? A transitional object can help the client remember important corrective emotional experiences after the goodbye. One example of a helpful transitional object is a list of all the learning experiences that the therapist and client have put together in the preceding sessions. Another example could be an object that the therapist gives to the client which represents the most important learning experience in the therapy, or the most important need that the client should keep in mind (see Box 12.5 for an illustration).

Box 12.5 Clinical Example of Using a Transitional Object when Saying Goodbye

In the last session, the therapist gives the client a phantom crystal; a piece of quartz in which you can vaguely see the shapes of the crystal that it had when it was growing.

THERAPIST: I would like to give you this. If you look closely, you can still vaguely see the shapes of the crystal when it was smaller. You're actually looking at the earlier generations of this crystal, the flawless crystal with smooth surfaces that it was in the past. But at a certain point, under the right conditions, a new layer starts to form on those smooth surfaces. At that time, it's a little rough; not as beautiful and shiny. But after some time, those shiny surfaces return; it is a beautiful crystal again, but bigger now, and more developed.

To me this is a symbol of your progress here: you came to me when things were a bit rough, and old forms – your old life – were all mixed up. That was a difficult phase for you. But you have persevered and grown over the past couple of years, and now there is more peace, more shine in your life. That old phase is still visible; there are vague memories of that difficult time. Whenever another intense period comes along, you will remember that growth may be a bit prickly and messy, but it also leads eventually to more shine.

What Will You Miss?

A topic that is often overlooked is to answer the question 'What will you miss?' Saying goodbye is letting go and it is important that the therapist pays attention to this pain of loss. Many clients have not received any support in dealing with pain of loss in their past. Acknowledging this pain, combined with an explicit understanding of it, is a healing form of compassion that allows the client to feel connected, understood, and seen. Within the professional framework of care, the therapist may indicate what they will remember best about the client.

Possible Problems and Challenges

In previous parts of this book, schema therapy has been referred to as a healing process in which stunted emotional development is released into motion, leading to a stronger, Healthy Adult part of the client who is capable of handling their various modes. The implicit expectation is that the client will develop with increasing stability into a Healthy Adult for whom a goodbye is prepared through mutual support.

The therapist should be prepared for the fact that clinical reality is often different. In the final phase, clients may appear irritated by the schema therapy model, the therapist, and the language of modes and basic needs. The contact with the client may therefore be difficult and it may seem as if the client is falling back into old patterns and making behavioural choices that seem unhealthy. A client may, for example, resume contact with an ex-boyfriend while many sessions in therapy have been spent trying to break free from this unhealthy relationship.

Such repetition of patterns that have taken so long to break through can easily evoke feelings of anxiety, frustration, and despondency in the therapist. The therapist must first of all be compassionate and understanding in recognising such feelings. Of course, it is frustrating or unsettling when contact with someone you care about seems to fall down again, and it is saddening when, for the umpteenth time, someone seems to be making choices that seem clearly unhealthy. Perhaps such feelings are better understood from the therapist's personal history and the schemas that developed from it and interact with it. Next, the therapist's thoughts of uncertainty, anger, or despondency need to be critically evaluated. This begins by recognising any modes within the therapist that may be influencing their reactions. Perhaps feelings of despondency arise from a critical, demanding side of the therapist believing that they should be able to take away all the client's problems. It is important for the demanding side of the therapist to recognise that with the client's increasing independence comes the client's right to make their own choices – even 'wrong' choices – just as adolescents who leave home make not-so-healthy choices while continuing to grow into healthy adults. Therapist supervision and self-reflective practice is especially important in evaluating these therapist reactions (see Chapter 18: Schema Therapy for the Schema Therapist).

When faced with clients who seem to be relapsing, it is tempting for therapists to abandon their plan to discharge the client and prolong therapy. This (understandable) urge should be resisted. Prolonging therapy does not guarantee that the client will resume making 'pleasing' life decisions. At this stage, it is usually best for the therapist to simply express their concern about the client's plans but leave responsibility for the choice with the client. At this stage of therapy – just as a parent might do with a young adult – the therapist supports the client's autonomy. The therapist can prompt the client to check whether their decisions are being generated by their Healthy Adult mode, something the client should be encouraged to continue to do when faced with decisions throughout their lives after therapy ends.

Concluding Remarks

The final phase of schema therapy rarely goes smoothly. The appropriate timing of when the end of therapy is announced and how this phase is handled makes a big difference in how successfully therapy is completed. The goals of the final phase are to strengthen the Healthy Adult mode, break through problematic behaviour patterns, and prepare the client for future problematic situations. The style of the therapist shifts more to coaching from the sidelines and pushing for actual behaviour change. Methods and techniques – often from traditional behaviour therapy – are used to strengthen the Healthy Adult mode and change schema-driven behaviour patterns. Imagery scripting can be applied to anticipated problematic situations in the future. Chairwork aims to strengthen the Healthy Adult mode via the therapist playing the role of parent and coping modes so that the client can practise their opposing arguments. The process of termination and working through a 'goodbye' means, on the one hand, giving attention to what has been learned and to what will be missed and, on the other hand, looking ahead to future problem situations. Transitional objects may be used to help remember insights and experiences.

References

1. Schacter D, Addis D, Buckner R. Remembering the past to imagine the future: The prospective brain. *Nature Reviews Neuroscience.* 2007;8(9):657–61.

2. Libby L, Shaeffer E, Eibach R, Slemmer J. Picture yourself at the polls. *Psychological Science.* 2007;**18**(3):199–203.

3. Van der Winjgaart, R. *Imagery rescripting: Theory and practice.* Pavilion Publishing & Media; 2021.

13

Schema Therapy for Chronic Depression and Anxiety Disorders

Introduction

In this chapter, we outline a schema therapy approach to mood and anxiety disorders wherein schema therapy may be considered a second-line treatment option for those cases in which (a) there is an inadequate response to first-line treatment (e.g., CBT) and/or (b) significant symptoms of personality disorder are assessed to be maintaining the severity or chronicity of illness, including treatment engagement and responsiveness. In most cases, schema therapy for depression and anxiety disorders is largely just schema therapy 'as usual'; however, there are several issues worth considering when applying the model to these problems and related disorders. We describe how schema therapy might be applied to the treatment of chronic depressive and anxiety disorders, either as a course of complete schema therapy or as a source of adjunctive components for a first-line approach.

When a Schema Therapy Approach to Anxiety and Depressive Disorders is Warranted

Due to its extensive research base, cognitive-behavioural therapy (CBT) is rightly considered a first-line psychological treatment for a plethora of psychological disorders. As discussed in Chapter 2, the evidence for schema therapy as a first-line treatment is strongest for personality disorders. With other high-prevalence disorders, once known as 'axis 1 disorders' (e.g., Major Depressive Disorder), evidence is now emerging for schema therapy as a second-line treatment in its own right [1, 2]. Proponents of schema therapy note that first-line treatments such as CBT for mood and anxiety disorders can have limited efficacy, especially among chronic sufferers [3]. Comorbidity and dropout is commonplace in everyday practice. Comorbid personality disorders and symptoms are also common [4] and predict treatment non-response [5, 6]. In his seminal book, Young noted that as many as 50–60% of clients treated with first-line cognitive therapy either do not respond satisfactorily to treatment or relapse within one year [3]. Meta-analytic studies have since shown that the efficacy of CBT for depression, for example, has been steadily decreasing over the three decades since Aaron Beck's seminal studies [7].

From a schema therapy perspective, treatments that focus only on presenting 'axis 1' problems often overlook patterns of avoidance and rigidity characteristic of underlying personality disorder pathology that can drive treatment non-response. This was – in no small way – part of the original motivation for the development of schema therapy: to address chronic treatment-resistant 'axis 1 problems' [3].

The application of schema therapy to mood and anxiety disorders can be approached in one of two ways. The first is to use schema therapy as a second-line treatment. Here, a complete schema therapy protocol is applied to a depressive or anxiety disorder; the disorder is conceptualised in terms of schemas and modes, the therapeutic relationship is characterised by limited reparenting, and the full range of schema therapy interventions is employed. For these situations, we refer to the rest of the book as an example of how to apply the model.

Alternatively, components of schema therapy can be used as adjuncts to first-line treatments to enhance their efficacy. For example, imagery rescripting targeting negative childhood memories has been proposed as a useful addition to the CBT treatment of social anxiety disorder [8]. Other CBT authors have also recognised the utility and promise of integrating chairwork dialogues into CBT [9]. In this case, the therapy remains a (relatively) short-term complaint-targeted treatment in which some of the language, concepts, and treatment techniques of schema therapy might be integrated without adopting a full schema mode conceptualisation or entering into an attachment (limited reparenting) relationship.

Schema Therapy Case Conceptualisation of Chronic Depression and Anxiety Disorders

As always, case conceptualisation is paramount to the idiosyncratic understanding and treatment of presenting concerns. In the following sections, we address conceptualising cases of depressive and anxiety disorders.

Depression and Related Syndromes

The types of psychological disturbance referred to as 'depression' or 'depressive disorder' share some core features (e.g., depressed mood); however, there is considerable heterogeneity between presentations. Some sufferers present as depressed alongside a seemingly intractable guilt, others with a sense of worthlessness or hopelessness. For some, there is strong suicidal ideation, while for others there is not. Another common experience is disconnection from positive affect such as interest, and low motivation. Some of these clients experience a loss of appetite, while others will overeat. Rarely will sufferers display all of the syndrome's criteria.

From a schema therapy perspective, the development and maintenance of depressive symptoms differs widely among clients. In one person, depression may be the result of being chronically overworked, whereas in another client the depression might have developed in the context of withdrawal from valued relationships and activities. We have seen other cases where some kind of grief reaction – long suppressed – is implicated in these set of symptoms. Therefore, there is no generic mode model that can be used with every depressed client. Clients who present as depressed will almost always present with their own combination of maladaptive modes. Case conceptualisation and mode mapping of depression is therefore idiosyncratic.

There is usually a unique combination of modes that interact as a causal *mode pathway* implicated in the development and maintenance of what we think of as depression. From this point of view, many of the modes described thus far in this book can be viewed as depressogenic risk factors. Consequently, we generally see little value in referring to depression as a separate mode – for example, 'your depressed side' – because it is unclear which mode or set of modes is being referred to. The critical maintaining factor in one client's depression could be the Punitive or Demanding Critic mode, whereas in another

Table 13.1 Common key modes and symptom/problem areas implicated in depression

Depression-Related Problem/Experience	Possible Mode(s)
Sadness, grief, loneliness, or isolation	Vulnerable Child
Mood irritability or anger	Angry Child, Angry Protector
Pathological guilt	Guilt-Inducing Critic
Self-criticism, worthlessness	Punitive Critic
Sense of 'pressure' or stress	Demanding Critic
Relationship problem – assertiveness	Compliant Surrenderer
Overworking	Overcontroller, Self-Soother
Avoidance and withdrawal	Avoidant Protector
Worry and rumination	Overcontroller (Over-analyser type)
Anhedonia, disconnect from positive affect, interest and motivation	Detached Protector
Helplessness and hopelessness	Helpless Surrender, Avoidant Protector
Stress/pressure/burnout	Perfectionistic Overcontroller mode, Demanding (Parent) Critic
Binge drinking (or other compulsive or addictive behaviour)	Detached Self-Soother, Impulsive Child
Suicidal ideation	Avoidant Protector

client it may be a strong Detached Protector. From the mode model, we also know that each mode requires differing treatment strategies, rendering the 'the Depressed side' mode less informative about what should be proposed in treatment. So, this is the heart of the schema therapy model of depression: depression can be understood as a toxic combination of modes. Schema therapists must work to map the unique set of modes, and their antecedents (e.g., developmental origins), as a part of case conceptualisation. Table 13.1 gives examples of links between specific modes and depression-related symptoms and problems.

Early Maladaptive Schemas in Chronic Depression

Specific schemas appear to be more common in presentations of depression [10, 11, 12]. Schemas hailing from the Disconnection and Rejection and Impaired Autonomy and Performance domains have been reported to correlate with depression severity [13]. The Emotional Deprivation, Self-Sacrifice, and Social Isolation schemas have been reported to mediate the relationship between physical abuse in the past and symptoms of depression in the present [14]. As a result of these schemas, the Vulnerable Child mode in depression will tend to present as lonely and isolated.

Depressed clients also commonly present to therapy in a very strong coping mode (e.g., Detached Protector, Helpless Surrenderer), and consequently it can be difficult for the therapist to make contact with the client's underlying needs and feelings (e.g., vulnerability). In this respect, there are similarities between depression and Cluster C personality disorders, which are also characterised by strong, rigid coping modes which sustain the pathology. In fact, many clients who present with chronic experiences of depression will be later assessed to have Cluster C (or other) comorbidity. The schema therapy approach to chronic depression thus mirrors that of Cluster C personality disorders. The therapist works within a pre-agreed treatment timeframe. In this way, having an explicit ending phase can provide additional motivation for the client to let go of their rigid coping modes and address their issues in therapy (see Chapter 12: Preparing for Termination and the End Phase of Schema Therapy for an overview).

Understanding and Conceptualising Elevated Mood States

Clients with depression and related problems will sometimes present with more elevated mood states characteristic of hypomania or outright mania – states that far exceed a mood improvement in response to treatment or recovery. Some clients will meet criteria for a bipolar disorder while others will not. Clients with severe mood elevation and bipolar disorder may require psychiatric evaluation as a first-line treatment and could be unsuitable for schema therapy. There is currently no evidence from randomised controlled trials demonstrating the safety or efficacy of schema therapy for clients with bipolar disorder. Yet, many clients with depression – and even personality disorders – will present with features of elevated mood states that do not feel full criteria for a manic or hypomanic episode. Beck, in his theory of modes, saw elevated mood states as somewhat the opposite of depression, which he called 'The Expansive mode' [15, 16]. In schema therapy, we often conceptualise such elevated mood states in the mode model as a kind overcompensation reaction to schemas typically responsible for depression (e.g., Failure, Defectiveness, Emotional Deprivation). Beliefs such as 'I am hopeless ... I should give up' are over-shadowed by overcompensatory beliefs such as 'I am superior ... I can do anything'. A mode characterised by grandiosity or superiority beliefs might be labelled as an 'Invincible Overcontroller mode' or a 'Superhuman mode' in a mode conceptualisation. Clients in this kind of mode might display expansive speech and over-productivity and present as overconfident and full of energy. This conceptualisation is consistent with studies reporting elevated EMS in bipolar disorder [11, 17] and risk for bipolar disorder [11], although, to date, a specific mode conceptualisation of bipolar disorder has not been empirically tested.

Anxiety Disorders

It is also possible to conceptualise anxiety disorders as a combination of modes, as we have demonstrated with depression. Anxiety disorders are characterised by both an overestimation of the risk of danger and an underestimation of one's capability to withstand or cope with danger [18]. Anxiety is often associated with the Vulnerability to Harm and Illness EMS, characterised by beliefs such as 'the world is a physically dangerous place, and I am particularly vulnerable to that danger' and the Mistrust/Abuse EMS (e.g., 'Others are out to harm, exploit or humiliate me'). Felt anxiety often presents as a Vulnerable Child mode. Beliefs associated with Unrelenting Standards, Failure, Defectiveness/Shame, and Dependence/Incompetence are also common and are often expressed as a Critic mode of one kind or another. The overestimation of danger can sometimes be conceptualised as a 'Warning or Alert coping mode', a subtype of the Overcontroller coping mode in which the client is alert to (or scanning) for disorder-related signs of danger in the environment. The client typically experiences the physiological signs of anxiety from the Vulnerable Child mode, which might also be more aptly labelled a Fearful or Anxious Child mode. Overt avoidance behaviour, characteristic of anxiety disorders, is conceptualised as an Avoidant Protector.

In obsessive compulsive disorder (OCD), overestimation of the risk of danger and the severity of that danger can also be framed as a Warning mode: a coping mode which functions to control risk, thereby protecting the Vulnerable Child against activation of the Critic. An overestimation of the personal responsibility (conceptualised as a Critic mode) for preventing danger is typical of this disorder, causing these clients to have developed extensive rituals to ensure that the specific risk has been controlled (the Warning mode). Box 13.1 lists examples of the overestimation of responsibility.

Feelings of guilt in OCD could result from the activation of a Guilt-Inducing Critic mode wherein the client takes a look at themselves in a problematic situation and blames themselves for potentially harmful outcomes. Themes of guilt and personal responsibility are of course common in OCD presentations [19]. An example of a complete OCD case conceptualisation is provided in Box 13.2.

Box 13.1 Examples of Overestimation of Personal Responsibility in OCD

'If I don't [description of compulsive behaviour], then:

- ... it will be my fault that my girlfriend becomes infected with AIDS/Coronavirus/[insert illness].'
- ... it will be my fault that there is a break in.'
- ... I might act on my aggressive or suicidal thoughts.'

Box 13.2 Example of OCD Case Conceptualisation

Child Mode:
- Scared of danger and the severity of the danger
- Scared of the guilt/responsibility

Guilt-Inducing, Punitive Parent Mode:
- Overestimation of personal responsibility

Control-Maintaining (Warning) Coping Mode:
- Overestimation of risk/severity of danger
- Scanning/hypervigilance behaviour for signs of danger or threat
- Ritualistic behaviour with the function of avoiding or reducing the perceived danger or the perceived responsibility.

Avoidant Protector:
- Avoids situations likely to trigger intrusive thoughts.
- Engages in distraction and thought suppression.

In social anxiety disorder, the sufferer is certain that they are defective because others find them strange. The belief 'I'm strange' can be conceptualised as having developed due to an (Other-Directed) Punitive Critic mode – which interprets other people's behaviour negatively – generating repetitive automatic thoughts such as 'they think you're weird'. These Critic-driven messages can then activate or maintain fear or shame, which becomes part of the network of the Child mode. When anxiety or fear is experienced or expressed by the client, this may in turn be judged negatively by the Critic mode, generating more fear or shame, and so forth. It is common for the Critic and Child modes to be stuck in a cycle of dysregulation that eventually ends in some form of maladaptive coping. Those with a diagnosis of social anxiety disorder will commonly employ an Avoidant Protector as a primary coping mode, perhaps alongside an Overanalysing Overcontroller mode (characterised by worry and post-event rumination).

The use of Mode Language and the Mode Model in Treating Depression and Anxiety Disorders

Use of mode language and creating mode awareness through identifying and naming modes is important for helping clients defuse from Critic mode activation and overwhelming child states. The rationale for using the language of modes is to help the client shift from viewing their thoughts as facts (e.g., 'I am stupid and worthless') to an observing perspective (e.g., 'I am suffering from that punitive voice telling me that I'm stupid and worthless'). Often the client's experience of anxiety or mood disturbance becomes their identity (i.e., 'I'm anxious'). Relabelling anxious thoughts and feelings as modes (which are, by definition, only a subset or component of, rather than the totality of, the person) helps clients reduce the dominance of these experiences and begins to build a sense of the self apart from those experiences. The mode model is – in a sense – a model of defusion. Symptom-related experiences are tagged, categorised, and sorted into their relevant 'modes', all of which aids in mode awareness. The client learns to inhibit or delay automatic patterns of responding and just notice or label aspects of their experience. Becoming aware of and learning to look at an experience first instead of simply undergoing that experience seems to be a necessary condition for a change process. In schema therapy, this is the first step towards building the Healthy Adult mode (see Chapter 10 for an overview).

The Importance of Conceptualising and Bypassing Repetitive Negative Thinking (Rumination, Worry, and Obsessive Thinking)

We have often spoken in this chapter in terms of 'disorders' as a way of clinical shorthand; however, schema therapy should be considered a transdiagnostic framework. The transdiagnostic approach of the mode model is very useful in conceptualising and intervening with comorbidity. One mode with central importance to the conceptualisation and treatment of chronic depression and an anxiety disorders is the Overanalysing Overcontroller. This is a truly transdiagnostic mode, responsible for symptom dimensions across depression and anxiety, including worry, rumination, and obsessive thinking. This mode, in its more extreme forms and when presenting as the primary coping mode, is implicated in generalised anxiety disorder [20]. This is an important mode to recognise and manage in the treatment of anxiety disorders in particular; therapists will struggle to apply schema therapy to depression and anxiety disorders where this mode predominates because it blocks access to the 'backstage' emotions (e.g., Critic, Anger, Vulnerability). Our definition of this mode taken from Chapter 1 is below for reference.

> *Overanalysing Overcontroller* (**OACM**): characterised by the predominance of verbal-linguistic processing of past- and/or future-oriented material (e.g., rumination, worry, or obsessive thinking), at the expense of attending to the contextual and emotional qualities of present-moment experience.

Chair Techniques for Depression and Anxiety Disorders

Chapter 8 explains that the use of chairwork supports the process of distancing oneself from unwanted psychological experiences. By placing a mode on a chair while the client literally occupies a distinct physical space from that chair, the mode can be viewed with a greater sense of emotional distance. For example, consider a case of a person with OCD who has rigid symptom-related beliefs about the risk of infection with AIDS/Coronavirus which block the cognitive examination of those beliefs. The Alert/Warning Protector mode could be placed on a chair and the client could interview the mode about those beliefs from the chair representing their Healthy Adult mode (see Box 13.3 for an illustration).

Box 13.3 Clinical Example of Using Chairwork Mode Dialogues in OCD: Healthy Adult Mode and Warning Protector Mode

THERAPIST: OK, so we are busy investigating the realistic possibility of you becoming infected with AIDS by touching the door handle, and we are at the point where we have mapped out that disaster scenario, the necessary conditions for potentially infecting your girlfriend with AIDS. First and foremost, for that to even be able to happen there has to be someone with AIDS who has touched that same door handle, and that must have happened on the same day as you are touching the door handle now. Then . . . *[the therapist goes through all the individual steps of the disaster scenario].*

So, now we know what actually has to happen, yet we still need to find out how likely it is that all of that will happen, but we would like to find that out so that we can see whether your precautionary measures, those compulsive actions, are also necessary in actual practice. In order to determine that, we first need to investigate the likelihood of each of these individual steps. Should we briefly examine that first?

[Client nods]

Good, so if we now step away for a moment and take a good look, what is the realistic chance of someone with AIDS having touched that same door handle on that same day?

CLIENT: Yes, it could happen.

THERAPIST: So the possibility of that happening, as you see it, is then . . .

CLIENT: Well, definitely, yes, so 100 per cent.

THERAPIST: And what makes you so certain of that then?

CLIENT: Well, just, just that it could happen. There are lots and lots of people with AIDS, so yes, that door handle could definitely be infected with it.

THERAPIST: . . . Let me just think about that out loud for a moment, because you may have noticed that I have gone a bit quiet. I wonder who I am listening to when you say that it is 100 per cent because that's just the way it is. Am I listening to that Healthy Adult side which I invited to conduct this investigation *[therapist points to the client]*? Or am

I actually listening to that Alert/Warning Protector of yours, who actually always shouts that there is a danger and is convinced of it too? *[In the case of the latter, the therapist gestures to a spot next to the client.]*

CLIENT: . . . *[pauses]*

THERAPIST: What do you think?

CLIENT: I don't know, that's just what I think.

THERAPIST: Yes, I understand that, but the question now is, if you say that you are certain of that, is it then that Healthy Adult *[therapist gestures towards the client]* or that Warning Protector *[therapist gestures once again to a spot next to the client]*?

CLIENT: Yes, maybe it's that Protector then.

THERAPIST: OK, but if he is still present, please take a seat in this chair *[therapist places chair in the spot that was gestured towards when the Protector was named]*.

Go and sit in that chair.
[Client goes and sits down on the Protector's chair.]

THERAPIST: Just be that Protector here. OK, Protector, I think that you're convinced that that entire situation with the door handle is dangerous, right?

CLIENT: Yes, it just is, and I don't want to be blamed for my girlfriend suddenly getting infected.

THERAPIST: I understand that, but that's why together with *[name of the client and pointing at the original chair]*, I would like to examine the realistic possibility of that actually happening. And if you keep yelling the whole time that it's 'just 100 per cent', we won't be able to examine that properly. Only then could I accept that you really think that, but then it's also certain that he *[pointing to the original chair]* will continue to be troubled by all the consequences of your compulsive actions. Couldn't you give us the opportunity to gain a bit of clarity, some certainty first?

CLIENT: . . . OK.

THERAPIST: Great! But then we also really need to be given the opportunity to do so, so I would like to ask you to just suppress your automatic reflex of saying '100 per cent' to everything just a little so that he *[pointing to original chair]* and I can explore this, OK?

CLIENT : . . . OK, that's fine.

THERAPIST: Great, now can you come and sit next to me again? But now that you're getting up, just remember for a moment that there *[pointing to the Protector's chair]*, you can say that everything is 100 per cent unsafe, but leave that conviction behind for a moment when you come and sit next to me here.
[Client comes and sits next to the therapist again in the original chair.]

THERAPIST: Good, he *[pointing to the Protector's chair]* will declare that everything definitely poses a danger, but you and I must first of all carefully consider, investigate, whether that is actually true. And when it comes to the question of how likely it is that an AIDS client has touched that same door handle that same day, how likely do we think that is?

CLIENT: . . . I don't know.

THERAPIST: I do know what that person there *[pointing to the Protector's chair]* would say, but what do we think? Is it really a certainty? How many AIDS clients are there actually?

CLIENT: . . . I don't know.

Table 13.2 Core fears in anxiety disorders with corresponding examples of target imagery and possible intervention

Disorder: core fear	Trauma memory/image	Possible intervention/message
Panic disorder: 'My bodily symptoms are an indication that I will go crazy.'	Image of little Jenny as a 14-year-old in a panicked state after taking THC: 'I'm going to die.'	'It's OK that you are anxious, this will pass. It is normal for your body to react this way to these kinds of substances.'
OCD: 'My sexual thoughts are a sign that I am bad and will go to hell.'	Image of Little Johnny, aged 13, on his bed struggling with intrusive sexual thoughts about his mother.	'A thought is just a thought … you are thirteen and going through puberty. It is normal to have sexual thoughts, even strange ones! They do not mean anything. You get to choose how you act. Thoughts are just thoughts.'
Social anxiety disorder: 'I will be humiliated'	Image of little Freddy, 9 years old, being shamed by a teacher in front of the whole class.	Confront teacher and send them away: 'What is wrong with you, treating a child that way?!' Address the child after.
Health anxiety: 'I will get sick and die'; 'I am physically vulnerable'	Image of little Lee, 6 years old, getting heart surgery, all alone in surgery without her parents.	'I'm here with you. I promise you that you will be OK. I will stay with you until this is all over. Your parents can come in too!'

Imagery Rescripting for Depression and Anxiety Disorders

The use of imagery rescripting in the context of depressive and anxiety disorders is, in a sense, 'business as usual' for the schema therapist. Imagery targets in the case of depression tend to involve themes of disconnection and isolation. Imagery targets for anxiety disorders tend to involve themes of vulnerability to harm, trust, and abuse. Of course, many cases will have all of these themes. In all cases, imagery rescripting can be used to process important events in the past that form the basis for experiencing the presenting problem. In the case of anxiety disorders, target images of the past often represent aspects of a *core fear* [18]. Table 13.2 provides some examples of core fears as seen across various anxiety disorders, and how imagery rescripting might address them, and Box 13.4 provides a clinical example of imagery rescripting with social anxiety disorder.

Behavioural Pattern Breaking for Depression: Learning to Identify and Connect with Core Emotional Needs

The aim of the initial phase of therapy is to make the client more aware of the modes and basic needs, while at the same time offering corrective emotional experiences. Depressed clients, however, tend to have a great deal of difficulty making contact with their feelings and needs. In the initial phase of the treatment, becoming aware of these needs must therefore be practised specifically. In addition, during this initial phase, behavioural change is also

---

Box 13.4 Clinical Example of Imagery Rescripting With Social Anxiety Disorder

The client reports that she has felt very anxious in the company of a few colleagues. The therapist suggested an imagery exercise to gain a better understanding of what made the client so anxious and to moderate that anxiety with the help of this exercise. The client has her eyes shut and has just described the situation with colleagues as she currently sees it.

THERAPIST: So, they are standing there next to you and you can see them laughing . . . how do you feel now?

CLIENT: Nervous, tense . . . they must be laughing at me because I am blushing . . .

THERAPIST: So, that's what you're scared of now?

CLIENT: . . . Yes . . .

THERAPIST: And where do you feel that anxiety, where do you mainly feel tension in your body?

CLIENT: [Points to her abdomen.]

THERAPIST: OK, now concentrate on that feeling, that anxiety that they are laughing at you because you are blushing . . . concentrate on this and allow the image to fade away . . . If you concentrate on this feeling, what images from your past appear to you then?

CLIENT: A particular situation at primary school, in the school playground and them bullying me . . .

THERAPIST: What do you see now?

CLIENT: Those boys, with that big kid in front calling me names and making fun of me . . .

THERAPIST: OK, OK, let's just pause that image for a moment, just press that pause button to make everything come to a standstill . . . I want to join in, because what is happening here isn't good. I want to help you . . . can you see me?

CLIENT: . . . Yes . . .

THERAPIST: Where can you see me? I would prefer to be standing next to you now.

CLIENT: Yes, next to me, to the left of me . . . [gestures to the left].

THERAPIST: Then listen to me when I speak to those bullies . . . [therapist turns his head away from the client so that, to the client, it sounds as if the therapist is actually speaking to someone else]. 'Oi! Stop that now! Stop being so mean to [name of client]! You wouldn't like it if someone did that to you, would you?' [To the client] Well, what do they say to that?"

CLIENT: . . . Yes, no . . . yes, that they understand it, yes . . .

THERAPIST: Exactly! How do they look?

CLIENT: A bit uncomfortable.

THERAPIST: How does it feel for you to see them feeling uncomfortable now instead of you?

CLIENT: . . . Yes, good . . .

---

encouraged with the aim of validating these needs. This kind of pattern-breaking closely resembles the behavioural activation phase in CBT for depression. The aims of behavioural activation are to instigate an initial reduction in some of the symptoms of depression and to gain access to the underlying modes. Thus, the encouragement of behavioural change happens earlier in the treatment of depression compared to schema therapy for personality disorders. Another issue that therapists often encounter in this context is that clients may be very detached from any sense of their needs. For these clients, the 'What do I want or need right now?' question and exercise can be used to give clients some gradual experiential contact with their needs.

Exercise: Activating and Reinforcing Needs 'In the Moment' With the 'What Do I Want or Need Right Now'? Question

This intervention consists of the following steps:

- Rationale
- Identifying needs
- Validating those needs
- Realising the healing power of attending to needs
- Homework

Rationale. The rationale clarifies why the client must practise asking themselves the question: 'What do *I* want/need NOW?' The emphasis in that question is on '*I*' and 'NOW'. The emphasis on 'I' is designed to draw attention to one's own needs, because clients who are depressed often primarily pay attention to the wishes and expectations of others or society, or are just disconnected from their needs.

The emphasis on 'now' is primarily to learn to focus their attention on smaller feelings which can be validated relatively easily this way. The question 'What do *I* need/want NOW?' is introduced as a behavioural 'medicine' against depression, which they must take regularly, several times a day.

Identifying Needs. After explaining the rationale, the client practises asking the question in the session right away. The therapist can help with this exercise, which many clients initially find very difficult. The therapist lets the client ask the question out loud, with the emphasis on the words 'I' and 'now', and then asks what the answer to this question is for the client at that very moment.

The most common answer given by depressed clients is that they don't know. The therapist stresses that there are always needs, but that the client is obviously struggling to make contact with them. The therapist can always help by making suggestions, as well as giving mainly small, practical examples, such as the need simply to take a look outside, to stretch or to relax and enjoy a cup of coffee. Thanks to this perseverance, often something is eventually mentioned, and although those needs are not always immediately practical or important, the client can nevertheless be praised for finding an answer to the question.

Validating the Identified Need. The next step is that action actually takes place in response to the identified need. The purpose of the exercise is to reach a form of counterconditioning: 'You've always had the experience that your needs did not matter and were brushed aside. Now you have identified your needs and we're going to take them seriously!' Here, the advantage of small, concrete examples such as 'look outside' or 'drink something' become apparent, because these needs are easy to validate during the session. The therapist pulls up the blinds or grabs a cup of coffee or talks for a moment about something completely different to what the client says that they need.

Box 13.5 Example of the 'What do I Want or Need Right Now?' Exercise

THERAPIST: How do you feel now, since you felt like simply looking outside and you are actually doing that now?

CLIENT: Normal, the same.

THERAPIST: Does it feel worse to do what you want, exactly the same, or does it feel a bit better to be doing what you want to be doing?

[The therapist moves her or his thumb slightly down then up as a kind of indicator, whereby making small subtle changes turns something negative into something positive.]

CLIENT: Well . . . yes . . . a bit better perhaps, but not much!

THERAPIST: I understand that. It is just a small difference compared to before, but it is a more positive feeling than what you previously had. Even though it's really small, it's still a very important difference all the same! That means that you feel a bit better if you listen to your needs . . . not much, perhaps, but it is just like digging for gold; it might be difficult and take a great deal of effort to find a speck of gold, but if you spend a while doing that, in the end you will end up with a little stack which is literally worth its weight in gold.

Becoming Aware of the Healing Power of Connecting With Needs. During the validation of the expressed need, the therapist pays attention to signs of any changes in mood. These signs can be subtle in severely depressed clients, which is why we recommend being extra alert to them: the beginning of a smile, a lighter tone of voice, a somewhat lighter mood in the conversation, or the client being slightly more physically active could all be potential signs of the healing power of the validation of identified needs. The therapist also draws the client's attention to any change in mood they might be experiencing by specifically asking about their mood and drawing the client's attention to the significance of that feeling. This exercise is illustrated in Box 13.5.

Homework. The homework consists of repeatedly practising 'The Question'. The rationale behind this is just like with a lot of medication: it only starts to work when it's taken regularly. Over time, this exercise can be linked to full behavioural pattern breaking explicitly connected to the client's stated needs domains (see Chapter 9 for an overview).

Conceptualisation with Cases of Adjustment Disorder

Mood and anxiety problems also commonly present for therapy in the context of an adjustment disorder. In these cases, mood and anxiety problems have developed in response to an identifiable stressor or difficult life event (e.g., relationship problems, work stressors). Schema therapy has an interesting perspective on the possible schema and mode processes underlying problematic adjustment reactions. In the midst of the COVID-19 pandemic, Brockman [21] described three pathways that might contribute to the onset and mainten-ance of adjustment problems. While these pathways are presented separately, in practice, clients tend to present with a combination of the three. These pathways are described in depth as follows:

1. **The Stressor Triggers Schema-Driven Distress.** Most often the stressor or difficult life event experienced directly triggers one or more relevant EMS, resulting in heightened activation of relevant schemas and core emotional 'back stage' modes (e.g., Vulnerable Child, Angry Child, Critic modes). For example, in a situation such as a pandemic, the inherent health crisis and surrounding media attention might trigger a Vulnerability to Harm EMS in combination with an Abandonment EMS (e.g., a fear that a family member might die), producing anxiety or fear in the form of a Vulnerable or Fearful Child mode. For individuals prone to taking excessive personal responsibility for negative events, if a family member becomes sick this might result in the activation of a blaming or Guilt-Inducing Critic mode generating repeated negative automatic thoughts (e.g., 'I should have done more to care for my loved ones'). The ongoing and uncertain nature of some difficult life events and stressors can prolong EMS and maladaptive mode activation. Conversely, resolution of stressors (e.g., improvement of a relationship) tends to reduce EMS and mode activation.

2. **The Stressor Overwhelms the Client's Usual (Primary) Coping Mode(s).** It is very common in cases of adjustment disorder to find that the client self-managed reasonably well before the onset of the stressor. They will often present as having previously been quite well adjusted, and successfully compensated (or overcompensated without causing any major problems) for any core EMS held over from childhood. For this group of clients, the stressor directly threatens the efficacy and workability of long-trusted coping modes. Picture the overworking 'perfectionist' who has overcompensated for unwanted emotions through work and perfection for thirty years but is suddenly retrenched. Clients exposed to such stressors often find themselves 'without a coping strategy' or 'de-compensating'. Such situations deprive the client of the ability to follow the if–then rules they developed to cope with their core EMS (e.g., 'If I am perfect then I am loved and "good enough"'). The client is then prone to being flooded by emotions associated with previously dormant schemas (e.g., Defectiveness, Abandonment) and modes (e.g., Vulnerable Child mode, Punitive Critic). These clients often present – understandably – with very high levels of distress (Vulnerable Child mode), blaming 'the situation' (Angry Child mode), and wanting therapy to 'fix' the situation or assist them to regain a sense of control. Because they are so 'in touch' with their distressing feelings, these clients often present as quite motivated to work on their issues, at least at the beginning of therapy. However, motivation can wane as therapy progresses and clients feel more 'in control' again. Therefore, therapists should take advantage of stressful 'crises' to build the client's mode awareness and motivate the client to redirect their focus away from their past overcompensatory habits and towards healing their schemas to pursue meeting their needs from this point on in their lives.

3. **The Stressor Activates Secondary or Historic Coping Modes.** Another relatively common adjustment reaction is that clients will inevitably pivot to some (secondary) form of coping. For example, a 'perfectionist' that is retrenched might resort to withdrawal and avoidance (Avoidant Protector), placing them at further risk of low mood and anxiety. A similar pattern might see clients resort to – or relapse into – historic coping modes (including any former addictive coping behaviours, e.g., binge drinking) to cope.

Perfectionist/Over-Controller Mode

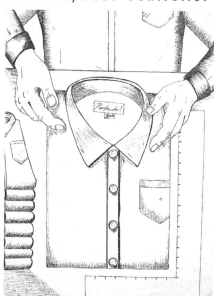

Illustration 13.1 Perfectionistic Overcontroller mode

Concluding Remarks

In this chapter we have provided more detail on how schema therapy might be adapted and applied to a range of presentations that fall into the category of 'high-prevalence disorders' such as depression and anxiety. While this chapter confined itself to a description of schema therapy for depressive and anxiety disorders, it provides a template for the transdiagnostic treatment of other high-prevalence 'axis 1' problems.

References

1. Renner F, Arntz A, Peeters F, Lobbestael J, Huibers M. Schema therapy for chronic depression: Results of a multiple single case series. *Journal of Behavior Therapy and Experimental Psychiatry.* 2016;**51**:66–73.

2. Renner F, DeRubeis R, Arntz A, et al. Exploring mechanisms of change in schema therapy for chronic depression. *Journal of Behavior Therapy and Experimental Psychiatry.* 2018;**58**:97–105.

3. Young J, Klosko J, Weishaar M. *Schema therapy: A practitioner's guide.* Guilford Press; 2003.

4. Friborg O, Martinsen E, Martinussen M, et al. Comorbidity of personality disorders in mood disorders: A meta-analytic review of 122 studies from 1988 to 2010. *Journal of Affective Disorders.* 2014;(**152**):1–11.

5. Newton-Howes G, Tyrer P, Johnson T, et al. Influence of personality on the outcome of treatment in depression: Systematic review and meta-analysis. *Journal of Personality Disorders.* 2014;**28**(4):577–93.

6. Reich J, Schatzberg A, Delucchi K. Empirical evidence of the effect of personality pathology on the outcome of panic disorder.

Journal of Psychiatric Research.
2018;**107**:42–7.

7. Johnsen T, Friborg O. The effects of
cognitive behavioral therapy as an
anti-depressive treatment is falling: A
meta-analysis. *Psychological Bulletin.*
2015;**141**(4):747–68.

8. Wild J, Clark D. Imagery rescripting of
early traumatic memories in social phobia.
Cognitive and Behavioral Practice. 2011
Nov 1;**18**(4):433–43.

9. Pugh M. Chairwork in cognitive
behavioural therapy: A narrative review.
Cognitive Therapy and Research. 2017;**41**
(1):16–30.

10. Halvorsen M, Wang C, Richter J, et al.
Early maladaptive schemas, temperament
and character traits in clinically depressed
and previously depressed subjects. *Clinical
Psychology & Psychotherapy: An
International Journal of Theory & Practice.*
2009;**16**(5):394–407.

11. Hawke L, Provencher M. Early
Maladaptive Schemas among clients
diagnosed with bipolar disorder. *Journal of
Affective Disorders.* 2012 Feb 1;**136**
(3):803–11.

12. Petrocelli J, Glaser B, Calhoun G,
Campbell L. Cognitive schemas as
mediating variables of the relationship
between the self-defeating personality and
depression. *Journal of Psychopathology
and Behavioral Assessment.* 2001;**23**
(3):183–91.

13. Renner F, Arntz A, Leeuw I, Huibers M.
Treatment for chronic depression using

schema therapy. *Clinical Psychology:
Science and Practice.* 2013;**20**(2):166–80.

14. Lumley M, Harkness K. Childhood
maltreatment and depressotypic cognitive
organization. *Cognitive Therapy and
Research.* 2009;**33**(5):511–22.

15. Beck A, Haigh E. Advances in cognitive
theory and therapy: The generic cognitive
model. *Annual Review of Clinical
Psychology.* 2014;**10**(1):1–24.

16. Beck A. Beyond belief: A theory of
modes, personality, and
psychopathology. In Salkovskis P, ed.
Frontiers of cognitive psychology.
Guilford Press; 1996. pp. 1–25.

17. Granger S, Pavlis A, Collett J,
Hallam KT. Revisiting the 'manic
defence hypothesis': Assessing explicit
and implicit cognitive biases in euthymic
bipolar disorder. *Clinical Psychologist.*
2021;**25**(2):212–22.

18. Beck A, Emery G, Greenberg R. *Anxiety
disorders and phobias.* Basic Books;
2005.

19. Stewart S, Shapiro L. Pathological guilt:
A persistent yet overlooked treatment
factor in obsessive-compulsive disorder.
Annals of Clinical Psychiatry. 2011;**23**
(1):63–70.

20. Stavropoulos A, Haire M, Brockman R,
Meade T. A schema mode model of
repetitive negative thinking. *Clinical
Psychologist.* 2020;**24**(2):99–113.

21. Brockman R. Schema Therapy in the Age
of COVID-19. Webinar published 2020;
schematherapytrainingonline.com.

Working with Complex Trauma and Dissociation in Schema Therapy

Introduction

In this chapter, we present a schema therapy conceptualisation of complex trauma and dissociation. Because the prospect of confronting historical trauma can be anxiety provoking for clients and therapists alike, the task can easily remain hidden or be avoided. Although a schema therapy approach to complex trauma follows the core principles of the standard model, several additional aspects of client presentations warrant consideration. Here, we present adaptations and alternatives for providing schema therapy interventions to this population.

The Schema Therapy Approach to Trauma: Balancing Trauma Focus with Meeting Core Emotional Needs

The experience of prolonged and repeated trauma in early child development (such as sexual or physical abuse) can have a broad and varied range of consequences [1]. In some cases, clients may present with post-traumatic stress disorder (PTSD) as described in DSM-5. Other clients may present with the increasingly recognised complex post-traumatic stress (CPTSD) [2, 3]. CPTSD includes difficulties in affect regulation, severe (stable) negative self-concept and interpersonal problems (where relationships are seen as problematic and to be avoided), and the core symptom clusters observed in PTSD: avoidance, re-experiencing, and hypervigilance/arousal [4]. Schema therapy is a model designed to address the impact of adverse childhood experiences and is well suited as a treatment framework for CPTSD cases.

Trauma-focused treatment approaches have historically been placed in two categories. The first views trauma processing as the focal ingredient of change [5]. Here, reducing trauma symptoms is the primary goal and sufficient to produce increased stability and change. The second category is phase-oriented trauma treatment [5], wherein the therapist aims to provide stability initially (in an extended 'Stabilisation Phase') before moving into trauma processing. There has been substantial debate as to which approach is the most useful for CPTSD [5, 6]. Trauma processing–focused supporters argue that an extended focus on stabilisation often prevents the client from processing trauma because the therapist usually manages extraneous factors that affect stability for very long periods [6]. Consequently, there is concern that some clients never achieve sufficient stability to process their trauma or that much time, energy, and (limited) therapeutic resources are taken up during this phase. In contrast, phased-oriented proponents argue that clients cannot successfully process trauma-related material while emotionally unstable and therefore require a careful and sometimes extensive phase of stabilisation [5].

Schema therapy can provide a middle path between trauma-focused and phase-based approaches. Rather than focusing on stability before moving to trauma processing (primarily via imagery rescripting), the focus is on the client's emotional needs. Schema therapy does not primarily focus on stability as a core treatment process. Instead, schema therapy encourages the early commencement of processing trauma-related imagery and other experiential exercises. Exercises focus on creating corrective emotional experiences of the client getting their needs (e.g., for safety or validation) met. A critical aspect that is different from phase- and trauma-focused approaches is the specific use of limited reparenting in schema therapy. The therapeutic relationship itself is considered to be a crucial contributor to change, in which the therapist seeks to directly meet needs for care, validation, limit setting, guidance, and encouragement. Schema therapists argue that it is the establishment of a limited reparenting relationship that provides the safety and containment required for the client to have an early focus on experiential work.

Differences in trauma therapies can be likened to different approaches to teaching a child to ride a bicycle. If the caregiver were to wait for the child to be emotionally resourced and stable before proceeding, the child may not ever learn to ride the bike. In turn, if the caregiver were to compel the anxious child to commence riding without managing the potential underlying needs of safety and encouragement, it may result in the child harming themselves and resisting further invitations to learn to ride. A schema therapy–informed caregiver aims to give the child cyclist a helmet, knee pads, and training wheels and runs alongside the child, ready to steady them if they should fall. In processing work, limited reparenting can be interwoven throughout the treatment or done in a block of work; however, this depends on the specific core emotional needs centred around trauma. The therapist may guide and encourage the client to do trauma-focused work (possibly in a block of sessions with a trauma focus). To do so, they may need to overcome modes that block change and model a Healthy Adult willingness via reparenting. There are two main ways to conceptualise schema therapy for complex PTSD: (1) As a ready-made approach that incorporates imagery rescripting as the primary trauma-focused treatment; and (2) a broader integrative approach, where a range of trauma-focused interventions (e.g., EMDR) can be embedded within a schema therapy case conceptualisation.

Therapist Confidence and Approach

Traumatic material can be complex for therapists to navigate with the client; some therapists feel anxious about re-traumatisation or getting techniques 'wrong' or applying them imperfectly. It is also typical for disclosures of childhood trauma among survivors to be delayed until well into adulthood [7]. Whether or not the client discloses traumatic experiences will be partially influenced by their assessment of how the helping professional will react to such content [8]. Therapists should project confidence that they can manage the disclosure of trauma experiences and trauma reactions and that clients will be believed and validated by the therapist [9]. This will provide the 'safe space' necessary for clients to discuss traumatic experiences. In addition, the therapist needs to display confidence in their conceptualisation of the client's difficulties, and in the delivery of techniques, to provide a sense of safety in the treatment itself [10].

Assessment and Trauma Work

Clients present to treatment for many reasons. In some cases, clients specifically seek help with traumatic events and related clinical symptoms. However, in many cases, individuals with historical trauma (particularly childhood sexual abuse) present for various reasons (e.g., relationship problems, work stress) that may initially appear unrelated to trauma [2]. Regardless of whether clients raise the subject, therapists need to assess whether the client has experienced significant childhood trauma. Often clients attend with an 'if they don't ask, I won't tell' mindset. It is essential for therapists to 'give permission' for this material to be shared by asking about the potential impact of any relevant traumatic events. Frequently, clients are not inclined to mention distressing childhood trauma in the initial assessment phase because they are ashamed of those experiences and/or present in strong coping modes. Therapists can utilise several screening tools to detect the possible experience of trauma. For example, the Life Events Check List [11] has items such as 'experienced ... other unwanted or uncomfortable sexual experience' with a range of responses such as 'happened to me', 'witnessed it', and 'doesn't apply'. At the screening stage, the therapist can affirm that they don't yet need to know the details of confirmed responses. It is essential to highlight that the client has control over if, when, and how much they disclose. Nevertheless, therapists should identify whether the client has a history of trauma early on, with the view to possible exploration later in treatment.

See Box 14.1 for details of themes in childhood trauma and aspects of schema healing.

Box 14.1 Themes in Childhood Trauma and Aspects of Schema Healing

Manipulation, Silence and Shame

Clients have often been silenced to keep neglect and abuse secret. As children, the child may have been encouraged to 'keep secrets' from supportive adult caregivers. Those abusing the child may have sought to undermine the child's confidence in speaking out, highlighting that 'no one will believe them'. This experience further disrupts the child's need for autonomy and control, thus compounding the effects of any initial trauma. Furthermore, as the child grows older, they may become increasingly aware of what it means to have been sexually abused. They will eventually develop an awareness that society views sexual acts with children as a shameful wrongdoing. The child may then incorrectly infer that they must have done something wrong for being involved, resulting in a profound sense of shame. This experience is linked to the core emotional need for unconditional acceptance and validation. In schema healing, the therapist aims to assist the client to increase their self-compassion, acceptance, and understanding of the context of maltreatment. Here, the therapist seeks to have the client rightfully attribute their abuse to the perpetrators rather than themself as an adult survivor.

The Influence and Reactions of Caregivers

The reactions of those caregivers not directly involved with abuse can also be pivotal. Failing to protect the child, denying abuse, or criticising or maligning a child for seeking safety and security may result in profound and long-term adverse outcomes. Such responses can significantly influence the meaning of abuse. In some cases, these acts can be as damaging as the abusive acts themselves, considerably impacting the legacy of the abuse in the adult's life.

Power, Coercion, and Control

Clients with childhood trauma often have difficulty being appropriately assertive and setting limits. They often harbour deep feelings of disempowerment and helplessness and can easily feel controlled or manipulated by others. Clients often did not have their basic need for autonomy met during childhood; they could not state their needs and preferences – typically, out of fear of consequences or reprisals. In schema therapy, it is essential to empower the survivor of abuse and increase their autonomy and agency. The therapeutic aims are to enable the client to overcome fear and mistrust and increase their capacity to set limits, be assertive, and hold their views and opinions.

Lack of Trust in Self

Clients may deeply feel that they are ill-equipped to protect themselves, 'make things safe', or stand up for themselves. Clients may simultaneously overestimate their threat of harm and underestimate their capacity to keep themselves safe. In schema mode terms, the Vulnerable Child mode is hypervigilant for the next episode of violence and continues to scan for danger into adulthood. The child then develops coping strategies that have manifested as coping modes into adulthood. The resultant coping modes (such as avoidant coping modes or Detached Protector) can undermine confidence in managing the threat of danger in adulthood. The mode interplay could be seen as follows:

Vulnerable Child mode: 'I'm afraid. I can't assert myself. I can't stick up for myself.'

Detached Protector mode: 'Saying what you need will overwhelm you, it's easier if we put it off.'

Healthy Adult mode: 'You have got this! You can do what you want now. It's not like it was when you were growing up.'

Schema therapy aims to strengthen the Healthy Adult and encourage the client's Vulnerable Child mode to trust their developing Healthy Adult to manage stressors and challenges.

Relationships: Re-Victimisation in Adulthood

Frequently, clients who experienced childhood abuse experience re-victimisation in their adult life [12]. Ongoing adult abuse may be related to the operation of coping styles.

Surrendering: taking a position of resignation and surrendering to others. The client perceives that 'this is how life is', and the best way to cope with it is to give in to others and give up on change.

Avoiding/Detaching: Avoiding 'rocking the boat' reduces the potential for distress and ramifications. Also, further abuse may act as a trigger for dissociation and numbing (which is comforting).

Overcompensation: 'If the abuse is going to occur, then it's on my terms, under my control.'

The therapeutic aim in schema therapy is to enable healthy, satisfying relationships where needs are met and there is an ending to further abuse and experiences reinforcing schemas and modes.

Case Conceptualisation: Key Modes and Schemas

As in all schema mode conceptualisations, the therapist working with complex PTSD is encouraged to consider the function and origin of the client's modes. The following sections provide a selection of commonly observed modes in complex trauma cases and how the schema therapist responds to them.

Abused/Vulnerable Child Mode

This mode typically 'holds' memories, emotions, and beliefs linked to trauma. In cases of PTSD, this is the mode that is most often responsible for holding the (unprocessed) trauma memories. When these memories and images are activated, it is as though the client is stuck in the child's experience, re-experiencing those events from the perspective of the (abused) child. Such clients also often present with deep feelings of shame, mistrust, humiliation, and betrayal related to abuse. Some trauma survivors experience child-like feelings of attachment allegiance and loyalty with abusive figures. As a result, the client may feel conflicted and confused towards the perpetrators of their abuse. This likely reflects a core conundrum the client has been experiencing since childhood: that the perpetrator (often a parent) both satisfies some needs (perhaps, for example, generally meeting needs for care) and at other times is abusive. This can lead to situations where the client may flip into a Vulnerable Child mode and attempt to retract statements about the abuse they received from caregivers; they may present feeling fearful, guilty, and undeserving. In the therapy relationship, the Vulnerable Child mode also fears further abuse, humiliation, and invalidation from the therapist. This is where Limited Reparenting is central; the therapist should consider and attune to the client's perception of potential threat and provide safety, stability, and unconditional acceptance and validation.

Detached Protector Subtypes

The Detached Protector mode often presents in a prototypical way: emotionally withdrawn, numb, detached, and 'disconnected' from affect. However, we have observed several specific subtypes of this mode that are worth consideration. In a Spacey/Dissociative Protector mode, the client experiences depersonalisation, derealisation, feeling 'foggy', 'spaced out', or 'numb' towards affect. Psychological denial and the slow accommodation of abusive behaviour may also drive the process of detachment. Knipe [13] highlights the fundamental attachment conflict that a child has towards abusive caregivers. He notes that children may develop ways to accommodate abusive acts to mitigate against distress and powerlessness from the relationship, such as blaming themselves for the abuse rather than face the overwhelming dilemma of what to do about a toxic home environment in which their caregivers can't be trusted. A therapist might encapsulate for the adult client how their child self may have rationalised the abuse they endured: 'Some children may take the view that "it's better to be a bad kid in a good family than a good kid in a bad family"'. The child's reframe can serve to deny or minimise the impact of the abuse, thereby preserving their fundamental attachment to the caregiver and seemingly securing their short-term or overall survival. The changes in emotion and thinking to accommodate an abusive relationship may often be the seeds of the Detached Protector mode or other coping modes (e.g., Compliant Surrenderer).

Angry Protector Mode

The Angry Protector mode serves to keep others away from vulnerability. The function of the mode is to push others (including the therapist) away. The tone can be defiant and hostile ('Didn't you hear me; I don't want to talk about it'). Non-verbal language can also act to provide a 'stay away from me' message to the therapist [14]. Clients ordinarily use avoidant coping modes and flip into this overcompensation mode when 'pushed into a corner'. This reaction may result from probing questions from the therapist or when the avoidant coping fails to prevent access to the Vulnerable Child mode.

Punitive Critic Mode

A conceptualisation of the Punitive Critic mode centres around introjection. The client may have been exposed directly to punitive caregiving and internalised this way of relating to the self. At some point, The Punitive Critic mode may have served an adaptive purpose for the child. For example, in the past the client may have been harsh and blamed themselves in an attempt to mitigate further abuse or blame ('Get a grip, stupid, or dad will go crazy'). However, schema therapists assume that typically the current form of the mode (in an adult client) no longer serves a function; it is an obsolete legacy of a traumatic childhood. The client needs to take an understanding but determined and firm position. Therapists can acknowledge the prior value of the mode (as helping in the past) but note that the impact of the mode is now damaging and wrong – for example (to the Punitive Critic): 'I don't agree with the rules you make for her, you may have once helped her; but now you are damaging, wrong, and you will stop.'

Healthy Adult

The therapist aims to strengthen and enhance the client's Healthy Adult mode. A critical sub-goal is to strengthen this existing mode enough to undertake specific trauma-focused interventions. Throughout treatment, therapists aim to help empower clients and provide them with a sense of mastery. Experiential exercises, rather than being delayed, can be used gently and titrated, building on increasing emotional capacities. Psychological 'resource development' [15] typically used in EMDR treatments can also be applied to enhance and strengthen such resources directly (e.g., specific skills and adaptive emotional capacities such as self-compassion).

Schemas

Therapists should also attune to specific schemas evident in the case conceptualisation and relate them to trauma-based memories. Key schemas typically observed in complex trauma can be seen in Table 14.1.

Complex Post-traumatic Stress Disorder Versus Borderline Personality Disorder

CPTSD clients can share similar symptoms to BPD, particularly concerning affect dysregulation, negative view of self, and difficulties maintaining a relationship [16]. In our opinion, a defining difference is that clients with CPTSD lack a pervasive Abandonment schema. CPTSD clients frequently do not exhibit distress related to 'endings' (e.g.,

Table 14.1 Common schema themes observed in PTSD trauma memories

Schema	Emotional themes	Key trauma cognitions
Defectiveness & Shame	Feeling of being at fault for abuse; feeling unacceptable as a result of abuse	'I'm to blame for what happened'
Subjugation	Feeling controlled; coercion applied in abuse context; lack of power and autonomy	'I'm powerless'; 'I can't stop this from happening'
Emotional Deprivation	Feeling caregivers are not attuned to basic needs or can't empathise or provide safety/guidance	'No one is there for me'; 'No one cares about what happens to me'
Mistrust/ Abuse	Unable to trust other's intention; assumption that the world is unsafe, and others will exploit and be harmful	'I can't trust anyone'; 'Nowhere is safe for me'

a therapist leaving for holidays or a session's ending) and do not interpret relationships ending as meaning they will be abandoned, which is typically very prominent in BPD.

Dissociation

Dissociative symptoms include depersonalisation (being detached from the body), derealisation (not feeling the world is 'real'), amnesia, identity confusion, and identity alteration [17]. Schema therapy considers dissociation to be the expression of extreme variants of modes and rapid changes in schema modes ('flipping' from one mode to another) [18, 19]. Clients typically have a dominant avoidant coping mode developed to manage extreme fear, shame, and distress, but occasionally flip into acute variants of Child and Critic modes when triggered.

Some clients (in childhood and adulthood) may have a propensity to dissociate [20]; however, typically a child will develop a sequence of survival responses to extreme threat. As a child, the client may not have been able to escape, avoid, or fight off repeated abusive acts. Instead, they implemented dissociation to cope with the ongoing abuse or lack of safety. Schauer and Elbert [21] note two major classes of dissociative states: Type 1, the 'Uproar', which is akin to Vulnerable and Angry Child activation, resulting in feelings of dizziness, palpations, unreality, and muscle tension; and Type 2, 'The Shutdown', which is associated with a drop in arousal, cognitive failure, immobility, and numbing of all emotion. 'The Shutdown' can be conceptualised as an extreme type of avoidant coping mode, usually some form of Detached Protector. It is activated by implicit or explicit reminders of traumatic experiences coupled with activation of the Punitive Critic mode, resulting in a cascade of distress which the avoidant coping mode serves to terminate.

Box 14.2 presents examples of methods that may be employed to manage dissociation in session.

Modes, Alters, and Identities in Complex Dissociative Cases

Treatments for complex dissociative disorders (e.g., dissociative identity disorder [DID]) have historically used models that describe 'structural dissociation' of the personality or dissociated 'ego states' [24, 25] to describe rapid fluctuations in states frequently observed

Box 14.2 Methods to Manage Dissociation in Session

It is not helpful for the client to remain in a dissociated state during a therapy session. The therapist should intervene to help the client reorient to the present moment. The 'window of tolerance' [22, 23] model can be a helpful idea to guide the therapist's assessment of the client's emotional experience. There is an optimal level of emotional arousal in which to participate in psychotherapeutic activities. This 'window' lies between hypoarousal (insufficient emotional experience) and hyperarousal (excessive or overwhelming emotional experience). The following suggestions can assist the client to manage the intensity of their emotional arousal.

Use of a shawl/blanket: The therapist can use a shawl or rug and ask the client to hold one end and the therapist the other. The therapist may tug on their end of the rug to gently capture the client's attention when they become too detached.

Grounding of senses: Clients can be encouraged to perceive their surroundings, engaging their senses within the room: 'What are five things you can see?'; 'What five sounds can you hear in the room?'; 'What are five things you can physically feel?' This sequence can be then counted down 5–1 using the same format.

Use of balls/pillows and playing catch: A small ball or pillow can be thrown between the therapist and the client. This 'playing catch' can be a method to orient the client to the present moment.

Use of smell: The therapist can use pleasant smelling scents, such as scented oils, mints, or coffee beans, to engage the sense of smell and orientate to the present moment.

Intense temperatures: Frozen cooler packs, oranges (or other frozen objects), drinking a glass of cold water.

in complex trauma. In such models, the therapist can separate trauma memories and related experiences into different components of the self. Furthermore, clients with complex presentations may present with many 'identities' or 'alters' of the self. Huntjens and colleagues [18], describing the model of schema therapy for DID clients, argue against the notion of separate 'identities' and compartmentalised identity states that operate as wholly dissociated aspects of the self. Instead, they suggest that clients with severe dissociation (and DID) may hold positive metacognitive beliefs about having 'identities' and keeping experiences separate. For example, 'If I keep these elements separate, then I can deal with the trauma that I've experienced'. Instead, they suggest utilising the mode model and encouraging a move from an 'identities' framework to one based on modes. This change is quite subtle but perhaps also profound. Rather than reinforce the notion of a family of personalities, the schema therapist uses mode language to introduce the idea that these are all 'parts' of one's self. In this way, the schema therapist simultaneously validates the client's experience of dissociation while slowly helping the client gain awareness of an overarching 'self', thus promoting integration over time. Therapists can collapse multiple compartmentalised identities into a mode that serves a common function within the conceptualisation. For example, several child-like parts could be collapsed into the Vulnerable Child mode and worked with in such a fashion. The primary aim is to provide a coherent, clear case conceptualisation and reduce the complexity of the presentation for the client and therapist.

> **Box 14.3** Key Treatment Themes
>
> - Increase self-compassion to self and the client's history.
> - Reattribute blame for the experience of trauma, manage Punitive Critic mode.
> - Increase control and sense of autonomy and power towards others.
> - Increase belief in self to 'make things safe'.

Our experience is that the dissociative processes in session – such as the client 'zoning out', being unresponsive, or being flooded with distress – are often linked to activation of the Punitive Critic mode. Often clients privately flip into a Punitive Critic mode that may activate intense feelings of shame and fear. If extreme emotional reactions occur in session, it may be helpful for the therapist to inquire whether such activation has just occurred. Mode work can then be used to manage the impact of the Punitive mode. Helping the client manage and ultimately reduce the activation of the Critic can be a crucial step in establishing enough safety to begin any trauma processing. This process also introduces the client to working on many themes that will come up later in memory-focused processing work (imagery rescripting). Box 14.3 summarises the key themes in treatment.

Preparation for Trauma-Focused Work

Trauma-focused interventions specifically for processing traumatic memories are seen to be more effective than approaches that do not focus on trauma but instead focus on increasing coping techniques, such as affect regulation and anxiety management [26]. Clients receiving childhood trauma treatment also recognise the importance of focusing on trauma memories [10]. Trauma processing interventions fit within the broader schema therapy model, which acts as a helpful framework. In our perspective, if the client is willing (i.e., they are open to doing trauma-focused work) and able (i.e., they have some capacity to tolerate trauma-linked emotion), the therapist should seek to proceed with trauma processing-based interventions. Boterhoven De Hann and colleagues [27] demonstrated that both imagery rescripting and EMDR were very effective in treating PTSD due to childhood trauma. Such treatment consisted of a block of twelve sessions that included trauma processing in each session. It may be helpful for the therapist to suggest a block of trauma-focused work for the client, thus creating an expectancy of the content of sessions and assisting with the management of avoidance of trauma material.

If the client is unwilling, the therapist should focus on mode work typically observed in non-complex trauma personations. Here, the therapist seeks to understand what modes are preventing the therapist from accessing trauma content. The conceptualisation of the avoidance in mode terms can be developed and should be communicated to the client (e.g., see Table 14.2). The therapist can then work with the client towards overcoming the block via cognitive, experiential, and limited reparenting techniques.

If the client cannot tolerate their emotions, the therapist is encouraged to slow their approach and titrate the intensity of emotion evoked during experiential techniques (again, keeping in mind the 'window of tolerance'). The therapist may wish to initially guide the client to complete imagery rescripting with neutral or positive imagery. For example, the client may access an image of them sweeping the floor up as a child (as a neutral image).

Table 14.2 Overcoming avoidance of trauma processing: Mode work and trauma

Mode	Potential sentiments towards trauma material
Vulnerable/ Abused Child	'I'm afraid of these memories and these feelings. I feel ashamed that this all happened, scared that others will do it again.'
Angry Child	'I'm sick and tired of this! Why do I have to go through it all? It's all painful and no one understands how bad it is for me!'
Detached Protector	'She can't handle these memories. It's better to forget all this and move on. This is too much for her.'
Angry Protector	'How many times do I have to say it! I don't want to talk about it! Why do you keep asking! I told you there is no vulnerable side.'
Punitive Critic	'She doesn't deserve to feel better'; 'She shouldn't be speaking about this childhood stuff; she's a bad daughter, a traitor.'
Healthy Adult	'These memories cause me pain, and It might be difficult to manage at times, but I can trust myself and can trust the therapist.'

They can initially learn to tolerate the therapist entering the image to help with the sweeping (or with the therapist bringing in a new vacuum cleaner). In separate subsequent exercises, the therapist may also seek to have the client join this neutral image and assist the child as an adult. Imagery can be adapted later to include marginally distressing images, such as a child feeling sad, with the therapist providing care and safety, without any negative antagonist present. In this way, the therapist can scaffold trauma-focused work (indeed, all therapeutic work) in ways that help the client 'get within the therapeutic window'.

The therapist can also utilise a mode conceptualisation to understand the mode interplay causing the client distress about trauma processing. For example, perhaps the Punitive Critic mode becomes activated when discussing traumatic experiences. Alternatively, the client may not feel they can trust themselves to manage the affect evoked by the traumatic memories and associated ideas. In this case, the Vulnerable Child and Detached Protector modes may work together to undermine the client's confidence that they can cope with their emotions associated with the trauma.

Box 14.4 presents a pseudonymous case study ('Katie') utilising various modes to address trauma.

Processing Trauma Memories

Clients presenting with complex trauma may have had many toxic experiences that contributed to their PTSD or that resulted in EMS. Lee and Boterhoven De Hann [27] recommend undertaking a process of 'trauma mapping', in which the therapist and client link trauma-related memories to corresponding EMS. The client and therapist can identify a distressing aspect of the trauma memory (e.g., sexual abuse from stepfather). The therapist then breaks the trauma memory into three main components: (a) the sensory component (someone coming into my room), (b) the affective/physiological component (feeling tense in my chest, feeling anxious), and (c) the meaning of the event (I'm powerless, I can't stop this: i.e., Subjugation schema). Following identification of the meaning (typically linked to an EMS), the therapist can explore other memories and images related to this schema

Box 14.4 Case Example: Katie

Katie would typically prefer to 'talk' about her recent triggers and seek general support and validation. When the therapist suggested the idea of doing some specific work on processing trauma memories using imagery, she initially appeared open to the process. However, the therapist had concerns about Katie's ability to tolerate the fear and shame central to the abuse she suffered growing up. She would become tearful and overwhelmed when talking about her childhood, and reported some self-harming after a session where she listed some of the trauma memories she wanted to process. In subsequent sessions, the therapist conceptualised the self-harm and pattern of dysregulation via modes. It became apparent that the disclosure of events and the possibility of change activated her Punitive Critic mode. The Punitive Critic mode deemed her discussion of childhood abuse an act of betrayal toward her family (particularly her stepfather). Furthermore, her Vulnerable Child mode was fearful of rocking the boat (key schema: Subjugation) and was overwhelmed with fear. Her typical coping mode, the 'Blocker mode', also doubted her ability to cope and generally advised her to 'just forget about this childhood stuff'.

Over several sessions, the therapist used mode dialogues (between the therapist and the Punitive Critic) to contain and mitigate the effect of the Punitive Critic and the view that Katie was 'betraying her family'. Later, the therapist utilised chairwork where the stepfather was placed in the empty chair to help the therapist provide protection and safety. Later, Katie used an empty chair dialogue with her stepfather to announce she was 'finished being afraid of him', resulting in empowerment and a greater sense of confidence. After several months, Katie was increasingly able to use a phase of imagery rescripting focusing on childhood trauma memories.

theme. Images related to these events can then also be used as 'targets' for imagery rescripting.

Imagery Rescripting

Readers can read detailed procedures for imagery rescripting in Chapter 8. Here, we reiterate some critical points about its specific application to childhood trauma. Therapists have attributed adherence to imagery rescripting protocols for enhancing their confidence and assisting them to stay 'on task' [26].

A typical imagery rescripting protocol consists of two phases of processing [26, 28]. In the first phase, an upsetting trauma event is identified, and the therapist enters the image, providing safety, validation, and care. In many childhood abuse and neglect cases, the adult has poor examples of care. Therefore, the therapist aims in the initial stage to model how the client can rescript the scene and reduce disabling feelings of anxiety and shame. During the second phase, the therapist encourages the client (as an adult) to enter the image and manage the abusive antagonist and situation. It is vital to highlight the rationale for this practice to clients: it is an essential step for them to take to increase their experience of empowerment, autonomy, and mastery.

The number of sessions within phases 1 and 2 can depend on case severity and the effectiveness of the imagery. In our view, after 6–10 sessions of imagery rescripting within phase 1, it may be helpful to ask the client if they feel prepared to stand up for their child self. For example, 'On a rating between zero ("no way") to ten ("let me in there"), where do you feel you stand regarding rescripting the image?' If a client states a level of three or above, it may be time for the therapist to encourage the client to rescript the image. Our view is that successful processing ultimately requires the client to rescript the memory and independently care for their younger selves. Also, imagery rescripting may be more successful if the client comes to the session expecting to work on imagery rescripting (or another form of trauma processing) rather than introducing imagery rescripting exercises periodically or spontaneously. A 'block' of work can significantly help with avoidance, bring greater momentum and increasing the focus on changing legacies derived from traumatic events.

Concluding Remarks

Schema therapy is well suited to assist in the treatment of CPTSD. The model is a flexible framework for conceptualising complex client problems and behaviour patterns. The model can help the client be 'willing and able' to complete trauma processing work. Specifically, a schema therapy approach to CPTSD aims to strengthen the Healthy Adult mode to allow the client to participate in specific trauma processing interventions. While imagery rescripting is a natural tool for trauma processing (particularly concerning childhood trauma), the model can complement other trauma processing approaches (e.g., EMDR). Schema therapy's focus on the therapy relationship and offering the experience of limited reparenting is a crucial factor that sets it apart from other approaches and can significantly enhance therapeutic outcomes for the client.

References

1. Felitti V, Anda R, Nordenberg D, et al. Relationship of childhood abuse and household dysfunction to many of the leading causes of death in adults: The Adverse Childhood Experiences (ACE) Study. *American Journal of Preventive Medicine*. 1998;14(4):245–58.

2. Herman J. Complex PTSD: A syndrome in survivors of prolonged and repeated trauma. *Journal of Traumatic Stress*. 1992;5(3):377–91.

3. Cloitre M. Complex PTSD: assessment and treatment. *European Journal of Psychotraumatology*. 2021; 12:1866423.

4. World Health Organization. International statistical classification of diseases and related health problems (11th ed.) [Online]. 2019 (cited July 2021). https://icd.who.int/.

5. Cloitre M, Courtois C, Ford J, et al. *The ISTSS expert consensus treatment guidelines for complex PTSD in adults*. 2012. www.istss.org/treating-trauma/istss-complex-ptsd-treatment-guidelines.aspx.

6. De Jongh A, Resick P, Zoellner L, et al. Critical analysis of the current treatment guidelines for complex PTSD in adults.

Depression and Anxiety. 2016;33(5):359–69.

7. Royal Commission into Invitational Responses to Childhood Sexual Abuse [Internet], Canberra. Final report. 2017. www.childabuseroyalcommission.gov.au/final-report.

8. Ullman S, Brecklin L. Sexual assault history and health-related outcomes in a national sample of women. *Psychology of Women Quarterly*. 2003;27(1):46–57.

9. Ahrens C, Stansell J, Jennings A. To tell or not to tell: The impact of disclosure on sexual assault survivors' recovery. *Violence and Victims*. 2010;25(5):631–48.

10. Boterhoven de Haan K, Lee CW, Correia H, et al. clients and therapist perspectives on treatment for adults with PTSD from childhood trauma. *Journal of Clinical Medicine*. 2021;10(5):954.

11. Weathers F, Blake D, Schnurr P, et al. *The life events checklist for DSM-5 (LEC-5) PTSD*. National Center for PTSD; 2013.

12. Barnes J, Noll J, Putnam F, Trickett P. Sexual and physical revictimization among victims of severe childhood sexual

abuse. *Child Abuse & Neglect.* 2009;**33**(7):412–20.

13. Knipe J. *EMDR toolbox: Theory and treatment of complex PTSD and dissociation.* Springer Publishing Company; 2018.

14. Bernstein D, van den Broek E. Schema Mode Observer Rating Scale (SMORS). Unpublished manuscript, Department of Psychology, Maastricht University, The Netherlands; 2006.

15. Korn D, Leeds A. Preliminary evidence of efficacy for EMDR resource development and installation in the stabilization phase of treatment of complex posttraumatic stress disorder. *Journal of Clinical Psychology.* 2002;**58**(12):1465–87.

16. Phoenix Australia Australian guidelines for the Prevention and treatment of Acute Stress Disorder, Posttraumatic Stress Disorder and Complex PTSD. 2021. www.phoenixaustralia.org/wp-content/uploads/2020/07/Chapter-7.-CPTSD.pdf.

17. Cloitre M, Courtois C, Ford J, et al. The ISTSS expert consensus treatment guidelines for complex PTSD in adults. 2012. www.istss.org/treating-trauma/istss-complex-ptsd-treatment-guidelines.aspx.

18. Huntjens RJ, Rijkeboer MM, Arntz A. Schema therapy for dissociative identity disorder (DID): Rationale and study protocol. *European Journal of Psychotraumatology.* 2019;**10**(1):1571377.

19. Lynn S, Maxwell R, Merckelbach H, et al. Dissociation and its disorders: Competing models, future directions, and a way forward. *Clinical Psychology Review.* 2019;**73**:101755.

20. Schauer M, Elbert T. Dissociation following traumatic stress. *Zeitschrift für Psychologie/Journal of Psychology.* 2010;**218**(2):109–27.

21. Siegel D. *Developing mind: How relationships and the brain interact to shape who we are, 3rd ed.* Guilford Press; 2020.

22. Ogden P. Modulation, mindfulness, and movement in the treatment of trauma-related depression. In: Kernan M, ed. *Clinical pearls of wisdom: Twenty one leading therapists offer their key insights.* Norton & Company; 2010. pp. 1–13.

23. Leutner S, Piedfort-Marin O. The concept of ego state: From historical background to future perspectives. *European Journal of Trauma & Dissociation.* 2021;**5**(4):100184.

24. Nijenhuis E, van der Hart O, Steele K. Trauma-related structural dissociation of the personality. *Activitas Nervosa Superior.* 2010;**52**(1):1–23.

25. Ehring T, Welboren R, Morina N, et al. Meta-analysis of psychological treatments for post-traumatic stress disorder in adult survivors of childhood abuse. *Clinical Psychology Review.* 2014;**34**(8):645–57.

26. De Haan K, Lee C, Fassbinder E, et al. Imagery rescripting and eye movement desensitisation and reprocessing as treatment for adults with post-traumatic stress disorder from childhood trauma: Randomised clinical trial. *The British Journal of Psychiatry.* 2020;**217**(5):609–15.

27. Lee C, Boterhoven de Haan K. Working with trauma memories and complex post-traumatic stress disorder. In Heath G, Startup H, ed. *Creative methods in schema therapy: Advances and innovation in clinical practice.* Routledge; 2020.

28. Arntz A, Weertman A. Treatment of childhood memories: Theory and practice. *Behaviour Research and Therapy.* 1999;**37**(8):715–40.

Chapter 15

Schema Therapy for Eating Disorders

Introduction

In this chapter, we illustrate a schema therapy approach to working with eating disorders via a detailed case study of a young woman with anorexia nervosa. The case exemplifies problems that commonly accompany eating disorders, including post-traumatic stress disorder and borderline personality disorder. The case also highlights how to manage providing schema therapy in the face of serious medical issues, the schema therapy conceptualisation of eating disorders, and the integration of coping modes into the client's Healthy Adult mode.

Challenges in Treating Eating Disorders

There are several factors that create particular challenges in treating eating disorders. First, eating disorders are often experienced as ego-syntonic (e.g., 'I don't know who I would be without my anorexia') and are characterised by ambivalence about changing eating disorder behaviours. Second, the physiological effects of eating disorders can hinder treatment attendance and engagement. Third, although eating disorders may cause high levels of distress, they also function as a 'solution' to underlying difficulties and suffering by providing a sense of coherence, achievement, mastery, control, identity, emotional regulation, comfort, safety, and connection to significant others. Encouragingly, though, due to an established track record in the effective treatment of entrenched difficulties, rigid personality traits, and complex trauma, schema therapy appears well placed to work with eating disorders which have not responded to first-line treatments.

Eating disorders are characterised by high levels of avoidance and/or overcompensation, so under-reporting of schemas, modes, and unmet needs is common. Eating disorders can provide a 'cocoon', which functions to protect and disconnect the person from awareness of deeper emotional suffering. Clients frequently present citing the eating disorder as the primary issue, without awareness that it has developed to protect them from underlying distress and low self-esteem associated with EMS.

In the assessment phase, the more obvious precipitants to the development of eating disorders and associated EMS, such as sexual, physical, and emotional abuse, are usually easier to identify than those areas where unmet needs represent a 'lack' of emotional 'ingredients' such as empathy and attunement. Furthermore, many clients, especially those with avoidant personality traits, struggle to recognise and describe the more subtle ways in which their basic emotional needs were not met. It is common for those with eating disorders to experience high levels of shame and guilt and to be fearful of blaming caregivers for their difficulties. Therefore, identification of unmet needs in this population

279

often requires a great deal of detective work, using hypothetical questioning (for further details, see Chapter 3) and asking for concrete examples. In particular, clinicians should be alert to any mismatch between the client's temperament and the parenting style and/or childhood atmosphere they were exposed to as children: for example, a child with a highly perfectionistic temperament matched with a highly demanding parenting style or pressurised schooling environment; or a sensitive, anxious temperament with a chaotic and stressed family environment. It is also important to reassure the client that even though there may have been unmet emotional needs such as empathy and attunement, this does not negate any positive events, love, and affection that were experienced during childhood. From this perspective, it can be helpful to begin by assessing the best aspects of childhood and which needs *were* met, before investigating missing ingredients. The following case example shows how schema therapy can be applied to work transdiagnostically with even the most severe eating disorders, alongside other complex psychiatric comorbidities (e.g., BPD). For more detail about a schema therapy approach to eating disorders, readers are directed to work by Simpson and Smith [1].

Assessment and Conceptualisation: Case Example of 'Amanda'

Presenting Issues

Amanda was a 21-year-old woman meeting diagnostic criteria for anorexia nervosa (restrictive), PTSD, panic disorder, and comorbid borderline personality disorder. She presented for treatment with low weight (body mass index of 15), suicidal urges, and a pattern of self-harm through cutting. Eating behaviours included severe dietary restriction and ritualised laxative abuse leading to episodes of stomach pain lasting 3–4 hours overnight, followed by further severe restriction. At intake she also described poor concentration and memory, flashbacks, and nightmares associated with sexual abuse that had taken place from the age of seven. At the time of intake, she was still living at home with her parents.

Mental State

At intake, Amanda presented as detached and unaware of her emotions. She seemed concerned about how her eating disorder affected her family, but indifferent to her own struggle. She described feeling undeserving of treatment and believed she should 'stop being so selfish and sort [her]self out'.

Predisposing Factors

Amanda was a shy, anxious child. She and her brother spent most of their childhood alone with their mother as their father worked long hours. Amanda's parents struggled to cope with their own emotional difficulties, and their capacity to provide emotional support, nurturance, empathy, and protection was limited. Her father was rule-bound and viewed relationships and the world in black-and-white terms (i.e., 'there is a "right" and "wrong" way to do everything'). Her mother was passive, compliant, and often overwhelmed with anxiety; she struggled to assert her own needs and set limits on others. From an early age, Amanda took on the role as intermediary between her parents, attempting to anticipate and reduce her father's criticism of her mother whilst acting as a confidante and providing emotional support for them both. In contrast, Amanda attempted to reduce any potential strain on her parents by minimising her own emotional and physical needs whilst striving to meet their needs and expectations.

Due to her parents' own unresolved schemas, their love was expressed in a manner which was, unwittingly, conditional on her meeting their emotional needs. On the one hand, she was praised for being self-sufficient and the 'good girl' by helping with parenting and providing emotional support for her mother when required, whilst at other times sensing that her mother needed Amanda to need her. This resulted in a confusing paradox whereby she learned to read the cues that signalled her mother's needs to ascertain whether her 'Hyperautonomous Good Girl mode' (Overcontroller), 'Enmeshed Nurturer' (Compliant Surrenderer), or her 'Rescue Me' (Helpless Surrenderer) mode would be the best fit. Amanda learned from an early age that she was praised and appreciated when prioritising her parents' needs (and thereby her need to stay attached to them) over the need for authenticity (i.e., to be and express her true self) by blocking emotions and needs which may inconvenience others.

The home atmosphere was grim and austere, with minimal opportunity for play and fun. Amanda's attempts at individuation, such as trying to arrange activities with her friends or to plan for future studies, were met with disapproval and the feeling that she was in some way hurting her parents by making choices that were 'wrong'.

Amanda was sexually abused by her grandfather between the ages of seven and nine. Her eventual disclosure to her parents resulted in further isolation. Her mother became highly emotional, leading to Amanda feeling significant guilt and responsibility for her mother's distress. Her father reacted angrily, dismissing the grandfather, but never mentioned the issue again. This experience further reinforced Amanda's Helpless Surrenderer mode: she was helpless to prevent both the abuse itself and her parents' responses. Further, there was no opportunity to process her own distress and anger in relation to the trauma.

Amanda's EMS and modes were assessed through a combination of interview, the Young Parenting Inventory, and the Schema Mode Inventory for Eating Disorders (SMI-ED). Her most prominent modes and the dynamics between them are displayed in Figure 15.1.

Highest Scoring Schemas

Emotional Deprivation – Others can never understand me or meet my needs (because my needs are 'too much').

Defectiveness – I am undeserving, worthless, 'wrong'.

Emotional Inhibition – My needs and feelings are a burden/threat to others. I must keep them to myself.

Enmeshment – I only exist and have worth when in the presence of significant others.

Self-Sacrifice – I am responsible for 'fixing' the suffering of others.

Punitiveness – I deserve to be punished when I make a mistake or get things wrong.

Mistrust/Abuse – Others will hurt and use me.

Origins of Modes Linked to Onset of Eating Disorder

Prioritising the family's well-being required self-denial – and anorexia provided the solution. It was hypothesised that Amanda's Overcontroller coping mode drove her dietary restriction and low weight, enabling her to ignore her physiological (interoceptive) signals

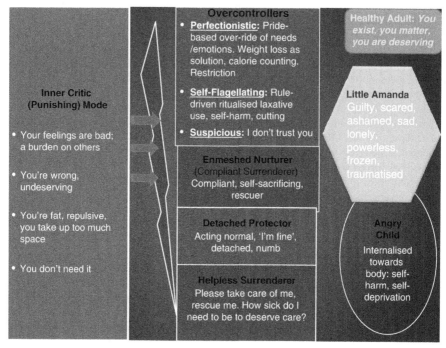

Figure 15.1 Example: Amanda's mode map

and emotions, thereby protecting herself from frightening trauma symptoms, loneliness, and shame. Amanda's Overcontroller (Perfectionistic, Invincible) mode was intermittently reinforced by a sense of achievement and invincibility by restricting her eating and the associated weight loss. She was later able to associate the onset of this coping mode to her experiences at age seven, when she felt overwhelming fear and helplessness in the face of sexual abuse. The Overcontroller mode generated the urge to engage in cleaning rituals, and later in dietary restriction, as a means of overcompensating for the feelings of powerlessness. It was hypothesised that early in childhood, after recognising her parents' extreme discomfort with anger, her (dissociated) Angry-Rebellious child mode was controlled and re-directed inward through a (Self-Flagellating) Overcontroller mode, manifested by laxative abuse and self-cutting. In this way, Amanda's Overcontroller also fulfilled a 'self-flagellating' role. Amanda described an evening ritual of taking large quantities of laxatives. This partially fulfilled a 'cleansing' function, which brought temporary relief from her inner sense of 'badness', but also led to painful stomach cramps, which she described as a type of ritualistic practice of self-inflicting pain as a means of increasing tolerance and sense of mastery over when and how she experienced pain. Self-harm through cutting fulfilled a similar function. Through the overcompensatory coping process of turning herself into the 'powerful one' who could control and inflict pain on her own body, she could temporarily eliminate the inner vulnerable, powerless, needy child whom she blamed for the rejection, loss, and abuse. By exerting control over her eating and weight and focusing on the sensations of emptiness in her body, Amanda described a temporary 'high', a rush of omnipotence associated with overcoming her basic human needs, and 'pleasure' associated with self-deprivation and punishment. Further, thinking of herself as the 'bad guy' provided a fantasy of control whereby through eliminating the bad aspects of herself, she could retain hope that she could someday be deserving of love.

Precipitants

Amanda's eating difficulties developed from age 12. As she reached puberty and gained weight and her body changed shape, she experienced a sense of being 'out of control' and 'exposed'. Her sense of herself as 'dirty', defective, and shameful became increasingly 'embodied'. She began restricting her diet and lost 10 kg over 8 months. Laxative abuse began at age 16. Each day became structured around episodes of taking laxatives and obsessional cleaning. Her regular admissions to the local inpatient facility always resulted in her discharging herself after 2–3 days due to high anxiety regarding weight gain. When she gained weight, her PTSD symptoms increased, leading to an increased urge to restrict and engage in laxative abuse.

Maintaining Factors: Vicious Mode Cycles

Primary messages associated with emotional neglect and abuse were internalised in the form of the Inner Critic. In childhood, this led to feelings of loneliness and powerlessness (Vulnerable Child), as well as a sense of unfairness and anger (Angry Child). The anger was repressed so as not to further threaten attachments with key caregivers. Amanda's eating behaviours and low weight provided an anaesthetising effect whilst she was engaged in these rituals (Overcontroller, Detached Protector), but afterwards she was overcome with a growing sense of shame and powerlessness (Inner Critic 'You stupid girl!' → Little Amanda [Shame]). Breakthrough flashbacks and nightmares continued to occur (Little [Abused] Amanda) and were largely controlled and numbed through laxative abuse and self-harm (Detached Protector; Overcontroller). Retaining the same level of numbness and the powerful 'high' required increasing levels of dietary restriction and self-inflicted ritualised pain via laxatives and self-harm (Overcontroller). Due to the time and energy required to focus on these rituals, Amanda became increasingly socially isolated (Little [Lonely] Amanda). Although her coping modes provided relief from emotional distress and avoidance of schema activation short term, over time the eating disorder itself increasingly became a source of secondary distress and shame (Inner Critic message: 'You're disgusting, unlovable').

By avoiding contact with others (Detached/Avoidant Protector), Amanda became increasingly reliant on her eating disorder as her only source of comfort, reinforcing her belief that she was inherently defective (Inner Critic 'You're so unlovable!' → Little Amanda [Shame]). On the one hand, her illness and low weight led to an increase in attention and concern by her parents (Helpless Surrenderer) but, on the other hand, they frequently remarked on the toll of her anorexia on them, reinforcing her sense that she was a burden on others (Inner Critic 'You're too much!' → Little Amanda [Guilt, Shame] 'I'm too needy, my needs are too much').

A flow diagram demonstrating the self-perpetuating pathways between these modes is presented in Figure 15.2.

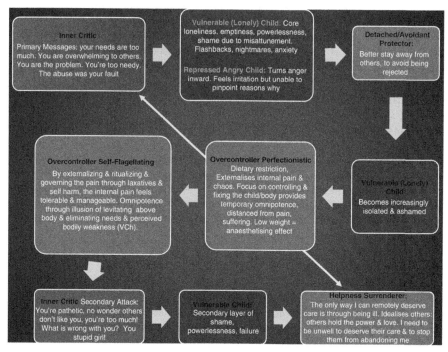

Figure 15.2 Self-perpetuating schema mode sequence

Treatment

Amanda attended 50 sessions over 18 months. Intermittent hospital admissions, fatigue due to insomnia associated with laxative abuse, and a very low BMI initially interfered with engagement and attendance. The treatment plan first prioritised reducing eating disorder symptoms, whilst addressing her schema-driven fears around connection and attachment to others, and, finally, resolving trauma symptoms.

Sequence of Therapy

○ *Bonding*: Developing trust, understanding and engagement, with an emphasis on limited reparenting as an antidote to childhood experiences.

○ *Weight gain and stabilisation*: Due to Amanda's low weight and inability to get any traction with weight gain in the community, treatment started with a 3-month admission to an inpatient unit to work on weight gain. It was explained that more than one admission may be needed, and she would be encouraged to work on weight gain in a step-wise fashion (increase weight, followed by consolidation, followed by further weight gain). In reality, this process is rarely linear, and setbacks in terms of weight loss are common. During this period, psychoeducation and stabilisation focused on identifying and interviewing the modes to discover how they were driving specific eating behaviours, body-image distortion, and self-harm. The therapist and the dietitian worked closely with

Amanda to manage high levels of anxiety and distress associated with preliminary weight gain. A mode map was developed collaboratively (see Figure 15.1).

o **Stabilisation continued after hospital discharge**: The therapist sought to activate and interact with the coping modes linked to laxative abuse and non-attendance. Through chairwork and imagery exercises, the therapist spent time getting to know these modes, validating their original intention and function, and gently reassuring them that the therapist was not trying to eliminate them, but rather work with them to care for and protect Little Amanda (Vulnerable Child).

o **Experiential mode work for increasing awareness**: Given Amanda's minimal awareness of her Vulnerable Child mode, experiential techniques initially focused on engaging with Little Amanda to increase her awareness of the underlying suffering driving her eating disorder. Chairwork was used to 'contaminate the chair' (for details, see Chapter 8).

o **Interviewing the modes**: Through a combination of chairwork and imagery, all modes were interviewed about their intention or function, as well as their hopes and fears about recovery. This was especially important because some coping modes were sabotaging her attendance at therapy sessions through: (a) interfering with sleep (due to laxative abuse); and (b) zoning out and telling her 'You don't need therapy'. Interviewing the coping modes revealed fears of getting in touch with difficult emotions, of being unsafe or at risk of further abuse and abandonment, and of being overcome by powerlessness and hopelessness. Her Inner Critic further sabotaged progress by telling her 'Treatment is a waste of time, you're not worth it'.

o **Empathic confrontation**: The first step to improving attendance was through gentle empathic confrontation with the modes via chairwork. Amanda was encouraged to change her routine so that laxative use did not take place at a time that interfered with attendance at sessions.

o **Getting to know the internal mode-family**: Imagery was used to set up 'mode meetings'. Amanda was guided to imagine a calm (safe) place where she could invite the modes that were driving her eating-disordered behaviours to meet. This was aimed at increasing co-consciousness: awareness of both the 'front stage' modes that she was already overidentified or 'fused' with, such as the Overcontroller modes, as well as the 'back stage' modes which had become rejected or dissociated, such as Vulnerable/Abused Child, Angry Child, and Impulsive Child. In the mode meetings, Amanda was asked to describe the appearance of each of the modes, and her feelings and reactions towards them from the perspective of her 'Adult self'. Through a series of meetings, it became apparent that there were alliances (e.g., Flagellating and Perfectionistic Overcontroller) and antagonism between some of the modes (e.g., Overcontroller [Flagellating, Suspicious] and Angry Child/Impulsive Child modes).

o **Increasing integration of modes by identifying common goals**: By having the modes meet and interact, common underlying goals and functions of coping modes could be identified, specifically to reduce suffering and increase safety, thereby beginning the process of gently encouraging them to work together. This is with the goal of eventually becoming a *Healthy Adult team* which retained all the positive traits and characteristics of even the most self-destructive coping modes (e.g., determination, conscientiousness, sensitivity, honesty). All modes except the Inner Critic were welcomed and engaged with.

o **Strengthening Healthy Adult mode**: Amanda's *Future Wise Self* was engaged as the part to take responsibility for attendance at sessions, holding hope that life could be different, and eventually coordinating the different modes that made up her 'self'. This part's role was to lead the Healthy Adult team (and move towards greater integration through resolving inner conflicts in the future).

○ *Reducing Dysfunctional Parent mode*: The origins of the Inner Critic were explored in terms of messages from the abuser, parents/family, and culture/media. Chairwork and imagery rescripting were frequently utilised to challenge this mode.

Experiential Mode Work for Healing Schemas and Increasing Internal Integration

○ *Chairwork to bypass coping modes*: Chairwork was used to highlight the role of Amanda's Inner Critic and coping modes in blocking connection with Little (Abused) Amanda. In one version of chairwork, the therapist played the role of the Vulnerable Child, whilst Amanda was invited to play the role of her Overcontroller mode, to promote emotion awareness. The therapist aimed to represent her suffering as authentically as possible, drawing on the client's previously reported (or 'hinted at') experiences of suffering and loneliness, in the hope that the Vulnerable Child part of her would resonate with this and feel 'seen' and heard. These exercises aimed to further increase schema and mode awareness through recognition that the different aspects of Amanda's 'self' and her eating disorder could be understood as 'modes' that were linked to EMS and unmet needs. Defusing from default coping modes and beginning the process of reconnecting with child modes was encouraged via chairwork. In Amanda's case, this internal awareness work allowed her to become aware of parts of the self that had become highly dissociated as a result of early traumatic experiences.

○ *Empathic confrontation*: When Amanda's coping modes felt threatened, such as when experiential techniques were suggested, they often attempted to block the work through debating, giving long detailed narratives, getting involved in power struggles, or protesting that it would be damaging and lead to self-harm. Empathic confrontation was used to validate their intention, whilst firmly reminding them that the goal of therapy was to heal Little Amanda, and that this would only be possible if they could allow access.

○ *Imagery rescripting*: Reparenting within imagery rescripting took place on a regular (at least fortnightly) basis, whereby Amanda's Wise (Healthy) Adult self and the therapist began to connect with Little Amanda to validate her needs and feelings. As she began to gradually increase her tolerance of revealing her vulnerability and getting her emotional needs met, the focus of this reparenting expanded to meeting a range of (previously unmet) needs related to her schemas, including emotional warmth, empathy, encouragement, guidance, play, and protection. Imagery rescripting was focused on challenging messages from childhood that invalidated Amanda's needs and emotions, whilst encouraging her to relinquish responsibility for her parent's emotional well-being (e.g., 'It's not your job to take care of the grown-ups. You're just a little girl'). Following 4–5 months of imagery rescripting sessions focused on early childhood experiences, Amanda's Wise Adult self was strengthened sufficiently to switch the focus of imagery rescripting to processing memories of sexual abuse, as well as the subsequent parental invalidation she experienced. When coping modes interrupted trauma-focused imagery rescripting – either directly through avoidance within sessions, or indirectly through increasing eating disorder and other risky behaviours outside of sessions – the focus switched to chair dialogues to reduce their interference through empathic confrontation.

○ *Transitioning Healthy Adult role to client*: Through imagery rescripting and chairwork, Amanda was encouraged to increasingly practise listening and talking to Little Amanda and her Angry Child (which were previously dissociated from conscious awareness) and to express distress and irritation at the schema-related messages.

○ *Imaginal mode meetings*: Through regular imagery and chairwork, the Overcontroller, Helpless Surrenderer, and other modes were gradually integrated via several 'mode meetings' in imagery, whereby Amanda's Healthy Adult side learned to acknowledge the messages, fears, and agendas of all the other modes, and to provide leadership, limit setting, and nurturance to her inner system. For example, the therapist might say 'Keeping your eyes closed, from your Wise Side, can you invite in the mode that is afraid to stop taking the laxatives? Which mode is it? Can you ask her what she is afraid of? What does that side need from you, as Wise Adult, to feel confident that she will be safe to take this step? Can you give her that?'

Between sessions, she was asked to notice which modes were underlying the thoughts and urges associated with her eating disorder, and to engage with Little Amanda (and/or other child modes) through imagery, enquire about her needs, and try to meet these in some way rather than 'acting them out' through disordered eating behaviours (see Chapter 11 for further details on working with coping modes).

Cognitive and Behavioural Interventions

Cognitive and behavioural work focused on defying schema messages and prioritising play, fun, and joy. Amanda was encouraged to 'rebel' against her Inner Critic and to set boundaries with others in her present-day life. Most importantly, goals were set to prioritise her nutritional needs and to learn to develop her proprioceptive and interoceptive awareness. She was encouraged to tolerate 'taking up more space', by both allowing herself to reach a normal weight and learning to openly ask for her needs to be met, and to reconnect with the felt sense of being in her body. This took place alongside experiential exercises to develop a stronger sense of an embodied (as opposed to intellectualised) self. This was developed through playful positive-reparenting imagery focusing on sensory experiences (e.g., 'feel the grass under your toes') and prescribed somatic mindfulness practices.

Final Phase

In the final phase of therapy, further integration was pursued via 'mode meetings', with the modes being encouraged to work together to fulfil their roles as a 'Healthy Adult team' to meet the needs of Little Amanda. As Amanda learned to express herself in more direct ways, the urge to communicate her needs through the Helpless Surrenderer mode (i.e., helplessness, being 'ill'), and to self-regulate through the Detached Protector and Overcontroller modes, lessened.

Concluding Remarks

This chapter illustrates the complex functions that eating disorder behaviour can take, including self-punishment, emotional avoidance, empowerment, mastery, self-regulation, and appeasement of others. The schema therapy approach encourages disaggregating these functions, personifying them, understanding them, and directing dialogues between them. A case study illustrates the way in which the schema mode model can be applied to work with eating disorder symptoms alongside complex trauma. A sufficient level of medical and nutritional stability (as indicated by blood tests and weight) must be reached to provide sufficient safety for therapy to proceed. A key component of schema therapy is to understand the unmet needs and schemas that have led to the development of an eating disorder. The mode map should be developed collaboratively to elucidate the client's internal world, with particular emphasis on increasing awareness of dissociated modes. The client gradually learns to reconnect with her/his inner child states and needs through extensive experiential work. Coping modes are not just bypassed, but, through imagery and chairwork, are actively acknowledged and integrated with the Healthy Adult, to form a Healthy Adult 'team' that works to prioritise the inner child modes and ultimately meet the client's nutritional, physiological, and emotional needs.

References

1. Simpson S, Smith E. *Schema therapy for eating disorders: Theory and practice for individual and group settings*. Routledge; 2019.

Further Reading

Edwards D. An interpretative phenomenological analysis of schema modes in a single case of anorexia nervosa: Part 1. Background, method, and child and parent Modes. *Indo-Pacific Journal of Phenomenology*. 2017;17(1):1–13.

Edwards DJ. An interpretative phenomenological analysis of schema modes in a single case of anorexia nervosa: Part 2. Coping modes, healthy adult mode, superordinate themes, and implications for research and practice. *Indo-Pacific Journal of Phenomenology*. 2017;17(1):1–12.

McIntosh VV, Jordan J, Carter JD, et al. Psychotherapy for transdiagnostic binge eating: A randomized controlled trial of cognitive-behavioural therapy, appetite-focused cognitive-behavioural therapy, and schema therapy. *Psychiatry Research*. 2016;240:412–20.

Pugh M. A narrative review of schemas and schema therapy outcomes in the eating disorders. *Clinical Psychology Review*. 2015;39:30–41.

Simpson S. Schema therapy for eating disorders: A case study illustration of the mode approach. In van Vreeswijk M, Broersen J, Nadort M, eds. *The Wiley-Blackwell handbook of schema therapy*. Wiley-Blackwell 2012, pp. 43–71.

Simpson SG, Morrow E, Reid C. Group schema therapy for eating disorders: a pilot study. *Frontiers in Psychology*. 2010;1:182.

Simpson SG, Slowey L. Video therapy for atypical eating disorder and obesity: A case study. *Clinical Practice and Epidemiology in Mental Health*. 2011;7:38–43.

Waller G, Kennerley H, Ohanian V. Schema-focused cognitive-behavioural therapy for eating disorders. In Rodin J, du Toit PL, Stein DJ, Young JE, eds. *Cognitive schemas and core beliefs in psychological problems: A scientist-practitioner guide*. American Psychological Association; 2007.

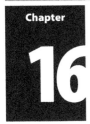

Chapter

Schema Therapy for Forensic Populations

Introduction

As an approach devised to better treat people with personality disorders, schema therapy offers a promising framework for addressing the psychiatric needs of forensic populations. In the past fifteen years, considerable progress has been made in conceptualising the personalities of those involved with violence and crime within the schema mode model [1, 2]. This has led to the identification of distinct modes and adaptations to treatment. In this chapter, we elaborate on the description and identification of schema modes characteristically seen in forensic populations and the adaptations needed to improve response to therapy.

Schema Mode Profiles of Forensic Populations

Research has shown a high prevalence of cluster B personality disorders (e.g., BPD, NPD, ASPD) in forensic populations [3], and a relationship between personality disorders and relevant schemas and modes [4]. Many, if not most, violent offenders are themselves the victims of childhood trauma or various other forms of maltreatment [5]. Coping modes such as Detached Self-Soother, Detached Protector, and Self-Aggrandiser were prevalent among these populations, but could not fully explain a wider range of forensic risk behaviour seen among offenders in the forensic system. This led to an expanded set of recognised schema modes to include the following, commonly seen among offenders: Bully and Attack mode, Paranoid Overcontroller mode, Conning Manipulator mode, and Predator mode [2].

The most striking commonality among schema modes found in forensic clients is the use of overcompensation as a coping style. Overcompensator modes occur when the person attempts to 'turn the tables' on others or 'take the upper hand'. Forensic clients often view the world in terms of victims and aggressors: 'top dog' and 'bottom dog'. The best strategy to avoid becoming a victim is to get on the offensive: dominate others, so they can't dominate you (Self-Aggrandiser mode); anticipate threats, so that you can attack before being attacked (Paranoid Overcontroller mode); manipulate others, so that won't take advantage of you (Conning Manipulator mode); bully and threaten others who might aggress against you (Bully and Attack mode); and use cold, calculated aggression to eliminate those who stand in your way (Predator mode). All of these modes employ overcompensatory coping for self-protection.

Early case studies demonstrated the relevance of the schema therapy model to understanding violent offenders, including psychopathic clients [6]. Interestingly, these studies confirmed that offenders may indeed present with Vulnerable Child feelings that could be reached and helped by a schema therapy. Recently, a large-scale randomised controlled trial was completed demonstrating the efficacy of schema therapy for violent offenders with personality disorders [7] (see Chapter 2 for an overview).

Schema Therapy Model of Forensic Risk Behaviour

The central tenet of the forensic schema therapy model is that criminal and violent behaviour (and the risk thereof) can be understood as an 'unfolding sequence of schema mode activation' [8]. The circumstances preceding criminal behaviour often involve the triggering of overwhelming child modes and related underlying schemas (e.g., Abandonment, Defectiveness, Mistrust/Abuse) that invariably lead to the activation of one or more coping modes that represent forensic risk behaviour (e.g., Bully and Attack, Self-Soother). The dominant question guiding forensic schema therapy assessment is: What mode, or sequence of modes, is activated during an offender's acts of crime?

The forensic schema therapy model (see Figure 16.1) provides a framework for understanding and treating forensic risk behaviour. Schema modes represent distinct 'pathways to offending' – internal vulnerability risk factors for offending behaviour [8]. Healthy schema modes (especially the Healthy Adult mode) are considered internal protective factors which decrease the likelihood of offending behaviour. While other developmental (e.g., history of trauma), situational (e.g., being incarcerated with antisocial peers), genetic, and temperamental factors will influence risk of offending, the likelihood of forensic risk behaviour at a given moment is determined by the relative activation of maladaptive and healthy modes for an individual [8].

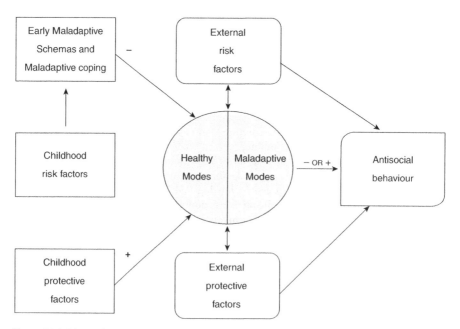

Figure 16.1 Schema therapy conceptual model of forensic risk behaviour
Adapted from Bernstein et al. (2019) [8]. **Note:** + increases forensic risk behaviour, – decreases forensic risk behaviour.

When forensic clients commit crimes or acts of violence, it is usually possible to reconstruct these events as an unfolding sequence of modes, with one state triggering another, culminating in criminal or aggressive behaviour. Research indicates that the events preceding crimes are often initiated by emotional triggers such as feelings of abandonment, loneliness, worthlessness, humiliation, mistrust, fear, anger, and frustration. Thus, child modes such as the Vulnerable Child, Lonely Child, Impulsive/Undisciplined Child, and Angry/Enraged Child, and associated EMS appear to play key roles in triggering a sequence of events that result in antisocial and violent behaviour. As events progress, the client's emotional vulnerability often becomes less evident, but their anger and impulsivity often escalate. Substance abuse often plays a major facilitating role in these events, as the client uses drugs or alcohol to quell any inner pain (Detached Self-Soother mode), further disinhibiting and emboldening them to carry out antisocial acts. During the crime itself, and the events immediately preceding it, the offender's overcompensatory modes tend to take centre stage. Here, the offender's use of dominance (Self-Aggrandiser mode), deceit and manipulation (Conning Manipulator mode), threats and aggression (Bully and Attack mode), hyper-alertness to threat (Paranoid Overcontroller mode), and cold, ruthless aggression (Predator mode) are evident.

It is not always the case that crimes are triggered by vulnerable emotions. In some cases, for example, crimes stem from entitlement, callousness, or impulsiveness; that is, some crimes arise from an insistence that one is entitled to get what one wants, with callous disregard for the rights or needs of others (Self-Aggrandiser mode), or a need for immediate gratification that overrides any inhibitions (Impulsive Child mode). Whichever way the crime is instigated, the therapist specifies the links between modes and crimes, giving them and the client clear and measurable targets, with the goal of reducing the client's risk of recidivism.

As with schema therapy for any population, the quality of case conceptualisation is critical to working with offenders. Schema therapy is indicated when specific modes are associated with particular criminal behaviours. Offence analysis involves understanding the mode sequence (e.g., Vulnerable Child → Punitive Critic → Bully & Attack mode) that propels the individual towards offending, as well as moments wherein healthy modes (e.g., Healthy Adult mode) have ascendance and offer opportunities for the individual to disengage from violent or other criminal impulses. Patterns of offending that do not fit well with a schema mode conceptualisation (e.g., violence driven by florid psychosis) are unlikely to be well suited to schema therapy. The internal risk factors for antisocial behaviour, their corresponding schema modes, the clinical manifestations of the modes, and the goals of schema therapy interventions are summarised in Table 16.1.

Forensic Schema Therapy: Considerations and Adaptations

The basic treatment approach is consistent with schema therapy generally as described in this book; however, a key objective for the treatment is to reduce the recidivism risk of offenders. Treatment ultimately aims to (1) help clients experience more satisfaction of basic needs, (2) heal underlying painful schemas, (3) reverse maladaptive coping behaviour, and (4) build the Healthy Adult mode. Schema therapy works across the central vulnerability factors for forensic risk behaviour (internal and external), while developing the Healthy Adult mode as a protective factor. Notwithstanding this, schema therapy with forensic clients also requires several considerations and potential adaptations from general clinical work [9], as discussed herein.

Table 16.1 Internal risk factors for antisocial behaviour, schema mode manifestations, and typical schema therapy intervention focus

Relevant Dynamic Internal Risk Factor	Schema mode	Clinical manifestation (Cognitions, Emotions and Behaviours)	Goals of Interventions
Early maladaptive schemas involving disconnection/ rejection and abuse	Vulnerable Child Lonely Child Punitive Critic Demanding Critic	Feels rejected, inferior, humiliated, anxious, isolated, excessive self-punishing, and self-critical	Healing painful emotions and underlying maladaptive schema Enhancing capacity for positive emotional states and healthy attachments to other people
Excessive anger, anger dysregulation	Angry/Enraged Child	Easily triggered to anger and rage; misperceives situations as threatening or unfair; rigid; 'all-or-nothing' control over anger	Experience degrees of anger; making realistic appraisals of situations; expressing anger in modulated, constructive ways
Behavioural disinhibition; low frustration tolerance	Impulsive Child	Acts quickly on impulses without thinking or planning; can't tolerate limits or delays in gratification	Increase frustration tolerance; stopping and thinking before acting
Addictive behaviours	Detached Protector, Detached Self-Soother/ Self-Stimulator	Uses drugs to self-regulate emotions, engages in addictive thrill-seeking behaviour	Improve emotional self-regulation; diminishing addictive behaviour; developing relapse prevention skills
Avoidant behaviours	Detached/Avoidant/Angry Protector	Excessive, inflexible avoidance of people and emotions	Increasing ability to experience and express feelings; make genuine emotional contact with other people; coping effectively with people and situations

Domination and exploitation of others	Self-Aggrandiser, Conning/Manipulator mode	Arrogant, condescending towards others; exploitative, uses other people; deceives and manipulates others	Approaching others as equals, and relationships as reciprocal; behaving honestly towards others, connecting with others
Threats and aggression towards others	Paranoid Overcontroller, Bully and Attack, Predator mode	Hypervigilant to (perceived) threats; 'hot' reactive aggression in response to threats; uses intimidation, aggression to achieve goals; uses cold, ruthless aggression to eliminate threats, obstacles, or rivals	Developing balanced, realistic appraisals of the intentions of other people; developing empathy for victims and remorse for previous offences; recognising and avoiding triggers for aggression; using healthy, non-aggressive methods of resolving conflicts and pursuing goals

The Forensic Treatment Context Is Considerably Different

First, schema therapy in forensic settings tends to involve clients who have been mandated to work on their risk of reoffending. Such clients will often be engaged for therapy while incarcerated or with considerable monitoring and oversight from some form of parole or supervision 'system'. This is important for at least two reasons. First, mandated clients tend to present as decidedly unmotivated for treatment. They present for treatment because they are obligated by the system in one way or another. This treatment context, and the loss of autonomy that it represents, will often result in clients presenting to therapy in very strong coping modes of one form or another. This contrasts from much general clinical work, where it is the client's Healthy Adult side that generally motivates them to initiate therapy. The mandated treatment context needs to be acknowledged and worked through in the initial stages of the therapy, where the therapist works to build safety and rapport and bypass the client's strong coping modes. While building rapport, the schema therapist works hard to build trust by being reliable and consistent, and following through on any agreements.

Second, the primary treatment goal in forensic settings is predetermined by the system: to reduce the risk of reoffending behaviour. While the schema therapist will, as in general schema therapy, be focused on healing the client's painful schemas and modes and apply a 'trauma lens', the offence analysis of risk and the client's offending behaviour must be on the agenda and be a primary treatment goal. Use of the emerging mode conceptualisation and mode map for the purpose of offence analysis is a distinctive feature of forensic schema therapy. Many forensic clients would be reluctant to engage in such analysis of their crimes and would employ coping modes to avoid or distract from this task. Some may come willing to work on their schemas, traumas, and 'pain' but would avoid anything that involves mode awareness of their offences. This is because reflecting and sharing details regarding one's pattern of offending can be very activating for offenders (e.g., shame, trust issues). Schema therapists need to be clients during this process, building up enough trust and rapport so that clients eventually feel safe to discuss and reflect on their offending pattern – but it cannot be avoided. The schema therapist works with the clients to understand their modes, and how they represent an offending risk pathway.

The Vulnerable Child Mode Can Be Hard to Reach in Offending Populations

Part of this is because forensic clients present in strong coping modes. These will need to be navigated and ultimately bypassed in the therapy relationship, as is usual in schema therapy. Another reason is that many forensic clients are not connected to this vulnerable mode and are not accustomed to expressing their needs through vulnerability. This is to be expected. Many such clients have come from backgrounds of abuse and neglect, wherein the expression of needs and vulnerability might have been punished or viewed as weakness. Schema therapists will be clients to bypass coping modes over time and look for opportunities to attune to and connect to any emerging vulnerable feelings.

At the same time, it is important not to push too much for vulnerability when other emotions are present to attune to. Many forensic clients are much more in touch with their Angry Child mode, or with feelings related to the activation of their Critic mode. It is worth remembering that both of these modes provide opportunity for attunement and corrective emotional experiences. One does not, for example, necessarily need to connect to the Vulnerable Child to do an affect bridge (imagery float back) exercise. Recent episodes involving the Angry Child mode provide a suitable experience from which to use an affect bridge and engage in imagery rescripting. Sometimes clients will retrieve memories involving themselves as a child in a state of frustration and anger, but on many occasions these memories will eventually link back to some feelings of vulnerability experienced as a child. When aiming to activate emotions in the client, it is more important to 'go with where the action is' (e.g., anger) rather than pushing too directly for vulnerability. In other words, the Angry Child mode, and indeed Critic modes, present as suitable initial targets for limited reparenting and experiential work.

Getting Comfortable Working With High Levels of Anger and a Larger Focus on Empathic Confrontation and Limit Setting

As already discussed, forensic clients tend to be much more able to express their needs through their anger than through vulnerability. Schema therapists thus need to get comfortable working with high levels of expressed anger. While schema therapists will seek to attune to, express, and validate Angry Child feelings in the therapy relationship, expressions of aggressive or destructive behaviour – often reflective of coping modes (e.g., Bully and Attack, Self-Aggrandiser) – should signal the therapist to instil more boundaries. Schema therapists working therapeutically with forensic clients thus become very good at providing empathic confrontation and limit setting and rely much more on these techniques than in general clinical work. Forensic clients are much more adept at pushing boundaries in the therapy relationship, perhaps reflective of some of their central problems. In the schema therapy model, boundary violations in the therapy relationship are seen as important opportunities for intervention, especially to heal schemas within the Impaired Limits domain. Bernstein and colleagues [8] describe this as limited reparenting with a 'here and now' focus. For some clients, therapeutic interactions may be one of a handful of times someone has tried to set a boundary and 'stick it out' in a caring and empathic way. Boundary violations in the therapy relationship thus reflect important opportunities for healing.

Working With the Conning Manipulator

Therapists not accustomed to forensic work are unlikely to have wide-reaching experience of being in a therapeutic relationship with someone with a strong Conning Manipulator mode. There can be a danger that therapists will fail to recognise this mode, with the result that the offender does not engage earnestly in therapy. Conversely, therapists who are too cynical about the possibility of change for offenders will struggle to provide a level of basic optimism in therapy. Forensic schema therapists are realistic about the high prevalence of Conning Manipulator among offenders, working directly with clients to build awareness of this mode when it is part of the case conceptualisation. For many clients, it is only natural that the Conning Manipulator mode presents itself at some stage during the therapy, especially at times of high distress or activation, or during impasses in the therapeutic relationship. Like with any coping mode, schema therapists seek to work directly with the coping mode, empathising with its adaptive value, but ultimately confronting and setting limits on this mode as it interferes with the client attaining their long-term needs

Conning/ Manipulation Mode

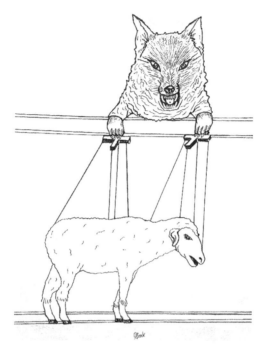

Illustration 16.1 Conning/Manipulation mode

(e.g., relationships) and increases their risk of reoffending. It can be disconcerting for therapists to work with modes that appear to have limited capacity for empathy for others; schema therapists need to be able to offer an alternative pathway to (operating in) this mode to enable connection to basic core needs (e.g., attachment and connectedness to others).

The Importance of Supervision and Self-Reflection

Having adequate supervisory support and reflective capacities are pivotal to working with offending client groups. Such client groups, with high prevalence of personality disorder traits, anger, aggressive behaviour, and impulsivity, can be very triggering for the therapist's own schemas. Transference issues are common and can be more intense in these settings (see Chapter 18).

The Need to Be Hopeful but Realistic About Change

Schema therapy offers a credible and evidence-based route to healing and reducing risk of reoffending, but it is not a panacea. The model suggests various factors within and outside of the person that are responsible for maintaining schemas and modes that present risks of offending behaviour. Several internal (e.g., motivation) and external (e.g., peer context) variables need to align to achieve optimal results and reduce risk of offending. A lot will also hinge on whether the therapist can engage the client in a limited reparenting relationship. Schema therapists will work hard to provide a therapeutic context for change, but remain realistic also about the challenges that lie ahead.

Working With Violent (Bully and Attack Mode) Urges in Imagery Rescripting Work

With aggressive antisocial clients, it is relatively common for violent urges to present themselves during imagery rescripting. In such imagery scenarios, clients may express the urge to be violent towards their antagonists and perpetrators, consistent with their Bully and Attack coping mode. Schema therapists need to be able to remain in control of the image and empathically decline the expression of such urges in imagery. Rather, the therapist seeks to find ways to meet the underlying childhood needs evident within the memory or image (e.g., safety) in a non-violent, but assertive (Healthy Adult) manner (see Box 16.1).

Working With the Impulsive and Undisciplined Child Modes

The Impulsive and Undisciplined Child modes are more common in offending populations and can represent a significant challenge for schema therapists who are not accustomed to regularly working with these modes. Intervening with these modes often involves working with underlying EMS in the Impaired Limits domain (e.g., Entitlement, Insufficient Self-Control) that can feel quite different for therapists in terms of the sentiment of any rescripting or reparenting interventions. The key here is that the care and limited reparenting offered in the treatment strategies with these schemas and modes involve the provision of limits and boundaries. These differences are exemplified in the script presented in Box 16.2 on Imagery Rescripting for the Impulsive and Undisciplined Child modes (ICM/UCM).

Box 16.1 Example of Violent Urges Within Imagery Rescripting with Forensic Clients

THERAPIST: What do you think Little Johnny needs right now in the image?
CLIENT: He needs someone to kill him (his father) . . . to smash his face in . . .
THERAPIST: Of course, you might feel that way . . . that is understandable given how he has been treating Little Johnny, and of course that is how you have learned to survive this.. But there is another way . . . another way to make it safe that does not involve being violent . . . let me show you. I will deal with dad now . . . Let's just have Little Johnny stay behind me I will protect him now.
CLIENT: . . . OK . . .
THERAPIST: (Takes care of the situation in an assertive manner consistent with a Healthy Adult)

Box 16.2 Therapist Instructions for Imagery Rescripting for the Impulsive and Undisciplined Child Modes

A. Select a Recent Episode and Tune in

Start with a discussion that involves a recent problematic episode when the Impulsive or Undisciplined Child mode (ICM/UCM) was being triggered. Spend some time attuning to this experience for the 'client' (e.g., scroll through specific triggers, feelings/bodily sensations, meanings/schema themes, and needs in that moment). It often presents as excitement or maybe frustration in being blocked in some way from acting according to their ICM/UCM. Once you and your client have a solid, shared understanding of the recent episode, invite the client to do some 'imagery work' on this recent trigger/feeling.

B. Connect to the Recent Episode in Imagery

Ask the client to . . .

> Close your eyes and get an image of yourself in this recent difficult situation. When you have the image tell me what you see . . . feel . . . also in the body.

Check for the meaning (i.e., slow things down again and help the client to 'tune in' to the image, with eyes closed). The goal is to put them 'in touch' with the feeling of this mode.

C. Invite the Affect Bridge/Imagery Floatback

> Now hold onto that feeling . . . the feeling of being xxxxxxx *[for example, being frustrated . . .that you should be able to do what you want]* . . . now take that feeling back as far as you can go . . . . . . *[pause]* . . . . . . even as far back as being a little boy/girl . . . *[pause]* . . . what's the first image that comes up for you connected to this feeling?

D. Tune in to the Child Experience in the Image

> When you have a childhood image tell me what you see as if you're there right now. Where are they? How old are they? What's happening in the image? What is Little [client name] feeling? What do they need or want?

Here we are trying to get an image of the child in the IC/UC state. Ensure the client stays in present tense.

If the client just goes to an image of the Vulnerable Child, just do a Vulnerable Child rescript as usual. This is relatively common. Underneath the ICM/UCM may be unmet Vulnerable Child mode needs such as neglect. However, if the client goes into an image of an ICM/UCM scenario then you will need to be ready to rescript those specific needs with some kind of boundary setting. So, tuning in here and understanding the child's needs here is crucial.

E. Therapist Enters the Image

> Can you bring me into the image with Little (IC/UC) [client name]?

When the client has you in the image, again ask what's going on for them, what are they feeling, thinking, etc. Your goal here is to keep the connection to the child feeling strong and build a solid understanding of the situation so that you can form an idea of what is needed for the child in this situation. What would a healthy parent do or have done in this kind of situation?

F. Therapist Rescripts. Step 1: Confront the Caregiver and Model Healthy Behaviour

Confront the caregiver with the need for limits, boundaries, and discipline:

> You think it's easier to let little [client name] do whatever they want, but it's not easier for them . . . when they grow up and you haven't given them the skills to control themselves and/or have the discipline they need.

Remember, you will need to meet the needs of the child in this moment so you must be attuned to their particular need(s). This may be a mixture of needs including boundaries, involvement, guidance, or stability. Continue until you 'win the exchange'.

G. Therapist Rescripts. Step 2 Child-Nurturing Image

> Turn to the Child. Ask Little [client name] 'How are you feeling now?' and 'Is there anything else you need from me to feel better [or the feeling that's most relevant to them, e.g. safe, content, peaceful]?'

If there are some residual needs, continue until the needs are met. If the client is now in their Vulnerable Child mode this will look more like child-compassion imagery. If the client is in their ICM/UCM, this will look more like empathic confrontation, as you would with a child who 'wants something' they can't have: 'I know it's frustrating for you when . . . but you can't have everything that you want.'

H. Finish the Image with Some Positive Activity/Involvement (If Possible)

When Little [client name] expresses feeling better, ask what they would like to do now. Engage in the imaginary activity for a few moments designed to help them feel your attention and connection. For example, you might take them to the park, read a book to them, or play catch. Note: It is likely this involvement/connection was missing, along with the limits.

I. Bring Back to the Present Moment and Prompt Some Reflection on the Process

Then say:

> When you're ready, slowly open your eyes and orient yourself to the room.

Ask them what it was like and what was most helpful in the image. Explain the concept of the relevant child modes (in which the primary feelings arising from unmet needs are felt) using the name, 'Little [client name]'. Suggest/discuss how they could bring what was helpful from the reparenting of Little [client name] in the imagery into the current situation when Little [client name] is triggered – i.e., how might Healthy [client name] take care of the needs in these kinds of situations? Tip: This might lead to a mode flashcard.

Additional Therapist Notes

1. In these ICM/UCM cases you are likely to land on an image of them getting what they 'want' or with a lack of boundaries/involvement or guidance. There can also be a significant Vulnerable Child mode element too in some cases. It is important to attune to, understand, and reparent both needs if they are present – a balance between warmth and limits. In some cases, you might decide to split the child feelings into its two parts – a Vulnerable Child mode and an ICM/UCM – and then address both parts.

2. In these cases, when addressing the parents, the classic scenario is that they will be under-involved or over-permissive. On occasion, you will encounter some more classic abusive, demanding, or controlling parents too, so be ready to provide safety and validation (or whatever else is needed) as with standard imagery rescripting protocols.

3. Sometimes there will be no parent involved in the childhood image at all. In these cases, just go straight to the child-nurturing image and provide a mix of care and attunement but also limits and boundaries, as required.

4. Remember: the chances of the child accepting your limits and boundaries in the image very much depend on the therapeutic relationship.

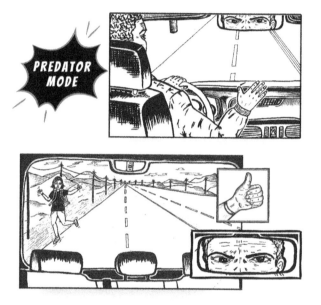

Illustration 16.2 Predator mode

Concluding Remarks

The schema mode model offers a nuanced understanding of offender behaviour that can promote deeper compassion for forensic clients. At the same time, the greater risks of harm to the client and others are real, so the forensic schema therapist, perhaps more than other schema therapists, must balance their nurturing abilities with their abilities to empathically confront and set limits. This is specialist work which we do not recommend undertaking in isolation, but, rather, with the supervision and support of forensic schema therapist colleagues.

References

1. Giesen-Bloo J, van Dyck R, Spinhoven P, et al. Outpatient psychotherapy for borderline personality disorder. *Archives of General Psychiatry.* 2006;**63**(6):649.

2. Bernstein D, Arntz A, Vos M. Schema focused therapy in forensic settings: Theoretical model and recommendations for best clinical practice. *International Journal of Forensic Mental Health.* 2007;**6**(2):169–83.

3. Blackburn R, Logan C, Donnelly J, Renwick S. Personality disorders, psychopathy and other mental disorders: Co-morbidity among clients at English and Scottish high-security hospitals. *The Journal of Forensic Psychiatry & Psychology.* 2003;**14**(1):111–37.

4. Keulen-de Vos ME, Bernstein DP, Vanstipelen S, et al. Schema modes in criminal and violent behaviour of forensic cluster B PD clients: A retrospective and prospective study. *Legal and Criminological Psychology.* 2016;**21**(1):56–76.

5. Schimmenti A, Di Carlo G, Passanisi A, Caretti V. Abuse in childhood and psychopathic traits in a sample of violent offenders. *Psychological Trauma: Theory, Research, Practice, and Policy.* 2015;**7**(4):340–7.

6. Chakhssi F, Kersten T, de Ruiter C, Bernstein DP. Treating the untreatable: A single case study of a psychopathic inpatient treated with Schema Therapy. *Psychotherapy.* 2014;**51**(3):447.

7. Bernstein DP, Keulen-de Vos M, Clercx M, et al. Schema therapy for violent PD offenders: a randomized clinical trial. *Psychological Medicine.* 2021;1–15.

8. Bernstein D, Clercx M, Keulen-De Vos M. Schema therapy in a forensic setting. In Polaschek D, Day A, Hollin C, eds. *The Wiley international handbook of correctional psychology.* John Wiley & Sons; 2019. pp. 654–68.

9. Madsen, L. Schema Therapy Crime Channel: Forensic schema therapy – Staring into the abyss [What's the Schemata: A Schema Therapist Podcast with Chris Hayes & Rob Brockman]. Perth, Australia. 24 July, 2021. www.schematherapytraining.com/podcast-whats-the-schemata/2021/7/23/schema-crime-channel-forensic-schema-therapy-staring-into-the-abyss.

Group Schema Therapy

Introduction

Group schema therapy has grown exponentially since the seminal 2009 paper by Farrell, Shaw, and Webber [1] demonstrating large effect sizes and low dropout rates in the treatment of BPD (see Chapter 2 for more details about research on group schema therapy). Given the current financial restraints on both public- and insurance-funded health services around the world, there is high demand for more efficient schema therapy protocols such as group-only schema therapy or group–individual hybrid models. Group schema therapy provides a wide range of corrective emotional experiences and greater opportunities for authentic rehearsal of new Healthy Adult mode behaviour than individual therapy can offer. In this chapter, a brief and general overview of group schema therapy is provided, emphasising the adaptations from individual schema therapy and drawing on foundational work by Farrell and Shaw [1] and van Vreeswijk and Broersen [2, 3, 4].

Adapting Schema Therapy to Group Delivery

Schema therapy groups usually consist of 8–10 members with two therapists leading. Some key aspects of the role of group therapists, particularly in the early phase of therapy, are summarised in Box 17.1.

In selecting group participants, therapists should ensure some homogeneity of EMS whilst allowing a mix of interpersonal coping styles. It is important that each member has some EMS and coping behaviours in common with other group participants to maximise opportunities for connection and minimise the sense of feeling 'different' from others in the group. Selecting a mix of ages and genders where possible can simulate a family environment which is thought to facilitate therapy.

At the start of the programme, therapists should set out preliminary expectations and shared limits, and they may wish to have members formalise their agreement through signing a group contract. A key commitment is to stay in the group (or at least the building) even when feeling triggered. However, even with an agreement in place, it is not uncommon for participants to become triggered and leave the group. In these instances, one group leader should attempt to reconnect with them to help identify the activated modes and bring the member back to the group. It can be helpful to emphasise to participants that their attendance is important not only for their own recovery but also for that of other participants. Absences can be discussed with the whole group in terms of schema-triggering and impact on the group 'family'. This facilitates learning about the importance of members' presence to others, challenging the notion that the therapists are the sole therapeutic ingredient of their recovery and highlighting their own value in others' recovery [5].

Box 17.1 Role of Group Schema Therapists

- Group schema therapists should be well-trained and access regular supervision.
- The two therapists model the role of 'parents' for the group as 'family'.
- Just as in a healthy parent team, group leaders must work together, alternating the role of leading the exercise and staying connected with the whole group.
- Therapists combine providing a source of fun and playfulness with setting limits and containment (i.e., an emotionally attuned safe space).
- Group leaders must develop ways of balancing the needs of individuals with the collective needs of the entire group.
- Some participants have schemas (e.g., Social Isolation) that leave them sensitive to feeling left out. Thus, while one therapist takes the lead on any given exercise, the co-therapist should attend to the rest of the group and look for opportunities to involve everyone.
- The co-therapist can highlight points of commonality between group members and challenging the tendency for specific individuals to self-exclude.
- Group leaders should model healthy expression of emotions, vulnerability, and needs, drawing on their own experiences when helpful.
- It can be helpful for group leaders to demonstrate healthy management of conflict as issues arise between them. Participants' attention can be drawn to these incidents, and they can be invited to reflect and comment on these from their own perspectives (drawing on how their schemas would have them interpret these situations). For example:

THERAPIST: Did anyone notice that Mary and I just had a little disagreement? I'm aware that sometimes this type of thing can trigger schemas, so I wonder what that was like for you to watch this mini-conflict? Did anyone notice any tension, or anxiety, or other reactions? Can you think about which schemas might have been triggered and how this might link with your own childhood experiences of conflict? From a healthy perspective, it is natural for relationships to have moments of conflict. One of the goals of this group will be for everyone to experiment with expressing annoyance or irritation in healthy ways, and learning when and how to set boundaries.

NB: Group work can activate therapists' own schemas, leading to conflict and/or competition between group leaders, burnout, and difficulty setting limits or taking a clear stance with overcompensatory aggressive coping modes or Angry Child modes. This area is expanded further in Chapter 18. Therapists' capacity to recognise and overcome their own schema 'clashes' provides a solid foundation that allows them to work together to manage difficult interactions within the group, provide containment and set limits as necessary, and provide a safe space for participants to fully express themselves.

As the group progresses, therapists should hand over increasing responsibility to group members to raise awareness of schemas and modes in each other, and to empathically confront and compassionately reparent each other.

Within the programme content there is a strong focus on helping participants learn to manage both their own and others' expressions of emotions and needs. Participants who are reticent about connecting to their Vulnerable Child mode are often encouraged by watching others, which can give them the courage to take risks and show this side of themselves to others. Group leaders must be prepared to set limits on outspoken modes, such as Angry

Child, Bully and Attack, or Punitive Inner Critic, which may cause harm to themselves or others. Depending on the level of threat this poses to other group members, the therapist may need to stand nearer to the client (between the client and others) and even hold up a hand to signal that a pause is needed. For example, a therapist might say 'Tony, I know that you are annoyed, but I need you to pause, take a few deep breaths, and take a step back until the feelings subside just enough for you to tell us what is going on just now for you. It's not okay to shout at others like that.' This facilitates confidence within the group that the therapists will keep them safe. Furthermore, even in the face of inappropriate expressions of emotion (such as may occur in Angry Child mode or Impulsive Child mode), the therapist must find ways to reassure the client that although we are setting limits on their behaviour, they continue to belong and be cared about by the group. For example, a therapist might say, 'I know this might feel a bit overwhelming for you just now, Tony, but sometimes when this angry side gets triggered, it's hard to hear what you really need. This side makes us all want to run for cover. In this group we will help you to find ways of expressing your needs in ways that others can hear you because that's what you need and deserve, just like everyone.' When one member is engaging in angry venting, other participants who are emotionally triggered can be offered the option of taking refuge behind a protective shield of cushions or pillows [6].

Stages of Group Therapy

Although the format and specific content of group schema therapy varies across settings and client groups [6, 7, 4], the stages of therapy remain largely consistent and similar to individual therapy. The first phase focuses on bonding and stabilisation. The middle phase is when the most concrete efforts to change client schemas occur, via a range of cognitive, experiential, interpersonal, and behavioural techniques. In this phase, therapists encourage participants to help each other to bypass their coping modes to reach their Vulnerable Child modes. Ultimately, as the group progresses, participants are encouraged to learn to compassionately reparent each other and themselves and to learn to overtly ask for their needs to be met. The final phase of therapy is based on consolidating gains, with exercises focused on embodying the Healthy Adult mode, making behavioural changes which heal rather than perpetuate their schemas. Sessions and homework tasks are focused on processing loss and endings, and, in particular, on preparing for schema triggers with cognitive strategies (e.g., flashcards, schema diaries, pie charts, reality testing) and experiential exercises (e.g., self-reparenting imagery, chairwork).

Bonding and Stabilisation Phase

The early phase of the group is focused on building and strengthening connections between group members and group leaders. Psychoeducation is provided about childhood needs, schemas, and modes and learning to recognise schema activation within and outside the group. Mode guessing games can be introduced whereby group leaders and/or participants can act out modes, with participants trying to identify them. This can lead to discussions about how the specific modes manifest across group members, including language, posture, function, and triggers. The Healthy Adult concept is also introduced, and psychoeducation is provided about ways of distinguishing it from coping modes. Participants can be encouraged to monitor these modes during and between sessions using simple mode diaries or monitoring forms. Group exercises at this stage are focused on establishing a group sense of belonging and emotional safety. Preliminary imagery work involves generating a group 'safe place' image, enhanced with individual elements to suit individual participants' needs. Participants are guided to focus on all of the sensory aspects of experiencing that place from their mind's eye.

Tangible representations of group connections can be provided through playful exercises such as throwing a ball of wool and/or holding onto scarves to create a visceral connection between group members [6]. At later stages of the group (especially BPD-specific groups), scarves can also be used as a mechanism for stimulating internalisation of object permanence, whereby the client uses transitional objects to facilitate capacity to generate a soothing mental image and sense of connection, even in the absence of key attachment figures. When the co-therapist notices a group member becoming detached or distressed, the scarf can provide a mechanism for drawing that person back to connect with the person who is holding on to the other end and, crucially, to the group. This also provides a gentle, de-shaming mechanism by which participants can learn to reconnect even in the face of coping mode activations that would normally drive disconnection. Exercises which enhance the Happy Child side are introduced early on in therapy, as this is often underdeveloped in participants, and such exercises provide an ideal opportunity for group bonding and breaking up the heaviness of working on schemas and difficult issues. Early groupwork also focuses on emotional famil-iarisation, through learning to identify bodily sensations and identify their accompanying specific emotion. Any method (including colours, facial emojis, and emotion-based apps) can be used to increase emotional awareness [6].

Mode Modification and Healing Phase of Therapy: Strategies for Change

The initial focus of mode modification sessions is to address schema modes shared by group members that are likely to sabotage progress. In the early phase of therapy, the Inner Critic tends to be ego-syntonic (i.e., participants believe its message to be true and find it almost impossible to challenge). By addressing the Inner Critic as a whole group, participants generally find it easier to challenge, especially when it is attacking fellow participants. This gradually empowers participants to begin to recognise and challenge their own Critic mode.

Changes takes place via a range of cognitive, experiential, and interpersonal strategies, including psychoeducation about universal needs, flashcards, schema diaries, schema monitoring forms, and exploring the pros and cons of modes. Schema healing takes place through limited reparenting of all participants' Vulnerable Child selves. Limited reparent-ing is provided within the context of a range of experiential techniques, including chairwork dialogues, imagery rescripting, empathic confrontation, and historical role-play/psycho-drama, in which all participants play a role. More detailed descriptions are available to provide guidance on working with specific modes [6, 7]. Some examples of specific tech-niques adapted to group therapy are described in the following sections.

Chairwork to Bypass Coping Modes. In the early phases of group therapy, it is important to address coping mode behaviours that block connection within the group and prevent participants from getting their needs met. An introductory exercise that illustrates the interpersonal consequences of coping modes involves one participant either placing a piece of paper in front of their face or turning their chair around to face outside the group, whilst the group continues to discuss a relevant issue. The participant is instructed to initially ignore attempts to draw them back into the discussion. After a few minutes, the designated participant returns to the group and is invited to reflect on what it felt like to be the one who was disconnected from others in the group. The remaining participants are invited to reflect on what it was like for them to try to connect and be ignored. This can be a useful psychoeducational exercise which is generally only carried out as a one-off, when first introducing the concept of the Detached Protector and helping participants to consider its impact on relationships.

Group members are encouraged to consider the ways in which their main coping modes (especially Detached Protector and Detached Self-Soother) may interfere with their capacity to get their needs met in the group and in other relationships through dissociation, addictive behaviours, self-harm, and so on. Group participants are encouraged to problem-solve ways in which the group can reconnect when any member is clearly in a coping mode. Furthermore, group members can be encouraged to become more aware of their own Detached Protector mode, such as by drawing it, monitoring physical and emotional signals as homework, and noticing how it affects their relationships and capacity to connect with others. In group work, a chair can be brought in to represent the whole group's Detached Protector, with another chair behind them which is covered in photographs of all participants as children (Vulnerable Child chair). The group's Detached Protector represents that part in each participant who wants to turn away, to block emotions, to disconnect from others in the face of suffering and distress. This exercise helps participants to learn that this is a common way of coping. The group Detached Protector represents a shared object onto which individuals project their individual protector modes. The group can then be encouraged to address this mode by showing appreciation for all of the ways in which it has helped them (from each individual's perspective). The group can then go on to remind the group Detached Protector that it is necessary to reach their Vulnerable Child mode to allow healing work to take place within the group. Participants can respond by moving to the Detached Protector chair and voicing any concerns or fears that their Detached Protector mode has. Group participants can then move to the Healthy Adult chair (i.e., all participants stand behind the chair) and offer healthy responses based on what they know their own (or others') Vulnerable Child part needs. Participants are encouraged to notice the sensations of the Detached Protector as it fluctuates in their life outside of sessions to develop conscious awareness and control of the mode. Members are encouraged to connect with their Vulnerable Child mode in group sessions and to allow themselves to hear the caring reparenting messages of the group. This exercise can be adapted and repeated when any specific group participant manifests a strong coping mode in group sessions.

Chairwork to Fight the Inner Critic. Fighting critic modes takes place via both chairwork and imagery rescripting. Instructions for group chairwork to fight the Critic are described in Box 17.2. All participants are encouraged to project their own Inner Critics onto the designated Inner Critic chair. In parallel, they are encouraged to observe as others describe their own Inner Critic messages. This process often triggers a natural sense of anger or irritation as they witness other participants being criticised by their own Critic, thereby facilitating the process of fighting back and setting limits on this side.

Imagery Rescripting. Mode-based imagery rescripting can be used to familiarise participants with the concept of reparenting their Vulnerable Child mode. In the first instance, participants are invited to close their eyes, visit their safe place, then connect with an image of their Vulnerable Child self for a few minutes (this time can be extended as the group

Box 17.2 Fighting the Group Inner Critic Through Chairwork

- Invite participants to reflect on the past week and share experiences of when their Inner Critic was active. Explore these incidents, reflecting on the impact on their inner child modes and their ability to make progress with their goals.
- Use the opportunity to draw parallels between similar experiences across participants.
- Group participants are invited to depict the tone of the Inner Critic via drawing on a large sheet of cardboard or cloth effigy.
- Identify one participant who is willing to allow the group to focus on their Inner Critic as a way of addressing all of the Inner Critics in the group.
- Chairs are allocated to the Inner Critic, the Vulnerable Child, and the Healthy Adult modes. The effigy is placed on the Inner Critic chair. Drawings or photographs of participants as children are placed on the back of the relevant chair.
- The chosen participant is invited to sit on the Inner Critic chair and voice the words of that mode, directed at the empty Vulnerable Child chair.
- The same participant is then invited to move to the Vulnerable Child chair and asked to reflect on how their child self feels when they receive this message. The co-therapist draws in the rest of the group to ask how they would receive this same message from their vulnerable side. Although participants usually note feelings of sadness and hurt, they may also remark that the critical voice feels 'right'. Therapists can explain that as these messages have been repeated over many years, they have become 'normal' and maybe even comfortable (in that the world makes more 'sense').
- Use a whiteboard to list alternative Healthy Adult mode messages generated by the group to fight these messages, with the goal of defending the Vulnerable Child mode. The confrontational tone is adjusted to the severity of the Inner Critic. For example, to a Punitive Critic, strong limits are required as if dealing with a bully, whereas with a Demanding or Guilt-Inducing mode, participants are helped to generate messages that unpick the logic and focus on unmet emotional needs.
- All participants are invited to stand behind the Healthy Adult mode chair and take turns to make one statement from their Healthy Adult mode, to set limits on the group Inner Critic.
- For homework, participants can be asked to reflect on the range of explicit and implicit messages they have internalised across childhood and adolescence from a range of sources: family members, teachers, peers, and siblings, as well as cultural/media messages. Participants are invited to note that often the Inner Critic messages are unwittingly passed down through the generations without being questioned. Clients who struggle with guilt when fighting the Critic can be reassured that we are not identifying the schema 'carrier' as a bad person; it is their destructive messages that we are targeting.

proceeds). Participants are instructed to focus on any image or memory (except trauma or abuse memories, which should be reserved for individual sessions). Participants are then invited to open their eyes and discuss their experiences as a group, drawing parallels between common experiences among participants. The co-therapist keeps an eye on any participants who need support with expressing their own experience of connecting to their little self. If any participants have been triggered, they can be invited to re-enter the image and identify their need, whilst the whole group generates creative solutions to meet these needs through imagery (see detailed instruction in Box 17.3). Over several weeks, all participants can take turns at being the focus of these rescripts, thereby facilitating ongoing reparenting experiences for the whole group. Participants are gradually encouraged to bring their own Healthy Adult side into the images to reparent themselves. Homework tasks can also be set to draw pictures of their Healthy Adult providing what is needed for their Vulnerable Child self. Furthermore, participants can be encouraged to notice triggers for these schemas within the group context (e.g., feeling left out when group therapists pay attention to others (Emotional Deprivation), or feeling unlovable when the group are nurturing towards another participant (Defectiveness/Shame) as a focus for diary entries, homework activities, and future-in-group session exercises. This can lead to further exercises focused on challenging those schemas and learning to get their needs met more directly.

Whole group imagery rescripting can be a powerful technique for fighting the Inner Critic, whilst also providing a valuable opportunity for reparenting. Ideally, every participant should have at least one opportunity to work through an early memory via imagery rescripting. One participant is invited to share a memory in which they received a critical message or didn't get their needs adequately met in some way. For an example of imagery rescripting in group schema therapy, see Box 17.3.

Box 17.3 Group Imagery Rescripting Illustration

Sally told the group that she had always kept others at a distance due to a longstanding sense that she wasn't good enough, and that once others saw the 'real me', they would not want anything to do with her. Over the course of her childhood, her parents were often busy and stressed with high work demands, and Sally's emotional needs for warmth and connection were largely unmet. Her sister was highly passive and compliant and was often praised for this. In contrast, Sally developed a sense that she was the 'problem child', as her expressions of distress and anger were interpreted as being 'over the top' and attention-seeking. Sally volunteered to be the focus of a group imagery rescripting, to work on a memory based on a recurring theme of rejection and emotional neglect.

Safe Place Imagery

The whole group was invited to close their eyes and guided to enter their safe place, imagining every detail, including image, sounds, smells, tastes textures, and felt sense. After 2–3 minutes, participants were encouraged to open their eyes.

Imagery Rescripting

1) *Identify core image*: Sally was encouraged to close her eyes and describe the image to the rest of the group, identifying feelings, thoughts, and unmet needs. She described herself as a 4-year-old who on her birthday had been in childcare all day and wanted to play with her parents but was told to go upstairs and quietly read in her bedroom. When she protested, her mother fiercely told her she was being naughty and to stop being so demanding. She identified her feelings as sad, empty, ashamed, and lonely; her thoughts as: 'nobody cares about me. I'm all alone. I'm a burden'; and her needs as a cuddle, someone to listen to me, and to matter.

2) *Group generates ideas for rescript*: Sally was invited to open her eyes and the whole group brainstormed constructive rescripting endings, which included a range of ideas

such as bringing her grandmother into the image to talk to her parents and provide comfort, arranging a birthday party with friends, and going to a trampoline park. The solution that resonated best for Sally was a combination of the ideas suggested by the group.

3) *Rescripting the ending*: Sally was invited to close her eyes again and the therapists guided her through this new ending to her memory, asking her to imagine that the therapists were there in the image, explaining to her parents that children need love and nurturance, and that like all little children, Sally needed to be cherished and celebrated, especially on her birthday:

THERAPIST: You're so lucky to have such a beautiful little girl. She is trying so hard to get your attention and it's not naughty to want to connect and play. All children need this. Although I know you are tired and stressed, you still need to find a way to be better parents to show your love and affection more openly. It's not good for young children to be left on their own for so long. Sally needs you to be present for her.

Group participants were invited to contribute to the Healthy Adult messages and to stand up for Little Sally.

4) *Group ending:* After further discussion and limit setting with the parents, the therapists invited Sally and all of her new friends to a trampoline party, with fun games, tasty food, and space to make lots of noise. The Vulnerable Child selves of group participants were invited to enter the image as 'friends' for the Vulnerable Child. All participants were guided to close their eyes and take in the reparenting messages that are directed toward the 'Vulnerable Children' of the whole group (i.e., 'Little Sally and all of the little children here, you are all precious and lovable. All children need care, love, and it's good to ask for what you need. We are here to take care of you and make sure that you get everything you need from each other and from us'). In the image, group members told Little Sally that they wanted to play with her. Furthermore, they imagined a group hug, with all of the children joining together to make Little Sally feel a sense of belonging.

5) *Debrief.* Group participants opened their eyes and debriefed. Sally was invited to reflect on how she could help Little Sally to get her needs met in the present, both through self-attunement and by learning to ask for her needs to be met more openly.

Empathic Confrontation. Empathic confrontation in group format is a powerful method for bringing attention to modes that block interpersonal connection with others and capacity to get emotional needs met. This begins with a gentle prompt by group leaders. For example, the therapist might say, 'Mary, something I noticed is that you have a natural inclination to want to help others, but that sometimes you get so drawn into trying to rescue others that your own little self doesn't get any airtime. This is no criticism at all, but I wondered if that might be an old schema pattern for you, taking care of others whilst neglecting your own needs?'

As the group progresses, participants are encouraged to gently confront each other to help overcome barriers to connection. Empathic confrontation can target any behaviours that prevent participants from getting needs met both in the context of the group and in what they report about their lives between sessions, including risky behaviours, non-attendance, and extreme attachment/clinging or overcompensation. Empathic confrontation is appropriate when group boundaries are violated (e.g., repeatedly verbally attacking other group members, or sending abusive emails to group leaders in Angry Child mode or Bully and Attack mode). Empathic confrontation includes suggestions that provide guidance on learning to self-regulate and switch modes to allow them to be 'heard' by fellow participants. On rare occasions when empathic confrontation is ineffective, this is followed by limit setting with natural consequences (e.g., losing email privileges).

We encourage group members to actively work on expressing vulnerability and asking for their needs to be met within the group rather than acting these out in a coping mode. It is of utmost importance that empathic confrontation is delivered skilfully; it should be made clear that the observation is not intended as a criticism, but a means of encouraging participants to learn more effective mechanisms for expressing their emotions and needs. A six-step process for empathically confronting behaviours within groups is described by Farrell and Shaw [8] (see Box 17.4), and an example of its application is presented in Box 17.5.

Box 17.4 Six-Step Process for Empathically Confronting Behaviours Within Schema Therapy Groups

1. Establish connection with the participant by making eye contact, leaning towards them, and using a warm, empathic tone. Reassure the participant that this is not intended as criticism, pointing out your concern that there is an issue that you want to highlight due to a concern that you have noticed a mode-/schema-driven behaviour that may interfere with them getting needs met in session.

2. Describe the interfering behaviour linked to schemas and modes.

THERAPIST: I am worried that when this side of you gets caught up with describing situations in such detail, it can feel a bit like our connection with you starts to waver, as we focus more on the facts and lose touch with your needs and feelings. While there is a side of me that gets it and is happy to go with the flow, there is another part of me that is concerned about the vulnerable part of you that needs emotional connection.

3. Point out that this coping behaviour probably emerged as a survival response in childhood, when there were limited options, but that life is different now and as a group we want to help them to get their needs met.

THERAPIST: I fully recognise that in the past, it must have been so confusing for you – you were criticised and given the message that whatever you said or did, it wasn't quite right or good enough. And I wonder if this side evolved as a way of trying to get things 'right'. The down-side is that when the details take centre stage, we lose sight of Little Peter and what he needs from us – even though it makes perfect sense as to why you learned to cope that way.

4. Offer an alternative that might show the participant how they could adjust to a healthier coping mechanism to get needs met in the present.

THERAPIST: I know that as a child, it wouldn't have been possible for you to show this vulnerable part of you, as you would have felt too exposed to the bombardment of criticism – you would have been put down for that. But it's different here ... we want to understand how you really feel. So, if you could maybe try a different way, by telling us a little bit about how you are feeling, that will help us to see that little part of you that has been neglected and to understand what you really need. This is really the most important goal of schema therapy – to take the risk of showing your vulnerability to others who care about you.

5. Consider options for change: help the participant to weigh up the pros and cons of the schema-driven behaviour and explore other possible ways to behave.

THERAPIST: I wonder if this mode might also have an impact on some of your other relationships, and whether it affects others' capacity to understand what you need? Although it has been a way of getting by in childhood, how might it be to experiment with reducing it for a short time?

6. Offer support with making changes: 'This old way of coping is totally understandable – but we are here for you and want to support you to get what you need in your life now.'

Box 17.5 Example of Empathic Confrontation in Group Schema Therapy

Merrin's Angry Protector mode would become triggered when she noticed other group members getting the group leader's attention. She would express this by withdrawing in a hostile manner, avoiding eye contact with others and responding to questions in an irritable manner.

THERAPIST: Merrin, I know that it might be difficult to talk about this just now, but I can see you are feeling hurt, and I think it's important that we try to understand what is happening just now. The tricky thing is that when this 'back off' part of you kicks in and you withdraw, we lose connection to you. It's difficult for us knowing that you are struggling, but it's hard to make contact with the vulnerable part of you when this part is so strong – it feels like this side is pushing us away. It's totally understandable that you have learned to cope this way, to protect yourself – in the past there were good reasons for that. One thing that many people find triggering in group context is seeing others getting the care that they crave. I know that this side kicks in and gives the message that it's better not to need others, that they don't care about your needs – this is what you learned as a child. But it's different here – we want to hear from you about your feelings. You're allowed to connect and to ask for what you need. Can anyone else in the group relate to this difficulty saying what they feel or need in direct ways when triggered . . . if so, could you share this with the group?

Empathic confrontation can also be used via chairwork dialogues to challenge coping modes common across the whole group. A chair can be brought in to represent the main coping modes within the group, with one chair as the child mode. Group participants can work in small groups to identify ways that the coping modes have helped them (past) but that also prevented them from getting their needs met and connecting with others (present). Therapists guide participants to present these perspectives to the coping modes as if they are talking to an old friend who needs to be updated about their role in their life. They are then guided to direct messages to the Vulnerable Child chair, finding words to represent what they now know that they needed but didn't get in the past.

Final Phase of Group Schema Therapy

In the final phase of the group – mirroring individual schema therapy – participants are encouraged to continue to work on consolidating behavioural changes that enable them to get their needs met and increase interpersonal connection in their lives. They actively practise self-nurturing and compassion as they crystallise Healthy Adult skills for self-care. This phase of therapy parallels the later stages of childhood: developing a sense of identity, individuation, and sense of autonomy. Group members are encouraged to connect to their own Vulnerable Child/Adolescent self to learn about their own needs, values, likes, dislikes, and wants. The group format provides a sense of belonging and acceptance within a peer group, a key healing ingredient often missing from their actual adolescence, which promotes identity development. In this phase, there is a focus on differentiating healthy from more 'addictive' or self-sabotaging mechanisms for getting needs met and learning ways of telling these apart.

Mode work becomes focused on looking forward to manage needs and anticipate difficult triggers that might lie ahead in the client's life outside the realm of the group. The focus is on firmly internalising the experience of the group as an 'alternate' childhood, whereby they have managed to get their needs met and can now take these forwards as an integrated Healthy Adult self that is capable of managing and meeting their own needs.

Concluding Remarks

Group schema therapy is well established as an effective format for the provision of schema-mode work. The group format appears to catalyse the effects of schema therapy through the context of a group 'family'. This microcosm of the outside world provides a foundational healing environment that imparts a sense of belonging and opportunities for vicarious learning. Participants learn to develop ways of getting their own needs met by internalising reparenting messages from the group and eventually through the evolution of their own Healthy Adult selves. Schema challenging thereby becomes more potent within a group context through the collective strength of the emerging group Healthy Adult, which can challenge out-of-date schema messages and provide the compassion, warmth, and connectivity that is needed for healing to take place.

References

1. Farrell J, Shaw IA Webber MA, A schema-focused approach to group psychotherapy for outpatients with borderline personality disorder: A randomized controlled trial. *Journal of Behavior Therapy and Experimental Psychiatry.* 2009;**40**(2):317–28.

2. Broersen J, van Vreeswijk M. *Brief schema therapy workbook: Experiential strategies for group and individual psychotherapy.* Available at: www.mfvanvreeswijk.com/downloads/brief-schema-therapy-workbook-experiential-strategies-for-group-and-individual-psychotherapy. Original Dutch edition: Werkboek kortdurende schematherapie; experiëntiële technieken/ copyright © 2017 Bohn Stafleu van Loghum, onderdeel van Springer media. ISBN: 9789082853902

3. Broersen J, van Vreeswijk M. *Brief schema therapy workbook: CBT techniques* (3rd ed.). (In Press).

4. Simpson S, Skewes S, van Vreeswijk M, Samson R. Commentary: Short-term group schema therapy for mixed personality disorders: An introduction to the treatment protocol. *Frontiers in Psychology.* 2015;**6**(609): 1–3.

5. Simpson S, Smith E. *Schema therapy for eating disorders: Theory and practice for individual and group settings.* Routledge; 2019.

6. Farrell J, Shaw I. *Group schema therapy for borderline personality disorder: A step-by-step treatment manual with patient workbook.* Wiley & Sons; 2012.

7. Farrell J, Shaw I, Reiss N. Group schema therapy for borderline personality disorder

patients: Catalyzing schema and mode change. In van Vreekswijk M, Broersen J, Nadort M, eds. *The Wiley-Blackwell handbook of schema therapy*. Wiley-Blackwell 2012, pp. 341–58.

8. Farrell J, Shaw I. Empathic confrontation in group schema therapy. In R. Vogel (ed). *Empathic confrontation*. Beltz; 2013. www .researchgate.net/profile/Joan-Farrell/publication/281108601_Empathic_ Confrontation_in_Group_Schema_Therapy/l inks/55d5e0cc08aed6a199a2a7aa/Empathic-Confrontation-in-Group-Schema-Therapy.pdf.

Chapter 18

Schema Therapy for the Schema Therapist

Improving Therapist Well-Being and Enhancing Client Outcomes Through the Awareness and Healing of Therapist Schemas

Introduction

Therapists are not immune to the effects of their own temperament and early child-rearing and socialisation experiences. Therapist schemas interact somewhat with client schemas such that certain client–therapist combinations make it harder for therapists to recognise problematic patterns or intervene to alter them early enough. Therapist schemas can have several other potentially pernicious effects, including propensity to burnout and boundary violations. Therefore, schema therapists are called to cultivate awareness of their own schemas. This chapter outlines some of the complications that arise for specific therapist EMS and provides guidance for managing their impact.

Early Maladaptive Schemas in Therapists

Since the beginnings of psychotherapy, therapists have had an inherent curiosity about their internal worlds and the factors that impede or enhance their own well-being. Indeed, therapists' own personal and family histories are likely to be motivational factors that draw them into psychotherapy as a profession [1, 2]. Research suggests that a substantial proportion of psychologists [3, 4, 5, 6], psychiatrists [7, 8, 9], and other mental health clinicians/psychotherapists [10] have experienced adverse childhood experiences. Whilst a prior experience of adverse experiences may increase our potential to understand and empathise with our clients, it may also increase the risk of schema-driven psychological difficulties, including burnout [3, 11]. Indeed, workplace demands can generate the 'perfect storm' by activating the very EMS that drew us into the profession in the first place [12, 10]. In this way, therapists' own schemas can simultaneously represent our superpower, driving empathy and understanding, but also our kryptonite, representing our blind spots and those aspects of the work that threaten outcomes as well as our own well-being [13]. There is also a core assumption within the schema therapy model that the therapist is the 'almost perfect' model of Healthy Adult attitudes, schemas, and behaviours. In other words, therapy proceeds as if the schema therapist has enough 'Healthy Adult' strength across all eighteen schema domains to be able to model this for clients. This, of course, is a problematic assumption. Although therapists usually experience less schema activation than clients, it is our observation – backed by research – that therapists are human beings too, and so come with all of the biases, struggles, childhood histories, schemas, and blind spots that can impact the therapy process. If those blind spots are not obvious in daily life, clinical work will often highlight them. And so, if we all have schemas and we accept that they can affect our work, it is important for the schema therapist to become aware of them and take steps to heal or manage their own schemas, to prevent them from becoming 'blind spots' in therapy.

Matches and Mismatches Between Therapist and Client Schemas and Modes

Therapists' own EMS can interact with those of their clients, commonly leading to blind spots and/or overidentification. For example, if both therapist and client have a Failure EMS, the therapist may not sufficiently actively encourage or challenge the client to reach their potential. On the other hand, if the therapist and client have opposite EMS (such as Failure and Unrelenting Standards), or the same EMS, with opposing coping styles (such as Defectiveness with a Self-Aggrandiser mode versus Defectiveness with a Compliant Surrenderer coping mode), the therapist might have difficulty identifying EMS-driven patterns because these seem 'normal'. When both therapist and client are in a Detached Protector mode, the therapeutic process can easily devolve into a 'chat-fest', whereby they merely talk about problematic issues without actively working on them or using experiential techniques for change. If both therapist and client are in Overcontroller mode, the therapeutic process can become stuck, whereby both are working through lists and agenda items in an attempt to be productive, whilst neglecting possibilities for emotional connection.

A particularly common and problematic therapist–client interaction can occur when the therapist has a strong Compliant Surrenderer mode and becomes too acquiescent in the face of their clients' overcompensatory modes; the therapist's EMS are likely to be activated by an Overcontroller or Self-Aggrandiser mode in the client. In this dynamic, the therapist may avoid addressing the client's unmet needs for boundaries and limits due to typical fears, such as being rejected or criticised (Defectiveness), conflict or anger (Subjugation), loss of approval (Approval Seeking), or being punished (Punitiveness). The client is therefore denied the opportunity to learn reciprocity and compromise within relationships. Although overcompensatory modes commonly trigger feelings of irritation and/or anxiety in the therapist, it is important to remain cognizant of the client's underlying fears that are linked to childhood experiences (e.g., 'showing my vulnerability will lead to humiliation') and to remain persistent in efforts to gain access to the Vulnerable Child that is hidden 'back stage', behind the coping mode. Keeping a photograph of the client as a small child in sight can help increase both therapist empathy and resolve to communicate with the client's vulnerable side. Therapists with EMS in the Disconnection and Rejection domain may be particularly prone to being blindsided by the charms of a Self-Aggrandiser mode in the early stages of therapy. For example, the client might flatter the therapist: 'I chose you as my therapist, as I heard you were the best in the practice ... I really admire your achievements and knew this would be a good match for me.' If the therapist does not recognise this as an overcompensatory strategy and slips into their own narcissistic coping mode, they become diverted from their primary goal of reaching the client's vulnerable side. When an over-compensatory mode is present, the therapist's attempts to engage in experiential exercises and make contact with the client's Vulnerable Child part may be met with cynicism, sarcasm, or claims that these methods are not appropriate for their problems. The therapist can thus unwittingly find themselves drawn into a relationship of 'friendly chat' or intellectualising, without providing the corrective emotional experience the client needs. Regular supervision and practice of empathic confrontation skills are essential, especially when working with clients with domineering coping modes.

Common Schemas Amongst Psychotherapists

Recent research has identified Self-Sacrifice and Unrelenting Standards as the two most common EMS amongst psychologists and psychotherapists, with Detached Protector and Detached Self-Soother as the most common coping modes [14, 11]. The strong drive amongst most therapists to sacrifice their own needs to meet the needs of their clients, and to set high standards for themselves, may enhance therapists' capacity to engage in the positive aspects of the reparenting approach (e.g., provide attunement, warmth, and empathy), but also reduce their willingness to engage in setting boundaries through empathic confrontation due to a fear of causing further distress for their clients. Other therapist EMS that may contribute to avoidance of the more confrontational schema therapist strategies include Subjugation (fears that the client will become angry), Defectiveness (fears that they will be rejected or criticised by the client), Emotional Deprivation (fears that they will be misunderstood), or Abandonment (fears that the client will leave).

The Self-Sacrifice and Unrelenting Standards schemas may also underlie the tendency amongst therapists to become overidentified with a 'rescuer' or 'Perfectionistic Nurturer' role. These roles blend Compliant Surrenderer, Overcontroller, and/or Self-Aggrandiser modes. The therapist gains a sense of self-esteem through being the one to find solutions for others' difficulties, which enables them to consistently avoid awareness of their own vulnerability and unmet needs. This may be particularly problematic when working with clients who have a strong Dependence/Incompetence schema (Dependent, Abandoned Child, Helpless Surrenderer modes); the therapist and client get locked in a cycle of triggering each other's EMS, with each remaining in their preferred coping mode, rather than addressing the client's underlying unmet needs. The therapist's 'Perfectionistic Nurturer' mode is gratified by being needed and designated as the 'chosen' therapist who is taking care of the client, whilst the client's Helpless Surrenderer mode (overcompensation for Abandonment EMS) is gratified by being rescued or 'saved' (see Box 18.1 for a clinical example). However, this 'dance of the coping modes' effectively prevents the client's underlying Abandoned/Dependent child from being authentically seen and healed, and the therapist's own Healthy Adult and Vulnerable Child remain out of the picture.

Furthermore, when clients have a strong Dependence/Incompetence or Abandonment/Instability schema, there is a high risk of therapy being stretched significantly beyond what would normally be considered an appropriate length, as the therapist unwittingly reinforces the client's fear of endings. As a result, the development of the client's Healthy Adult self becomes stalled. If the therapist pushes for autonomy, the Helpless Surrenderer coping mode (driven by Abandoned/Dependent Child) uses protest behaviours (e.g., pleas to be rescued through statements of helplessness and increased reporting of suicidal urges or illness behaviour) and guilt-inducing statements (thereby triggering the therapist's Self-Sacrifice schema) as a means of drawing the therapist back into the rescuer role. It is not uncommon to become stuck within this 'rescuer–victim' dynamic, creating an environment whereby the client has little opportunity (or incentive) for change. Alternatively, the therapist may become frustrated by feeling trapped within this dynamic, and flip into

Box 18.1 Therapist–Client Schema Chemistry: The Case of Franca

Franca (client) grew up in an environment where her basic needs for love, stability, and consistent care were not met. Her parents were mostly emotionally absent. Her mother frequently passed out on the sofa after alcohol binges and would also go missing for days at a time. Furthermore, she would threaten to leave if Franca did not behave perfectly. Her sister was treated better, and Franca learned that she had to work hard to earn 'crumbs' of affection. Although she was closer to her father, he was often away with work. Franca's upbringing was a key factor in the development of severe Emotional Deprivation, Abandonment and Dependency EMS.

When she first attended therapy, she presented with a primary presenting problem of obsessive compulsive disorder. Her predominant coping modes provided a means of attempting to deny the existence of her emotional needs through detachment and distraction (Detached Protector), and using rituals, perfectionism, and achievement as a means of gaining a sense of control and self-sufficiency (Overcontroller). In the initial sessions of therapy, Franca remained emotionally detached and avoidant. However, over time, as she allowed herself to become attached to her therapist, she began to 'thaw out' and express her needs and emotions more openly.

Her therapist Maria's main EMS were Emotional Deprivation, Unrelenting Standards, Subjugation, and Self-Sacrifice. In line with the schema model, Maria worked to meet Franca's unmet emotional needs through providing consistent emotional care, nurturance, and warmth. Although Franca appeared to benefit from this, she began demanding increasing amounts of care on weekends and evenings. It was hypothesised that this was a manifestation of Franca's Abandoned/Dependent Child mode, with an overcompensatory coping style. Maria found herself stuck in a cycle of feeling that whatever she gave, it was not enough. She sacrificed increasingly greater amounts of her personal time to provide on-demand care for Franca, sometimes leading to email conversations late at night, arranging extra sessions, and additional telephone calls. When she went away on holidays, this would be met with angry and demanding email messages, accusing Maria of abandoning her. Maria then increased her efforts to provide the 'perfect care'. Attempts to take a break led to feelings of guilt (Self-Sacrifice) and fear of being punished (Subjugation), alongside pressure to get the therapy 'right' and provide the perfect care (Unrelenting Standards). This pattern, alongside Maria's tendency to override her own emotional needs (Emotional Deprivation), led to increasing feelings of emotional and physical exhaustion.

Franca and Maria found themselves locked into a schema-perpetuating dynamic, wherein Maria found herself feeling increasingly burned out and frustrated by trying to provide the perfect care, and Franca became increasingly dependent and clingy, reluctant to take on a Healthy Adult role in her own recovery. Maria's own EMS prevented her from setting realistic limits in terms of the level of care that she was able to provide, with the result that Franca could continue to avoid emotionally processing the pain and grief associated with her EMS.

With supervision and personal therapy, Maria was able to recognise these EMS-driven processes and find a balance of providing nurturing care alongside healthy limit setting. Limits on the frequency and length of emails were introduced as a first step, and when these were overridden by Franca, natural consequences were introduced (i.e., emails would not be read by the therapist for the following week). Franca was also strongly encouraged to form relationships with peers that involved a healthy balance of learning to respect and support others' needs, whilst also learning to show healthy vulnerability to get her own needs met. Although the limit setting was met with a strong Angry Child response, thereby triggering Maria's Subjugation EMS, her resolve to create a healthier therapeutic environment gradually provided Franca with both opportunities to get her needs met and moments of frustration that began to stimulate growth of her own resilient Healthy Adult self, capable of meeting her own needs and forming healthy relationships with others.

a punitive-critical (Bully-Attack mode) or passive-aggressive (flipping between Compliant Surrenderer and Angry Protector mode) stance, thereby reinforcing the client's EMS and being drawn into a re-enactment of their early childhood relationship dynamics. In this way, the mode-flipping resembles Karpman's Drama Triangle, whereby participants move between the three roles of Perpetrator, Rescuer, and Victim [15]. This pattern is further reinforced by medical-model mental health systems which reinforce the notion of the client as a passive recipient of treatment that is 'administered' by the therapist. Schema therapists must work towards overcoming their own EMS that increase the risk of being drawn into this pattern, to allow them to bypass the client's coping modes and reach the Vulnerable Child mode, whilst also stimulating growth of their clients' Healthy Adult selves. For further reading on the Drama Triangle and links to the schema therapy model, see Edwards [16].

Schemas Associated with Therapist Burnout

Concerningly, research indicates that between 21% and 67% of mental health clinicians report high emotional exhaustion [17, 18]. More than 49% of clinical and counselling psychologists in a recent study reported moderate–to-high levels of burnout [19]. Burnout, driven by the underlying EMS and coping modes, may be characterised either by excessive involvement (e.g., Overcontroller mode) or disengagement (e.g., Detached Protector, Detached Self-Soother modes), or alternation between some combination of these [20, 21, 11]. Although all EMS and dysfunctional modes appear to be correlated with burnout, those schemas and modes identified as the strongest predictors are Emotional Deprivation [12], Abandonment, Emotional Inhibition, Mistrust/Abuse, and the Detached Protector mode [19].

In the case of Emotional Deprivation, therapists may overcompensate for their own lack of childhood nurturance through providing 'ideal' care for their clients whilst continuing to neglect themselves. This lack of awareness of their own needs may increase the risk of emotional exhaustion and reduce the opportunity for their clients to develop skills in dealing with minor frustrations (i.e., of not having all their needs met all the time). Indeed, therapists risk 'killing with kindness' by solely focusing on meeting clients' needs for understanding, safety, and nurturance at the expense of supporting them meeting their need for autonomy. As noted earlier, if the therapist has a Self-Sacrifice EMS, this can further exacerbate the pattern because the therapist is reluctant to set limits out of a fear of causing distress, reducing opportunities for the client to gradually strengthen their own resilient Healthy Adult self. Overidentification with clients' Mistrust/Abuse and Abandonment schemas risks reducing opportunities for schema challenging and healing. When both therapists and clients have unhealed Mistrust schemas, they may become mutually suspicious, reducing opportunities for corrective emotional experiences of honesty and connection. When both therapist and client have unhealed Abandonment schemas, they are at risk of clinging to each other (surrender), mutually keeping their distance (avoidance), or engaging in some combination of these, reducing opportunities for corrective experiences of stability within relationships. For therapists with an Emotional Inhibition schema, there is a propensity to quash emotional expression due to fears of rejection, disapproval, or loss of control. For the therapist, this may lead to increased risk for burnout due to reduced opportunity for mutual sharing of difficulties with colleagues and friends, thereby increasing emotional isolation.

Impact of Therapist Schemas on Capacity for Empathy and Schema Healing

Research indicates that emotional detachment (i.e., Detached Protector coping mode) appears to both operate as a risk factor for, and a consequence of, burnout, thereby functioning as a negative feedback loop, reducing job satisfaction and ultimately capacity for empathy [22]. Perhaps more than in many other 'manualised' treatment models, schema therapy requires the therapist to make a substantial emotional investment in the therapeutic process. It is common in schema therapy to be working with clients who describe harrowing life stories, including significant abuse and trauma. The limited reparenting approach requires a high level of attunement and empathy, with an emphasis on 'being with' rather than 'doing to'. Given that different authors frequently give contradictory definitions and distinctions to the terms *empathy, sympathy,* and *pity,* we'll leave these terms aside and describe the quality of attention and experiencing that good schema therapists adopt: therapists pay attention to their own Vulnerable Child mode, recognising the feeling that the client is describing, and share the client's emotional experience as much as possible. This is distinct from simply adopting a cognitive understanding in which the therapist protects themselves from their own vulnerability through creating emotional distance [23]. Therapists might avoid sharing client emotional experiences via a Detached Protector (e.g., 'I'm so sorry you feel that way. Shall we think of some distraction strategies together?'), Self-Aggrandiser ('I feel sorry for you'), or Overcontroller ('Let's see if we can help you find a solution for these feelings') coping mode.

More so than achieving empathy or sympathy, schema therapists strive to feel compassion towards clients. In a study where people were trained to respond to an image of a suffering person either through empathy or compassion, both groups experienced high levels of emotion in relation to seeing another person suffering, but those with empathy training more acutely experienced emotional pain (activating the anterior cingulate cortex). In contrast, those who received compassion training experienced a positive sense of reward from being able to help (activating the medial orbitofrontal cortex and ventral striatum). Whereas empathy involves one task – focusing on the other person's suffering – compassion involves an additional step, through connecting with their own and their clients' inner healing resources. In this study, those in the empathy group described the task of watching another person's suffering as emotionally uncomfortable, whereas those in the compassion training described greater motivation to be present and to help, which enabled them to tolerate the empathic-emotional pain. In schema therapy terms, empathy that is reflexive and unconscious can easily become entangled with EMS. *Entangled empathy* may be driven by EMS that drive overinvolvement (e.g., Enmeshment, Subjugation, Self-Sacrifice, lack of coherent self). In these cases, there is a lack of differentiation between self and other, and the therapist is at increased risk of emotional exhaustion. For example, in the case of the Self-Sacrifice EMS, the therapist can become overidentified with the client's emotional pain, taking responsibility for it, leading to a merging of self and other and increased risk of compassion fatigue. Research supports this notion, such that feelings of depression and lowered motivation are linked to this type of entangled empathy [24]. Furthermore, with entangled empathy we can feel weighed down by the suffering of the other but be less able to actually provide attuned support in the way that the other person requires. In contrast, Healthy Adult compassion involves a healthier version of empathy: 'feeling with' another, whilst retaining a differentiated, coherent self. Feelings of empathy are followed by a 'turning outwards', generating motivation to provide help in constructive ways.

Whereas the entangled empathy is emotionally exhausting, healthy compassion is restorative [25]. These findings lead us to consider ways in which therapists can address their own EMS and child-self needs, to best meet the needs of their clients.

Impact of Therapist Schemas on Boundary Crossing

The deep level of attunement and emphasis on emotional connection in schema therapy can create a greater level of emotional intimacy than many clients have ever experienced. As previously mentioned, clients with strong Abandonment/Instability and Dependence/Incompetence schemas may be more prone to misinterpreting the meaning of this therapeutic intimacy, and may entertain fantasies of being rescued or even 'falling in love' with the therapist. The schema therapist must be alert to these possibilities, and address them directly and empathically whilst acknowledging the unmet needs that the client is trying to satisfy through these fantasies. By using boundary transgressions as an opportunity to explore the role of EMS and unmet needs, the schema therapist's role is to maintain healthy boundaries whilst helping their clients to translate these into healthy relationship dynamics within their 'outside' lives. An example of healthy limit setting in the context of a client idealising or romanticising the therapeutic relationship is provided in Box 18.2.

The therapist's role is to validate the unmet needs associated with the client's history, to normalise the transference or 'schema chemistry' being played out within the therapeutic relationship, whilst sticking to their methods and holding the therapeutic boundaries. In the case of the example in Box 18.2, the therapist could follow this discussion with a chairwork exercise where the 'longing' or 'romanticising' part is interviewed, to find out how old it is, what memories are associated with it, and, in the case of a coping mode, what its function is. Furthermore, feelings and somatic sensations that arise in the client towards the therapist can be investigated through an affect bridge, whereby the client is encouraged to 'Focus on those sensations and feelings until they are as intense as possible, then let your mind drift back to an early memory when you experienced the same or similar sensations and feelings. Just allow your body (not your brain) to make any connections with anything at all that comes up for you.' The purpose here is to clarify exactly what the client's feelings and needs are. The feelings may represent developmentally appropriate healthy emotions that are emerging as healing occurs in other aspects of the client's life. On the other hand, the client may be mis-labelling or mis-identifying emotions that reflect child-like needs that the client hasn't been able to properly identify. Imaginal assessment and mode mapping can help the client better understand their experience.

It is worth noting that a client's tendency to sexualise the therapeutic relationship can often be traced to confusion caused by a history of childhood sexual abuse. For example, a child who was ignored by a parent except in the context of sexual abuse may have learned that the only way of being seen and valued is through being sexually attractive or provocative. The therapist's role is to be transparent in facilitating an authentic connection with the client, whereby they can learn that they are worthy of love for who they are as a person. The therapist needs to make space for the client to grieve for the losses of their childhood; it is typical for clients to realise what they have missed out on after some exposure to getting needs met in schema therapy. The therapist must also help the client update the information on which their old ways of coping and connecting were founded; even though it may have been necessary for them to play a prematurely sexualised role as a child to survive, as an adult they can now set clear, healthy boundaries to protect themselves from being 'used' or manipulated by others.

Box 18.2 Clinical Example of Limit Setting When the Client Romanticises the Therapeutic Relationship

Kerrie (client) had been attending regular therapy sessions with Sam (therapist) for five months, when Sam became aware of signs that Kerrie may be romanticising the relationship. She increasingly asked questions about how he would be spending weekends and what he was doing in his free time. She brought small gifts, but when Sam tried to explore the meaning of this behaviour, she dismissed it as 'Oh, I just wanted to show my appreciation for all you have done for me'. Sam sensed that there were several times that she was gazing at him for too long, suggesting that she was longing for a more romantic connection with him.

THERAPIST: Kerrie, I know that we have been meeting for a while now, and I want you to know that I'm really proud of what you've accomplished over that time. You're working so hard, and I'm noticing real shifts in the way you have been coping and relating to others in your relationships. One thing that I'd like to explore with you is that sometimes the various ages and unmet needs associated with different modes can lead people to have confusing feelings about their therapist. I wondered whether that is something that you might have noticed at all?

CLIENT: *[awkwardly]* I don't know what you mean . . . .ok, well maybe . . . this is hard to talk about . . . maybe I do have some unexpected feelings.

THERAPIST: Well, I want you to know that it's perfectly normal to experience confusing feelings in the context of therapy, and I really want you to feel comfortable to be able to tell me about what you have noticed, if anything in that regard. For example, it's very common to have fantasies of the therapist, such as an ideal parent or romantic partner. I don't know if I'm perceiving this correctly, but some of the things you have mentioned have made me wonder if there might be a side of you that maybe wishes or imagines our therapeutic relationship could go beyond that of therapy?

CLIENT: Well . . . I don't know. Maybe. It's hard to talk about. I feel a bit embarrassed, but I do sometimes wonder what it would be like to live with you. I know that sounds crazy, but I feel so cared for when I am with you, that sometimes I do wish it was more . . .

THERAPIST: The last thing I want you to feel is embarrassed. In fact, I think it's great that you have the courage to talk about this stuff. Therapy can be very confusing to the different modes . . . the different sides of you who are looking for opportunities to be cared for and to get your needs met. As a little child, you didn't get the care or the nurturance that you needed. You were dismissed and cast aside. And in therapy, for the first time in your life, we have been talking about very personal and intimate details of your life. There is a little child part who is lonely and longing to be loved . . . that's Little Kerrie. And then there is an adult part of you who is emerging, and perhaps more interested in adult version of love . . . I wonder if we might explore the thoughts and feelings of these different modes? I want you to know that it's safe here to explore these feelings – as your therapist, I can help you to make sense of these different modes, and the unmet needs behind these longings and desires. How would you feel about that?

Whereas clients with other-directed EMS, such as Self-Sacrifice, Enmeshment, and Approval Seeking, may have unmet needs for attuned care, they will also need more encouragement to enable them to develop a separate sense of identity, and greater autonomy. The therapeutic relationship provides a template for the client to learn how to function as a differentiated and authentic self, to make their own decisions and choices and to prioritise and balance their own needs alongside those of others to attain a healthy state of interdependence. Therapists with EMS in this domain may also be prone to boundary violations such as excessive self-disclosure, sharing of personal anecdotes, or answering emails/messages during their personal time as a means of gaining clients' acceptance or approval. Therapists are advised to explore and recognise their own personal boundaries alongside their professional boundaries, to ensure that they do not offer more than they can realistically manage. This may include availability outside of normal working hours, frequency of sessions, arrangements for crisis contact, and so on.

It is healthier to set realistic expectations from the outset rather than offering more than is manageable, thereby leading to resentment and later withdrawal of contact. For clients with an Abandonment schema, this pattern is likely to be particularly damaging, reinforcing previous relationship patterns whereby others have withdrawn contact with them, thus conveying the message that they are 'too needy'.

Clearly, the interaction of therapist and client EMS has the potential to raise ethical issues which can threaten the integrity of the therapeutic work. For further exploration of this issue in a schema therapy context, the following resources are recommended: Roediger and Archonti [26]; Simionato, Simpson, and Reid [27]; and van Vreeswijk and Zedlitz [28].

Addressing Therapist Schemas in Schema Therapy

The importance of therapists addressing their own EMS has been integral within schema therapy training since the inception of the model, with a proportion of supervision sessions within the certification programme allocated to this work. Furthermore, schema therapists are actively encouraged to seek out their own personal therapy to gain greater insight into their own unmet needs and EMS, and the ways in which these may play out in the context of both work and personal circumstances. Schema healing work is likely to reduce the incidence of schema therapists inadvertently making therapeutic decisions or reacting to meet their own needs rather than the needs of their clients [27].

Schema training and supervision already provides a key opportunity for schema therapists to reflect on their own EMS and well-being. We propose a range of strategies that enhance self-care amongst schema therapists, thereby enhancing their capacity to be authentically present and available for their clients (See Figure 18.1).

- **Continuing professional development** By taking advantage of regular professional trainings, schema therapists can prepare themselves for working with more complex clients; this will help them improve and maintain healthy boundaries in the face of their EMS triggers. When therapists are aware of their own vulnerabilities and strengths, they will have greater capacity to focus on the areas of practice that provide the most joy and sense of mastery, whilst improving their competence and practising self-reflection on the influence of their own EMS.
- **Seek support and connection:** One of the most important protective factors against burnout is social support. Schema therapists can enhance their connection with peers and mentors through involvement in peer supervision groups, ISST special interest

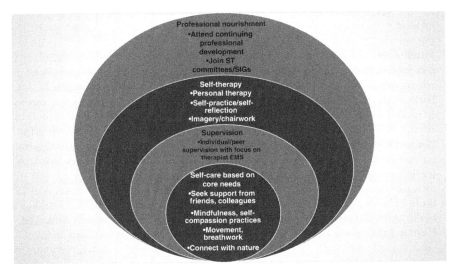

Figure 18.1 Model for the enhancement of schema therapist well-being

groups, and committees. These activities also create space and opportunities to connect socially.

- **Personal therapy:** Personal therapy provides an ideal opportunity for schema therapists to work specifically on their own EMS that manifest both at work and in their private lives. Well-being is enhanced as schema therapists learn to bypass their coping modes and to focus on their own Vulnerable Child modes, whilst learning to direct their energies towards getting their own emotional needs met. There is a culture of acceptance and encouragement among schema therapists that personal therapy can be immensely helpful.

- **Self-Practice/Self-Reflection (SP/SR):** The concept of 'self-therapy' has expanded exponentially over recent years and has been recognised as key to the effective practice of schema therapy. The SP/SR programme by Farrell and Shaw [29] is both a workbook and an experiential group learning programme for therapists to 'look at their own stuff'. It has been taught, practised, and evaluated extensively over recent years, and is currently being researched in terms of outcomes for therapists.

- **Schema techniques for exploring therapist-client chemistry:** Chairwork methods for working on therapist EMS both in the context of supervision and within live therapy sessions have been previously described [26]. Indeed, chairwork can provide powerful methods for challenging the therapist's Inner Critic mode and nurturing their own Vulnerable Child self.

- **Supervision:** Supervision is a valuable process for identifying and working through the interactions, or schema chemistry, between therapist–client EMS [26]. Schema therapy supervision provides multiple functions that contribute to therapist competence and well-being [30]. These include teaching and skills coaching, providing mentorship, and allowing thinking space when schemas have been triggered within sessions. Further, in schema therapy supervision, the supervisor can also fulfil the role as a reparenting agent by identifying unmet needs linked to EMS activations, and providing unmet needs through imagery rescripting, chairwork, and role-plays.

- **Mindfulness and self-compassion training:** In order to supercharge our capacity for compassionate empathy and reduce the risk of compassion fatigue, mindfulness and self-compassion training may be of particular benefit for schema therapists [28, 31, 32]. Further research is needed to explore ways in which compassion-based practices can be integrated within the schema therapy model, and to evaluate the effectiveness of these in strengthening therapists' Healthy Adult mode and capacity for compassionate empathy.
- **Get moving!** Integrated Healthy Adult well-being amongst schema therapists requires not just our heads, but, just as importantly, connection with our own bodies. Working for long periods of time, sitting at our desks, without moving and standing can lead to increased disconnection from the felt sense of our Vulnerable Child self that resides in the body. Body awareness and movement [33] and breath control [34] have clear links to health and well-being, providing a clear pathway to strengthening our own embodied Healthy Adult selves. Further, our bodies are a clear pathway to providing a joyful environment for our own Contented Child modes, through music, dance, running, climbing, or any movement that connects us with our life force.
- **Connection with nature:** Connecting with nature has been described a basic human need and has been shown to be a major predictor of well-being, vitality, and life satisfaction [35]. In fact, studies indicate that connection to nature may predict happiness over and above connection with family and friends [36]. Spending time outdoors and actively practising engagement with nature (flora and fauna) is arguably a missing piece in the puzzle of enhancing well-being both in ourselves and our clients.

Concluding Remarks

Schema therapy is built on the assumption that we all have schemas. Just as our clients are caught in self-perpetuating lifetraps that prevent them from getting their emotional needs met, so too are we as schema therapists. Within the context of our therapeutic work, our schemas can function as blindspots, potentially leading to reduced empathy and misattunement in our therapy sessions, as well as putting ourselves at risk for suffering from emotional difficulties, including burnout. Over the past twenty years, as the schema therapy model has expanded, so have opportunities for us to explore and work on our own schemas and access both professional and emotional nourishment. In this chapter, opportunities for building therapist well-being are explored through professional opportunities for awareness, growth and connection, personal and self-therapy, supervision, and self-care practices.

References

1. Bamber M. *CBT for occupational stress in health professionals: Introducing a schema-focused approach*. Routledge; 2006.

2. Bamber M, Price J. A schema focused model of occupational stress. In Bamber M, ed. *CBT for occupational stress in health professionals: Introducing*

a *schema-focused approach*. Routledge; 2006. pp. 149–161.

3. Barnett J, Baker E, Elman N, Schoener G. In pursuit of wellness: The self-care imperative. *Professional Psychology: Research and Practice.* 2007;**38**:603–12.

4. Elliott D, Guy J. Mental health professionals versus non-mental-health professionals: Childhood trauma and adult functioning. *Professional Psychology: Research and Practice.* 1993;24(1): 83–90.

5. Pope K, Feldman-Summers S. National survey of psychologists' sexual and physical abuse history and their evaluation of training and competence in these areas. *Professional Psychology: Research and Practice.* 1992;23(5):353–61.

6. Wise E, Hersh M, Gibson C. Ethics, self-care and well-being for psychologists: Reenvisioning the stress-distress continuum. *Professional Psychology Research and Practice.* 2012;43(5):487.

7. Firth-Cozens J. Emotional distress in junior house officers. *British Medical Journal (Clinical Research Ed.).* 1987;295 (6597):533–6.

8. Paris J, Frank H. Psychological determinants of a medical career. *Canadian Journal of Psychiatry.* 1983;28 (5): 354–57.

9. Rajagopal S, Rehill K, Godfrey E. Psychiatry as a career choice compared with other specialties: A survey of medical students. *Psychiatric Bulletin.* 2004; 28:444–6.

10. Galvin J, Smith AP. Stress in UK mental health training: A multi-dimensional comparison study. *British Journal of Education, Society & Behavioural Science.* 2015;9:161–75.

11. Simpson S, Simionato G, Smout M, et al. Burnout amongst clinical and counselling psychologists: The role of early maladaptive schemas and coping modes as vulnerability factors. *Clinical Psychology & Psychotherapy.* 2019;26(1):35–46.

12. Bamber M, McMahon R. Danger – Early maladaptive schemas at work! The role of early maladaptive schemas in career choice and the development of occupational stress in health workers. *Clinical Psychology & Psychotherapy.* 2008;15:96–112.

13. Phipps A. Self-sacrifice in schema therapists: 'Superpower or kryptonite?'

Conference presentation: Schema Therapy at The Coalface; 20 Feb. 2019; Sydney.

14. Kaeding A, Sougleris C, Reid C, et al. Professional burnout, early maladaptive schemas and the effect on physical health in clinical and counseling trainees. *Journal of Clinical Psychology.* 2017;73(12):1782–96.

15. Karpman S. Fairy tales and script drama analysis. *Transactional Analysis Bulletin.* 1968;7(26):39–43.

16. Edwards D. Self pity/victim: A surrender schema mode. *Schema Therapy Bulletin.* 2015;1(1):1–6.

17. Morse G., Salyers MP, Rollins AL, Monroe-DeVita M, Pfahler C. Burnout in mental health services: A review of the problem and its remediation. *Administration and Policy in Mental Health and Mental Health Services Research.* 2012;39(5):341–52.

18. McCormack HM, MacIntyre TE, O'Shea D, Herring MP, Campbell MJ. The prevalence and cause(s) of burnout among applied psychologists: A systematic review. *Frontiers in Psychology.* 2018;16(9):1897.

19. Simpson S, Simionato G, Smout M, et al. Burnout amongst clinical and counselling psychologists: The role of early maladaptive schemas and coping modes as vulnerability factors. *Clinical Psychology & Psychotherapy.* 2019;26(1):637.

20. Leiter M, Maslach C. Areas of worklife: A structured approach to organizational predictors of job burnout. In Perrewe P, Ganster D, eds. *Research in occupational stress and well-being.* 3rd ed. Elsevier; 2004. pp. 91–134.

21. Schaufeli WB, De Witte H. Work engagement: Real or redundant? *Burnout Research.* 2017;5(C):1–2.

22. Wilkinson H, Whittington R, Perry L, Eames C. Examining the relationship between burnout and empathy in healthcare professionals: A systematic review. *Burnout Research.* 2017;6:18–29.

23. Brown B. *Daring greatly: How the courage to be vulnerable transforms the way we live, love, parent, and lead.* Penguin; 2012.

24. Tullett AM, Harmon-Jones E, Inzlicht M. Right frontal cortical asymmetry predicts empathic reactions: Support for a link between withdrawal motivation and empathy. *Psychophysiology*. 2012;**49**(8):1145–53.

25. Singer T, Klimecki OM. Empathy and compassion. *Current Biology*. 2014;**24**(18):875–8.

26. Roediger E, Archonti C. Transference and therapist–client schema chemistry in the treatment of eating disorders. In Simpson S, Smith E, eds., *Schema therapy for eating disorders: Theory and practice for individual and group settings*. Routledge; 2019, pp. 221–241.

27. Simionato G, Simpson S, Reid C. Burnout as an Ethical Issue in Psychotherapy. *Psychotherapy*. 2019;**56**(4):470–482.

28. van Vreeswijk MF, Zedlitz A. Schema therapy for eating disorders: Therapist self-care. In Simpson S, Smith E, *Schema therapy for eating disorders: Theory and practice for individual and group settings*. Routledge; 2019, pp. 242–251.

29. Farrell JM, Shaw IA. *Experiencing schema therapy from the inside out: A self-practice/self-reflection workbook for therapists*. Guilford Publications; 2018.

30. Supervisory Skills Development Committee. Schema therapy supervision skills development. International Society for Schema Therapy; 2019.

31. Finlay-Jones AL, Rees CS, Kane RT. Self-compassion, emotion regulation and stress among Australian psychologists: Testing an emotion regulation model of self-compassion using structural equation modeling. *PloS one*. 2015;**10**(7).

32. Zarbock G, Lynch S, Ammann A, Ringer S. *Mindfulness for therapists: Understanding mindfulness for professional effectiveness and personal well-being*. Wiley; 2014.

33. Zubala A, MacGillivray S, Frost H, et al. Promotion of physical activity interventions for community dwelling older adults: A systematic review of reviews. *PloS One*. 2017;**12**(7):e0180902.

34. Zaccaro A, Piarulli A, Laurino M, et al. How breath-control can change your life: A systematic review on psycho-physiological correlates of slow breathing. *Frontiers in Human Neuroscience*. 2018;**12**:353.

35. Capaldi CA, Dopko RL, Zelenski JM. The relationship between nature connectedness and happiness: A meta-analysis. *Frontiers in Psychology*. 2014;**5**:976.

36. Zelenski JM, Nisbet EK. Happiness and feeling connected: The distinct role of nature relatedness. *Environment and Behavior*. 2014;**46**(1):3–23.

Chapter 19

Supervision and the Supervisory Relationship in Schema Therapy

Introduction

Supervision is essential to developing competence in schema therapy. Supervision to gain accreditation in schema therapy is a significant undertaking; it requires considerable time, money, cognitive effort, and emotional openness. In this chapter, we describe the style and activities of schema therapy supervision. We present common challenges that arise for supervisors and supervisees and how these may be overcome. In doing so, we hope to encourage more therapists to undertake supervision and go on to become schema therapy supervisors.

An Overview of Schema Therapy Supervision

Schema therapy supervision is an essential ingredient in the journey towards confidently and competently working with the schema therapy model. The primary aims of schema therapy supervision include providing good treatment adherence, as with all treatment models but in practice, supervision can offer so much more to the schema therapist. Schema therapy supervision supports the clinician to understand nuances in the model and its practical application that are difficult to convey in training contexts. Supervision also assists clinicians in understanding and formulating a wide range of presentations. Clients will invariably present with a range of complexities and backgrounds. Here, expertise is required in supporting the clinician to formulate an accurate case conceptualisation and develop the relevant treatment objectives. Supervisors also share and model how the treatment might unfold flexibly across time, including any decision points that come up in the process. It is hoped that there is a kind of knowledge transfer, with the supervisee internalising any useful information and attitudes conveyed. In this way, there is a bit of cultural transmission too; the supervisee acquires a 'feel for schema therapy' as it is practised. Schema therapy supervision is where the therapist learns the 'process' aspect of the model. It is here that they gain the contextual knowledge that enables them to 'join up' the different skills and aspects of the model in a coherent manner, as opposed to treating them as a 'set of tools' to be used in a rigidly prescribed manner.

In many ways, schema therapy supervision can mirror the therapeutic process; supervision will invariably help the supervisee develop professional as well as more personal capacities. Clients will inevitably present to treatment with modes and schemas that challenge the supervisee, which can symbolise central aspects of the client's presenting issues. Supportive supervision also aims at helping therapists gain awareness of any transference issues in their therapy relationships and understand their own schema activation with clients. In supervision, therapists are encouraged to engage with and develop their

'Healthy Therapist' mode, developing skills in managing areas of the therapy relationship that are challenging. Thus, schema therapy supervision takes a developmental view, just as in the therapy, supporting the development of confidence and skills that may typically lie out of the therapist's comfort zone.

The International Society of Schema Therapy (ISST) has led the way in developing the schema therapy supervision model that provides guidelines to those providing and engaging in schema therapy supervision. The ISST now requires suitably trained and certified schema therapists to attend specific training in this model to become schema therapy supervisors (enabling them to provide supervision for the purposes of accreditation or certification). The model and style of supervision defined by the ISST will be the foci of this chapter and are based on the latest ISST model and training materials [1].

The Supervisory Relationship and Three Roles of the Schema Therapy Supervisor

The general supervisory style of the schema therapy supervisor is largely consistent with the schema therapy therapeutic approach; the supervisory relationship is seen as an agent of change and development. Specifically, limited reparenting approaches evident in schema therapy are seen as an important aspect of training and supervision. Aspects of the schema therapy approach such as being authentic, genuine, and 'real' are central to the overarching style of the supervisor relationship. Despite often being in a position of influence, the supervisor, in our view, should present as a regular fallible clinician with appropriate self-disclosure (e.g., modelling the existence of their schemas and modes).

The schema therapy supervisor holds three specific roles within the supervisory relationship depending on the supervision needs at any given point:

1. **Supervisor as Educator/Coach.** The schema model can be complex, and clients can, of course, present with complex problems. In this role, the supervisor takes on a teacher or educator role, educating the supervisee to deepen their knowledge of the model and its application. The supervisor typically centres learning around a handful of clients and initially assists the supervisee to develop a thorough schema therapy case conceptualisation for these clients. In this role, the supervisor guides discriminating between various schemas and modes, allowing for more accurate assessment and conceptualisation of modes and schemas. In this role, the supervisor seeks to give feedback on the supervisee's skills. The Schema Therapy Competency Rating Scale (STCRS) is used by the supervisor to rate and give feedback on videotaped examples of the therapist's sessions. The Schema Therapy Case Conceptualisation Rating Scale (STCCRS) is similarly used to provide clear feedback on the therapist's case conceptualisation work. Based on this feedback process, skills competencies may be enhanced in supervision through the use of skills role-plays or demonstrations. While the other roles to be discussed are also important, in practice, the role of the supervisor as educator and coach is conceptual as the central role, charged with conveying the complexity of the model and building the requisite skills.

2. **Supervisor as Mentor/Role Model.** The schema therapy supervisor is aware of their role as a role model and mentor in the schema therapy model and their role as a therapist. Instead of appearing as an expert or an authority, the supervisor conveys a more egalitarian stance, modelling a level of warmth and openness about the inherent

struggles we all face as therapists. The focus in this role is on establishing a culture of openness, authenticity, and feedback within the supervisory relationship. This provides the safety for a focus on identifying and dealing with schema and mode activation in both the supervisee–client and supervisee–supervisor relationships. This includes the use of self-disclosure by supervisors of related challenges they have encountered in life and in clinical work. The aim here is to provide a supervisory space that is empathic and validating of the inherent struggles faced by therapists, and to show how therapists can approach common struggles with a level of openness and flexibility. It is hoped that this provides the supervisee with a working model of the stance of a 'Healthy Therapist Mode' that can be conceptualised and adopted into their own work.

3. **Supervisor as (*Limited*) Therapist and Agent of Limited Reparenting.** As we have discussed thus far, the tasks and general relationship style of schema therapy supervisors often mirrors that of the schema therapist. This is exemplified in the *limited* role schema therapy supervisors play for supervisees as a therapist and agent of limited reparenting. If schema therapists engage in *limited reparenting* approximating a parental role in therapy, schema therapy supervisors will at times employ a *limited therapeutic role*, including the provision of appropriate reparenting. It is important for schema therapists to develop a robust Healthy Adult/Therapist mode; schema therapy supervisors are charged with providing some *limited* opportunity to schema therapists to gain awareness of and heal schemas and modes that may otherwise be a hindrance to their work with clients. The aim here is to help therapists to become aware of and overcome their own internal obstacles (schemas, modes) to effective schema therapy. The schema therapy supervisor will thus employ some limited focus on providing a level of care, attunement, and guidance and, at other times, boundaries and limits as might be appropriate. At times, supervisors and their supervisees will become aware that these obstacles are of a nature and strength that will require some limited therapeutic focus. In these circumstances, schema therapy supervisors can offer some limited therapeutic focus, including conceptualisation, working to lessen the intensity of maladaptive modes at play (e.g., Critic, Surrenderer), reassure the Vulnerable Child, and ultimately strengthen the Healthy Adult mode. This limited focus on the therapy role should be offered collaboratively and as optional within the supervision relationship, and is most relevant when the problems the therapist identifies have clear relevance to their clinical work (e.g., therapist putting high unrelenting standards/ pressure on the client). Such a focus should not generally be undertaken for more than six supervision sessions within the advanced certification programme (or three in the context of standard certification) or for problems that are more relevant to the personal context than the supervisee's work context as a therapist (e.g., relationship problems/breakdown in the therapists personal life) [1]. If problems are identified that are of a severity or intensity beyond the *limited* scope of what should be provided within a supervision context, disproportionately distract from other tasks of supervision (e.g., conceptualisation and skills building), or that represent bona fide psychopathology (e.g., borderline personality disorder, clinical depression), supervisors will strongly encourage referral for personal therapy. Even outside this context, accessing personal therapy is encouraged for all schema therapists, as an opportunity for developing personal insight and awareness, healing schemas, and strengthening healthy modes.

Common Supervisory Issues

Just as clients often present to therapy with commonly seen schema-based patterns (e.g., depression related to Avoidant Protector and Punitive Critic), we have found several frequently observed patterns among supervisees that represent a risk to the development of confidence and competence in the model. Such patterns can and should be understood with regards to their underpinning schema and mode patterns and will become a central focus within supervision.

Therapists Avoiding Experiential Work

Experiential exercises within schema therapy can be anxiety-provoking for those learning the model. Therapists are typically concerned about making mistakes, or that clients will either experience an adverse reaction or will become defensive or rejecting of the therapist's work. Therapists may avoid experiential work and focus on themes or interventions (e.g., cognitive work) where they feel more confident. As a result, sessions can become overly cognitive or drift into supportive psychotherapy that from time to time 'mentions' schemas and modes without necessarily engaging them experientially for change. Experiential work is a central element of schema therapy. Supervisors should encourage supervisees to work outside of their immediate comfort zone, nurturing their skills while acknowledging and validating the challenges. Supervisors will assess the degree to which the avoidance is due to deficits in supervisees' knowledge and experience with the technique (requiring increased knowledge and skills coaching) or might be due to the therapist's own schema or mode activation (perhaps requiring a switch into the roles of supervisor as mentor or agent of some limited therapy focus). A common culprit here is the therapist's Unrelenting Standards schema: the therapist holds the belief that a new technique (e.g., chairwork) should only be attempted once it has been (perfectly) mastered. Here, the supervisor is likely to work closely with the therapist's Demanding Critic mode and related Unrelenting Standards schema.

Therapist Avoids Recordings of Clinical Work

Many clinicians have not been in the position of receiving direct feedback on their clinical skills, either by peers or supervisors, for quite some time (if ever). For therapists, providing examples of their therapeutic work for the purpose of evaluation is generally quite triggering. Notwithstanding this, setting the expectations early in the process of supervision that video-recorded sessions will need to be submitted for feedback is helpful. The supervisor will take a supportive and validating/normalising stance that sessions are never 'perfect'. Normalising feelings of insecurity can enhance a sense of safety and trust in the supervisory relationship. The core issue for these therapists is that without feedback on video recordings, they are missing out on important information relevant to their performance. Sometimes this is painful for the therapist, such as hearing that some aspects of their work can be 'improved'. Such negative aspects should be normalised as a part of the journey, and advice given on how to improve these aspects. In fact, to counter this, clinicians undertaking the certification process can be specifically invited to submit recordings which represent some kind of difficulty or 'stuckness' in the therapeutic process in preference to sessions which demonstrate their competence. Submitting these 'less perfect' recordings will often provide greater opportunity for the supervisor to offer clinically useful feedback regarding the treatment of specific clinical issues, thereby serving a dual purpose: (1) to provide feedback on the clinician's competence in specific aspects of the application of schema therapy and (2) to provide ideas and guidance regarding the treatment of specific clients and/or clinical presentations based on seeing their schemas and modes 'in action'. More often than not, therapists who lack confidence and who systematically avoid recordings tend to significantly underestimate their session performance because of schema-related biases (e.g., Failure schema). Accurate feedback based on video recordings for these therapists, handled supportively, can thus increase their confidence by providing some objective (and experiential) feedback on the positive aspects of their performance too. Video-recording feedback is therefore a characteristic feature of schema therapy supervision.

Supervisor's Unrelenting Standards Schema Impacting on Therapist's Confidence

Supervisors need to be aware of their own schemas in the supervision domain too, particularly regarding how these might impact on the supervisees' learning. In our experience, it is common for a supervisor's Unrelenting Standards schema to have a detrimental impact on the confidence of the developing clinician. Whilst it is important to meet a minimum level of competency and knowledge, it is important for the supervisor to adopt an encouraging and supportive approach rather than appear critical or demanding. Supervisors that have very strong Unrelenting Standards generally need to remain aware that supervisees generally have their own Demanding Critic modes, and thus tend not to benefit from that kind of modelling of unrelenting standards. Rather, in these cases the schema therapy model suggests quite the opposite: supervisors need to approach such supervisees with capacity from the Therapist as Agent of Limited Reparenting role and aim to engender a sense of relenting standards and healthy self-care.

The Aggrandising and/or Overcompensating Therapist

By way of their education, training, and work ethic, many if not most therapists might be considered 'high achievers'. A subset of therapists learning the model may indeed have a long list of achievements as therapists and in other areas of practice, making the role of 'supervisee' novel and, in some circumstances, uncomfortable. Some of these therapists may adopt some form of overcompensation or aggrandising in navigating the supervisory relationship to manage or regulate underlying feelings of discomfort. Therapists learning the model and engaging in supervision from the position of an Aggrandiser mode are in danger of overestimating their competency with the schema therapy model. In these cases, as in therapy, supervisors will work hard to build awareness of this mode and when it can be a hindrance to therapy and learning the model. This will perhaps be aided at times by the use of some form of empathic confrontation and limit setting. Video-recording feedback in this context is also very important in providing an objective method for the supervisor to rely on to provide accurate feedback. The goal here is to help supervisees engage in a more accurate reflection of their performance, from which they may be able to benefit.

Concluding Remarks

In this chapter we have introduced some of the latest ideas in the theory and practice of schema therapy supervision. Schema therapy supervision in many ways parallels much of the processes encountered in the therapy context. Accordingly, the interpersonal style and demeanour of the supervisor often reflects the supportive limited reparenting relationship seen in schema therapy. Notwithstanding this, the goals of supervision are different to those of therapy: supervision is ultimately focused on development of both the professional knowledge and skills and the personal capacities of the 'Healthy Adult Therapist'. This involves the supervisor becoming adept at switching between the three roles of a schema therapy supervisor. Following certification, schema therapists are encouraged to continue to seek expert and/or peer supervision in more focused ways that enable them to apply the approach in specific contexts (e.g., group, couples, individual), with specific populations (e.g., adults, older adults, children), and across a range of clinical presentations.

References

1. Supervisory Skills Development Committee. Schema Therapy Supervision Skills Development Document. International Society for Schema Therapy; 2019.

Chapter
20

Schema Therapy in the Online World

Introduction

There was a growing demand for therapy services to be delivered remotely online prior to COVID-19, which has increased exponentially since. Specific guidance on fundamental skills for adapting therapy and developing and enhancing the therapeutic bond via video-conferencing is available from other publications [1, 2]. In this chapter, we will explore specific ways in which technologies can be adapted for delivering schema therapy, with a particular focus on videoconferencing.

Technology Available for Remote Schema Therapy Delivery and Its Advantages

There is increasing demand to provide therapeutic services remotely via a range of tech-nologies. Online modalities such as videotherapy, telephone, email, synchronous/asyn-chronous chat, online forums, and coaching sites have accumulated a substantial evidence base over recent years and have demonstrated equivalence to in-person therapy in terms of both clinical outcomes and therapeutic alliance [3, 4, 5, 6, 7]. As new possibilities for working creatively with technology are embraced in schema therapy, opportunities for intimacy, play, and spontaneity can be greatly enhanced [8].

Hindrances to accessing services – such as geographical remoteness, disabilities/mobil-ity problems, incarceration, or illness/pandemics – can be overcome as online therapies become increasingly available. Online therapies provide a range of advantages, including reduced travel time and expenses, reduced disruption to work and childcare duties, greater access to specialist expertise or language/culture appropriate care, and greater continuity of care when either therapist or clients relocate. For schema therapists, the exponential growth of psycho-technologies provides significant opportunities for engaging new clients, as well as for extending our services beyond what was previously possible through combining technologies to match client need [8, 9, 10]. Due to the nature of some clinical presentations, technology-based treatment modalities may be preferable and the therapeutic bond may in fact be enhanced. For example, many clients experience video therapy as less confronting and distressing than in-person contact, so video delivery facilitates the expression of their needs and emotions [11, 5]. For some, online therapies can provide a level of perceived privacy and confidentiality beyond that experienced in in-person settings. Online modal-ities frequently lead to greater disinhibition and openness, resulting from a heightened sense of safety and a more neutral power balance [12, 13]. Clients who indicate a preference for video therapy describe feeling less self-conscious and less 'scrutinised', and having a greater sense of personal control, which may be particularly important when dealing with shame-related issues (e.g., sexual abuse, eating disorders, body-image disorders) [11, 5].

Schema therapists across the world have begun to find ways to draw on the strengths of online therapies to enhance the core therapeutic processes. Recent innovative developments in schema therapy that have harnessed technological advances include Secure Nest, a unique technology-enhanced framework for schema therapists [14]. This platform provides a 'meeting place' which allows therapists to provide rich opportunities for psychoeducation, connection, and emotional containment, thereby enhancing the limited reparenting experience without requirement for additional (costly) therapeutic sessions. Other innovations include a social media-based treatment programme for binge eating disorder [15], as well as videoconferencing-based individual [9, 10] and group schema therapy [16].

Adapting Schema Therapy Delivered Online

Strategies for Enhancing Limited Reparenting in Online Settings

The limited physical presence in online settings reduces opportunities for visceral connection, such as by touching a client on the arm when distressed or handing them tissues. Technical disruptions can potentially trigger a range of schemas, such as Failure/Incompetence ('If I wasn't so stupid, I could figure this out'), Subjugation ('My therapist's voice keeps fading in and out but I had better not say anything'), Entitlement ('There's no way I am putting up with losing part of my session – I'm not paying for that!'), Approval Seeking ('I need to monitor my own picture closely to ensure I portray myself in my best light), or Emotional Deprivation ('My therapist isn't looking directly at me, she thinks I'm too much'). With an accurate case conceptualisation, these activations can become 'grist to the mill', whereby therapists can use these opportunities to provide real-time corrective emotional experiences via experiential exercises and limited reparenting [17]. Schema therapists need to be mindful of the full range of limited reparenting tasks within the online environment. Whilst providing a nurturing, warm, and secure therapeutic space is the priority, therapists must also maintain professional 'Healthy Adult' boundaries, by being clear about confidentiality, time, and financial requirements, maintaining a professional therapeutic tone and manner when communicating via video or text-based messages, and maintaining consistency in time and location of sessions where possible.

The active ingredients of limited reparenting, including emotional presence and attunement, can be adapted to maximise connection through a range of strategies, some of which are described in Box 20.1.

Adapting Experiential Techniques in Online Settings

In our experience, imagery rescripting, chairwork, and even historical role-play can be highly effective within online settings with the help of minor adaptations. In this section we will explore some of the ways in which experiential techniques can be applied and creatively adapted within an online environment.

Imagery Rescripting and Historical Role-play. Imagery rescripting is ideally suited to the online environment. Clinical experience suggests that many clients prefer the experience of imagery in online settings due to the enhanced privacy of being in their own homes. In some cases, especially in instances of trauma processing, therapists may be advised to begin by

Box 20.1 Adaptations to Get the Most from Video-Delivered Schema Therapy

- Explain the technical aspects of videotherapy in advance to build confidence, adjusting the level of explanation to the needs and experience of the client. Explain contingency plans for when the technology fails, such as back-up videoconferencing platforms and/ or telephone contact. Explain the security limitations of technologies and provide opportunities for any questions clients may have in relation to this. Brief information sheets can be used to summarise these details.
- Use a quality web-camera that adequately conveys facial expressions and maximises eye contact.
- Eye contact is key to providing synchronised mirroring and attunement. Position the picture of the client on full-screen and make the picture-in-picture box as small and close to the webcam as possible. You can also stick a small photograph of the client above the webcam which can have the dual effect of drawing the therapist's eyes toward the webcam, heightening the experience of eye contact, whilst literally keeping the client's Vulnerable Child mode within the therapeutic focus.
- Provide verbal feedback in terms of positioning and remind clients that they can switch off their own picture-in-picture self-view if desired. Clients can be encouraged to experiment with distance and closeness to the screen and to notice the level of intimacy they feel most comfortable with. Those with schemas from the Other - Directedness domain can also benefit from being encouraged to experiment with taking control of their experience, such as by adjusting the size of images on their screen, the volume, and the distance of therapist and client from the screen. This can also be a useful way of experimenting with recognising their own interoceptive signals linked to boundaries and intimacy. For example:

THERAPIST: Just notice if anything changes in terms of your bodily felt sense when you move closer or further from the screen ... what comes up for you, if anything? As we talk, just notice any sensations, or urges. Notice whether there is any discomfort when we have eye contact. Notice if it feels forced or easy.

These explorations can help to unpack the body-based experiences associated with attachment disruption linked to core EMS. These can be more easily explored in the context of the close-up facial view offered by videoconferencing and the nuances of communicating at a distance via a screen.

- Clients working from home could be encouraged to separate their therapeutic space from their work environment. For those who access their sessions within a work environment, ensuring a private, bookable space where they will not be interrupted is essential. Ideally, their sessions should take place at the end of a work shift to allow space for emotions to emerge.
- Take clients on a virtual tour of your office space to enable them to visualise the therapist's surroundings. If clients are willing, they may also provide a virtual tour for the therapist, which can enhance the therapist's understanding of the idiosyncratic challenges faced by the client and provide valuable information about cues for coping behaviours (e.g., obsessional checking rituals, binge eating/drinking). For clients with a Mistrust/Abuse schema, taking this step can also help to provide additional trust and security, and allay any fears that others might be listening or watching the session.
- Virtual backgrounds and headphones are useful, especially when either party requires additional privacy, such as when sessions take place in private settings such as the bedroom.

- Invite clients to collate their own therapeutic resources to be available during sessions, such as a box of tissues, a soft fleece or blanket, a cosy (and sound-proof) therapeutic space. This can be particularly beneficial for clients with Emotional Deprivation and Abandonment schemas who feel deprived by the physical distance of online therapy. For clients whose Abandonment and Emotional Deprivation schemas get activated by the ending of sessions, these items can also be used as transitional objects, thus facilitating the development of object permanence.
- When audio recording sessions (e.g., to allow clients to listen to the session again for homework), ensure that files are stored confidentially (not within unprotected cloud files).
- Clients' pets can provide an additional soothing presence, enhancing feelings of security and connection.
- *Risk Management*: Ensure the client is in a safe location that facilitates their capacity to concentrate and communicate openly. Collaboratively develop a written risk management plan that details the steps required to ensure client safety. For clients with conditions that involve a high level of medical or psychiatric risk, ensure that they have access to local in-person contact with medical/psychiatric professionals who can provide additional support and hospitalisation if required (e.g., severe anorexia nervosa, addictions, acute suicidality).

Therapist Self-Care

- To allay potential 'zoom-fatigue' – the additional cognitive impact of extended periods of working via screens – therapists need to build in regular breaks and prioritise opportunities for connecting with nature and the outdoor environment each day, to prevent burnout.
- Prior to switching on the computer each day, stand, breathe, and shift your focus to your body, feeling the connection of your feet with the earth, and inviting yourself to notice this feeling of being 'in' the body. Take a few moments to move your fingers, toes, ankles, wrists, knees, hips, shoulders, and head clockwise and anticlockwise [18].
- Draw on your 'active' schema therapy skills, and use your body to stand, sit, and move about within the scope of the camera view, as you would in an in-person setting, to address the Inner Critic, reparent the Vulnerable Child, and so on [18].
- Schema therapists can increase their capacity to be fully present for clients through initially being present for and with themselves. Check in regularly with your own body and internal sensory experiences. What are you feeling, thinking? What images do you see? Notice the space around you, with your skin as the boundary that separates you from the world around you. Notice your position in the room, the building, the wider world. Notice yourself being 'held' by Mother Earth. Therapists can also talk clients through this grounding process early in the session, modelling a healthy process of reconnecting to the embodied Healthy Adult self [18].

pacing the work more slowly, and to titrate processing of traumatic memories with soothing calm/safe place imagery work. As in an in-person setting, to build a sense of confidence and reduce any anxiety regarding imagery work, the therapist can begin with simple reparenting imagery, meeting some of the client's needs from childhood. These can usually be audio recorded via the videoconferencing platform (e.g., Zoom) so that the client can listen to these between sessions, providing further experiences of getting their needs met. Imagery exercises can also be used to begin strengthening the client's Healthy Adult self, even before beginning any processing of traumatic memories. Preparatory practice of grounding techniques, including focusing on visual and physical sensory experiences and breathwork, can provide additional stability before undertaking trauma-based imagery rescripting. A simple orienting strategy for responding to a client who is activated is to suggest that they gently scan their room (away from the screen) and allow the gaze to rest wherever it naturally lands. Then invite them to close their eyes and turn their attention inward to notice the feelings associated with 'being' in the body. Both client and therapist take a deeper breath and notice the sensations of settling into the body. Moving through this process together facilitates a parallel process of co-regulation whilst providing an opportunity for the client to learn to manage their own schema-driven activations as they manifest in the body [18].

Enlisting the active involvement of the client's Healthy Adult self, a part which can take a self-observer stance and take responsibility for actively engaging in therapy, appears to be even more important in online settings than in in-person sessions, and is essential for effective processing. Schema therapists are advised to advance slowly with experiential work, ensuring that clients are grounded and embodied (i.e., have a felt sense of being in touch with sensations in the body) before moving into trauma work [17, 18].

Once the therapist is confident with the technology, they can draw on a range of creative adaptations. Puppets or peg-dolls and drawings can be used to represent the characters to re-enact the early memories associated with schema development. Incorporating innovative technologies such as avatar-based virtual worlds which can be shared and viewed simultaneously can also provide opportunities for experiential growth. Avatars can represent both the client's internal mode dynamics and important external relationships with others in their lives. This provides unique possibilities to explore how they currently interact, whilst learning new ways of operating in Healthy Adult mode and meeting the needs of their own Vulnerable Child. Online virtual platforms such as Pro Real (www.proreal.co.uk/) allow the client to explore ways in which they can rescript old memories, with significant characters represented by avatars and the range of mental states, emotions, choices, and dilemmas represented by a range of landscapes (e.g., cliffs, waterfalls, castles, pathways, crossroads) and symbols (e.g., mirrors, clocks, bridges, boulders, barriers). Such technologies can introduce a playfulness and fantasy that can enhance experiential techniques, allowing the client to experiment with previously unimagined options and ways of coping. They can also provide new possibilities, as clients begin to construct novel ways of envisaging their lives and future goals [8].

Chairwork Online. Online therapy makes it more difficult to use techniques involving physical movement and the use of physical objects such as chairs. However, the chair technique actually lends itself to online therapy too [19, 20]. It is highly preferable that the client has a laptop or tablet when this technique is being used online so that movements can be followed more easily by the client taking the laptop or tablet with him or her when making those movements in the physical space.

There are three versions of use of the online chair technique:

1. The therapist asks the client to move in front of the camera from one side of the screen to the other to adopt the position of a mode.
2. The chairs in the therapist's room are used. This form of online chair technique is particularly suitable for adapting work with parent modes during the initial phase of therapy.

3. Different chairs are used in the room where the client is located. This form of online chair technique is particularly suitable in working with coping modes or when working with parent modes. In the latter case, however, this occurs at the end of the therapy. The three versions are explained in further detail:

1. **Moving in Front of the Camera.** In this version, different chairs are not literally being used, but rather different positions in relation to the camera. While naming the active modes, the therapist may gesture to a specific side of the screen before asking the client to move to the side indicated. That specific position in relation to the camera then becomes the place of the active mode. Therapists should not describe this movement across the screen in terms of left or right, because the image is sometimes a mirror image, which can cause confusion as to which side is being referred to.

   Box 20.2 illustrates the use of video screen positions to simulate physical chairwork. In this example, the negotiation with the coping modes results in the client being asked to move to the other side of the screen. In this position, the therapist tries to make contact with the client's emotional side. Use of the camera here can provide opportunities to intensify contact by moving closer to the camera, for example, and looking directly into the camera whilst the therapist speaks directly to the client's emotional side using a gentle voice.

2. **Use of the Chairs in the Therapist's Room.** This version of the online chair technique is particularly helpful in addressing Critic modes during the initial phase of the therapy. In this initial phase of therapy, the healthy part of the client is either absent or barely present. The presence of a chair in the client's room which symbolises punitive messages from the past might therefore be difficult for the client to bear. It might be even more difficult for the client to put away this punitive side now that there isn't a Healthy Adult present and the therapist can only help through the screen. By using a chair in the therapist's room, the therapist can still symbolise a healthy parent fighting the punitive messages and putting the chair away.

Box 20.2 Clinical Example of Moving in Front of Camera to Simulate Physical Chairwork

THERAPIST: In the state you're in right now *[gestures to the right-hand side of the screen as well as looking at that spot next to the screen]*, you seem not to be feeling very much. I know that you *[gesturing to the camera]* can feel an awful lot, but in the state you're in right now *[gestures once again to the right-hand side of the screen]*, this is not the case and you seem to be feeling rather flat. I believe there is a reason for this. Shall we do a quick exercise to find out why that is?

[Client nods]

THERAPIST: I now want to ask you to move to that side *[gestures to the right-hand side of the screen]*.

[Client moves to the side indicated]

THERAPIST: *[looks directly into the camera]* In this position, I want you to be that non-feeling *[name of client]*. Just be the non-feeler here. I believe that for you *[gestures towards the camera]*, the non-feeler, this is more comfortable than if the emotional *[name of the client while simultaneously gesturing to the left-hand side of the screen]* were to be there, is that correct? How would they *[gesturing to the left-hand side of the screen]* feel if you *[gesturing to the camera]* were not there?

Box 20.3 Clinical Example: Using Chairs Within the Therapist's Room in Video Schema Therapy

THERAPIST: How have you felt over the past week?

CLIENT: Bad, stupid, I am doing everything wrong and I am a total failure . . .

THERAPIST: OK, I'll just interrupt you here for a moment.

The therapist identifies the punitive experience and asks the client to move in front of the camera to express this criticism about themselves from the right-hand side of the screen, making this position the location of the punitive side. The therapist then asks the client to move back to their original position and to explain from their emotional part how it feels to hear all that criticism about themselves.

THERAPIST: If I listen to all that criticism coming from that corner *[gestures to the right-hand side of the screen]*, it is just as if someone is sitting there pouring out all that criticism about you.

At this moment, the therapist turns the camera a little to the right so that an empty chair becomes visible next to the therapist. This is the moment that the punitive voice from the client's room is moved to the chair in the therapist's room. However, this is not so much discussed explicitly as suggested by the movement and the obvious nature by which the therapist indicates the punisher in the chair.

THERAPIST: I am therefore wondering who is actually sitting there? Who do all those punitive messages come from?

CLIENT: *[softly]* My father . . .

THERAPIST: I was thinking of him too. So, it is actually your father sitting there *[pointing to the empty chair which is still visible in view]*, raging at you like that. But I don't want you to have all that anger poured out over you, so I want to say something to him. *[The therapist turns towards the empty chair and challenges the imaginary father with a decisive voice].*

Fighting these punitive messages may result in the therapist removing the empty chair from the room. During this intervention, the therapist grips the laptop against their upper arm or shoulder with one hand and removes the chair from the room using their other hand. This way, the client is looking over the therapist's shoulder, so to speak.

In this version of online chair technique, the punitive side is moved out of the client's room into the therapist's room. It is recommended that this movement is not explicitly or expressly discussed during the exercise so that the exercise itself remains an emotional experience rather than expecting the client will develop a rational, explicit understanding of its purpose. Box 20.3 illustrates the use of chairs in video schema therapy.

3. **Use of the Chairs in the Client's Room.** During the final phase of the therapy, the client can learn to fight the punitive messages themselves by using chairs in their own room. After identifying the punitive side, the therapist asks the client to choose a chair or other object in the client's room which can symbolise these punitive messages. In this exercise, the therapist coaches the client in fighting that punisher. It is also important that the therapist continues to keep a close eye on what is going on in the client's room and must therefore give clear instructions as to where the camera is pointed.

Box 20.4 presents an example of chair use in the client's room during video chairwork, and Box 20.5 gives some tips for online chair technique.

Box 20.4 Clinical Example: Fighting Parent Modes via Chairs in the Client's Room During Video Chairwork

THERAPIST: What side can we recognise when you speak so negatively about yourself?

CLIENT: . . . Yes, that Punisher again . . .

THERAPIST: Exactly! Very good that you are able to recognise that so clearly. Are you now able to see an object or a chair in your room which can symbolise this punisher? And let me take a little look into your room too by turning your laptop around a bit.

CLIENT: *[grabs the laptop and turns the camera so that the therapist can see an empty chair]* That chair there, I think . . .

THERAPIST: Very good! Now place that chair so close, or so far away from you, that it matches how strong you feel the punisher is. If that chair is very close by, then it is as if that punisher is criticising your every move. Is that how it feels? Or was it not as strong and is that chair fine as it is, at this distance?

CLIENT: *[Stands up and moves the chair a little closer]* 'Well, here then I think, because I did feel it strongly, that feeling as if I wasn't worth anything . . .'

THERAPIST: Very good. Now I want you to stand up to that Punisher, to tell him why he isn't right. But that means that you have to get into that Healthy Adult part of you first. So, close your eyes and try to visualise that image of that Healthy Adult again, that captain of your ship . . . What can you see now?

This is how the therapist coaches the client: make contact with the healthy side first, and then, like those healthy adults, challenge the crime and remove the chair from the room if necessary.

Box 20.5 Tips for Online Chair Technique

- Use a laptop or tablet (both therapist and client)
- Avoid talking about 'left'/'right' and use gestures to indicate the direction
- Look straight into the camera when speaking with the mode
- Ensure short distance to the camera when making contact with the client's emotional part, a little further away for coping and parent modes

---

Concluding Remarks

As clients increasingly choose to access schema therapy remotely, it is essential for schema therapists to become digitally competent. Online settings provide multifarious opportunities for therapists to adapt schema therapy techniques in innovative and creative ways. In this chapter, a range of adaptations are described which can be utilised across a wide range of technologies. We encourage schema therapists to tap into their own creativity as they learn to adapt to online settings.

References

1. Simpson S, Smith E. *Schema therapy for eating disorders: Theory and practice for individual and group settings.* Routledge; 2019.

2. Simpson S, Richardson L, Reid C. Therapeutic alliance in videoconferencing based psychotherapy. In Goss S, Anthony K, Nagel D, Sykes-Stretch L, eds., *Technology in mental health: Applications for practice, supervision and training*. Charles C. Thomas; 2016. pp. 99–116.

3. Simpson S, Richardson L, Pietrabissa G, Castelnuovo G, Reid C. Videotherapy and therapeutic alliance in the age of COVID-19. *Clinical Psychology & Psychotherapy*. 2021;**28**(2):409–21.

4. Backhaus A, Agha Z, Maglione ML, et al. Videoconferencing psychotherapy: A systematic review. *Psychological Services*. 2012;**9**(2):111.

5. Simpson SG, Reid CL. Therapeutic alliance in videoconferencing psychotherapy: A review. *Australian Journal of Rural Health*. 2014;**22**(6):280–99.

6. Varker T, Brand RM, Ward J, Terhaag S, Phelps A. Efficacy of synchronous telepsychology interventions for people with anxiety, depression, posttraumatic stress disorder, and adjustment disorder: A rapid evidence assessment. *Psychological Services*, 2019;**16**(4):621–35.

7. Batastini AB, Paprzycki P, Jones AC, MacLean N. Are videoconferenced mental and behavioral health services just as good as in-person? A meta-analysis of a fast-growing practice. *Clinical Psychology Review*. 2020;**83**:1–22.

8. Simpson S, Francesco V. Technology as an invitation to intimacy and creativity in the therapy connection. *Schema Therapy Bulletin*. 2020;**17**:14–18.

9. Simpson S, Morrow E. The use of alternative technology for conducting a therapeutic relationship on videoconferencing. In *The use of technology in mental health: Applications, ethics and practice*. Charles C. Thomas Publisher, Ltd; 2010, pp. 94–103.

10. Simpson SG, Slowey L. Video therapy for atypical eating disorder and obesity: A case study. *Clinical Practice and Epidemiology in Mental Health: CP & EMH*. 2011;**7**:38–43.

11. Simpson S, Bell L, Knox J, Mitchell D. Therapy via videoconferencing: A route to client empowerment? *Clinical Psychology & Psychotherapy*. 2005;**12**(2):156–65.

12. Fletcher-Tomenious L, Vossler A. Trust in online therapeutic relationships: The therapist's experience. *Counselling Psychology Review*, 2009;**24**(2):24–34.

13. Roy H, Gillett T. E-mail: A new technique for forming a therapeutic alliance with high-risk young people failing to engage with mental health services? A case study. *Clinical Child Psychology and Psychiatry*. 2008;**13**(1):95–103.

14. Skewes S, van Vreeswijk M. How online tools can enhance schema therapy beyond the therapy room. *Schema Therapy Bulletin*. 2020;**17**:19–25.

15. Skryabina M, Borisova M, Kudrjasova N. The efficiency of schema therapy interventions for binge eating disorder using social media platforms. *Schema Therapy Bulletin*. 2020;**17**:3–5.

16. van Dijk SD, Bouman R, Folmer EH, et al. (Vi)-rushed into online group schema therapy based day-treatment for older adults by the COVID-19 outbreak in the Netherlands. *The American Journal of Geriatric Psychiatry*. 2020;**28**(9):983–8.

17. Feldman H, Liu X. Schema anywhere: The opportunities and pitfalls of delivering schema therapy online. *Schema Therapy Bulletin*. 2020;**17**:6–9.

18. Guiffra M. Strategies to mindfully integrate the missing element in online therapy. *Schema Therapy Bulletin*. 2020; **17**:26–9.

19. Pugh M, Bell T, Dixon A. Delivering tele-chairwork: A qualitative survey of expert therapists. *Psychotherapy Research*. 2020;**31**(3): 843–58.

20. Pugh M, Bell T. Process-based chairwork: Applications and innovations in the time of COVID-19. *European Journal of Counselling Theory, Research and Practice*. 2020;**4**(3):2020.

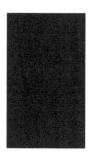

Epilogue

Continuing the Journey

The recent surge in research evidence supporting the efficacy of schema therapy has led to exponential interest in this model by therapists across the globe. Schema therapy is becoming increasingly applied to a wide range of clinical populations, including adults, children, and families with personality-related difficulties, chronic mood disorders, complex trauma, addictions, eating disorders, forensic settings, and relationship difficulties. Randomised controlled trials have supported its effectiveness with borderline and Cluster C personality disorders, forensic populations, and eating disorders, in individual and group settings.

The International Society of Schema Therapy (ISST) was founded in 2008, and now has over 2,500 members from more than sixty countries worldwide. Further, more than 100 schema therapy training programmes are now operating, increasing accessibility and applicability to a wide range of global cultures and languages. Training guidelines for ISST certification at standard, advanced, and auxiliary levels have been published for schema therapy, as applied to individual and group therapy settings. Separate certification pathways are available for those working with individuals, groups, children/families, and couples: see www.schematherapysociety.org/Certification.

A range of online schema therapy training options have become available over the past two years, prompted by the COVID-19 pandemic. This has resulted in increased accessibility and affordability of training and has been especially beneficial to those in geographical areas without access to local training programmes. In parallel with these changes, innovative adaptations to the way in which skills and techniques are practised in online settings have developed, leading to increased flexibility and creativity in practice.

Schema therapy training assumes that professionals are already qualified either as psychotherapists and/or allied health professionals, and have a foundational training in another approach, such as cognitive-behavioural, person-centred, or psychodynamic therapy. Following certification, further training is available to enable schema therapists to become ISST certified trainer-supervisors. Members are also encouraged to familiarise themselves with and become involved in the numerous ISST committees (https://schema therapysociety.org/ISST-Committee-Structure) and special interest groups (i.e., couples, online settings, clinical sports psychology, trauma, OCD, organisational development). Specialist training and supervision is also becoming increasingly available for a wide range of clinical presentations and difficulties and is ideal for those who have already completed the certification training.

We hope that you have enjoyed reading this book as much as we enjoyed writing it. It is truly a representation of teamwork and collaboration. Our mission has been to provide a roadmap for those new to schema therapy, as well as expert guidance for those who are already experienced in the model and are seeking new angles and creative adaptations. In our view, one of the most wonderful aspects of schema therapy is that it is forever evolving and integrating new material and understandings from developmental, neurobiological, and attachment-based research and literature. Schema therapy is based on the notion that, as humans, we all have schemas, modes, and unmet needs. The more we are in touch with our own Inner Child feelings and Healthy Adult selves, the more genuine and authentic we become as therapists and human beings. We therefore wholeheartedly encourage you to embark on your own lifelong journey of nurturing your own inner Vulnerable Child, and strengthening your Healthy Adult self, in parallel with your evolution as a schema therapist.

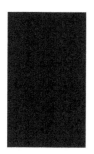

Afterword from Jeffrey Young, PhD, Founder of Schema Therapy

Recent times have seen the schema therapy approach exponentially expand in recognition and acceptance. It is now a gold-standard treatment that is recommended by national and international treatment guidelines and is evolving and flourishing throughout the world. The schema therapy model has been richly developed, allowing the approach to be utilised for a wide-ranging array of clinical problems and difficulties. Most importantly, it has dramatically assisted the lives of many individuals who were struggling with emotional challenges that therapists previously found difficult to address in therapy.

I'm very excited to see Rob Brockman, Susan Simpson, Christopher Hayes, Remco Van Der Wijngaart, and Matthew Smout collaborate to create a new comprehensive resource to assist those learning the schema therapy model. These authors are longstanding members of the schema therapy global community and have been at the forefront of treatment, training, and research.

At the core of the schema therapy model are unmet emotional needs. The treatment aims to help clients get their needs met and to develop healthy adaptive coping patterns. The authors have extrapolated the needs model to consider the learning requirements of the practitioner. The schema therapy trainee has specific educational and training needs, both in terms of understanding the key elements of the model and in learning how to put them together in a coherent way. This book aims to meet those needs. The authors have a unique understanding of the questions, concerns, and typical challenges facing the practitioner.

The book is a thorough resource for the practitioner learning the rich nuances of the schema therapy approach. The material has been carefully designed to assist in learning and understanding the model, and to provide practical guidance to bypass typical roadblocks and 'what do I do now?' therapeutic moments.

This text is an essential resource for those learning and developing skills for understanding and applying schema therapy, as well as for those advanced practitioners who are interested in innovative developments in the model in recent years. I am confident that readers will benefit from learning and practising this treatment approach. Furthermore, I wish all trainees and clinicians success in effectively assisting their clients with challenging emotional problems.

Appendix   Interview Questions/Guidance for the Assessment Process (Chapter 3)

Opening General Questions for Exploring Unmet Needs

- Invite client to describe their relationship with both parents and other significant caregivers throughout childhood. Identify differences in relationships with each parent (linked to possible unmet needs). Did the relationship change at any point? For example, as a result of divorce, parents re-partnering, parents moving away, death, or, in the case of a narcissistic parent, choosing a sibling to take on the role of the favoured or 'golden child'.

  Can you tell me about your mother?

  How would you describe her as you were growing up, compared with now?

  If she was a character in a book, how would she be described?

  If you had a basket right here, and I invited you to throw in some random words to describe your mum, what words would come to mind to include all of her different traits, positive and negative?

- Ask clients to describe their parents' personalities and to consider the ways that they are similar/different to each of their parents.

  How are you similar to your mum?

  And in what ways are you different?

  And how are you similar and different to your dad?

  Who do you think that you are more similar to: your mum or your dad?

- It is essential for therapists to maintain an empathic stance, recognising that often our clients' parent's intentions were good and that reduced capacity for interpersonal closeness and connection are largely a result of intergenerational trauma and neglect. In particular, reduced parental emotional presence and capacity for attunement is likely to be a legacy of intergenerational emotional neglect. It can be helpful to think of this as an emotional 'ingredient' that has dropped out of the family recipe at some point in the past.

- When asking about childhood experiences, it can also be helpful to explore possible links between these and adult patterns. It is important to explore any patterns within intimate relationships that have developed during and since childhood. Clients often recall having a 'crush' during childhood and may have been involved in intimate relationships in some capacity since adolescence. How long have these relationships generally lasted? Who ended the relationships, why, and how? How did the client cope at the time? If possible, ask enough questions about relationships across the client's life to understand the type of person they are attracted to, and recurring relationship dynamics which may be linked to EMS and coping modes.

- Over the course of the assessment, at a macro-level the clinician can explore the client's capacity for self-reflection: do they recognise any association between their relationship patterns in adulthood and their relationships with caregivers during childhood? Can they identify any missing emotional ingredients in their early relationships? Are they able to describe ways in which they would have liked their parents to be different and/or ways that they might consider parenting their own children differently, either currently or in the future (i.e., are there any aspects of their own childhood that they would do differently for their own child)?

Questions to Explore Need for Safe and Secure Attachment

- Enquire about significant disruptions to attachment during childhood, including loss of significant caregivers due to divorce, death, mental or physical illness (including personality disorders, and narcissistic traits), addictions, parents working away for long periods, being cared for by multiple (sequential) nannies, being fostered, or being adopted. Explore the client's understanding of how these events unfolded, how they affected them in the past (and now), and whether they believe that they hold any sense of responsibility or shame in regard to these events. Enquire about this at a cognitive and emotional level:

THERAPIST: Sometimes when people have experienced something like this (i.e., adoption, fostering, losing a parent), they might know in their minds that they weren't to blame, and yet another part of them still carries a sense of responsibility or self-blame, as though things might have turned out differently, if only you had been better or different in certain ways – is this something you have ever noticed?

- Enquire about the level of attunement the client received from caregivers: did parents spend time listening, showing an interest, emotionally connecting? How much explicit affection/nurturance was expressed, including affectionate physical touch? What 'language' did parents use to communicate love and affection (if at all): was it through overt affection or other external mechanisms (e.g., preparing food, expensive gifts, working long hours to put me into an expensive school, doing my washing/ironing)? Did parents have the capacity for emotional attunement and nurturance, and was this direct and developmentally appropriate, or indirect (e.g., through general reassurance, comfort eating).

Were your parents and other family members able to express love in an open, expressive way (e.g., hugs, telling you they loved you)?

How was love expressed in your family?

Did this change at different stages when you were growing up (e.g., baby, toddler, teenager)?

Did your parents suffer from any difficulties that might have interfered with their capacity to show affection in the way they would have wanted to (e.g., high anxiety levels, obsessive compulsive disorder, depression, eating disorder, addiction)?

Did your parents express love in different ways, or were they similar in the ways they showed affection? If different, how?

Did you do things together, and spend time connecting, such as through playing together and spending time together?

When you were together, to what extent were your parents able to shift their focus from their own duties and priorities to really listen to you and be available to you?

Did you feel like anyone really 'got' you and understood you? What were you going through then?

Did you ever feel like you were under the radar, as though no one really had time to pay attention to you because of how busy they were (with work responsibilities, etc.)?

Who would you have sought help from if you were upset (e.g., about being criticised at school, losing a good friend, your cat dying)? How would they have responded? (if the answer is 'no one', then ask 'Why not? What would you have been afraid would happen if you had told your mother/father about your anxieties? Just close your eyes and imagine yourself telling them and that fear coming true . . . what happens next?')

How did your parents find comfort for themselves? Did they comfort each other, and themselves, through affection, or were they more likely to find a way to shut down their needs and feelings?

- Use hypothetical questions to identify patterns of emotional neglect or conditional expressions of love.

What would have happened if you were distressed about something upsetting that happened at school? Who would you have gone to for support?

Who would you have approached if you needed a hug?

What would your parents have felt if you had openly asked them for affection (e.g., a hug)? Would it have come naturally, or felt awkward in any way?

Did you ever feel that you would have been more lovable if you had been different in some way?

Did you ever feel that you were missing important character traits that would have made you more lovable in your parents' eyes? Which traits do you feel were missing?

Looking back, if there was one thing that you could have done to change yourself as a child to make yourself more acceptable/lovable, what would it have been?

- Did the client experience any traumas/threats to their sense of safety during childhood, including domestic violence or aggression, death of significant others, and natural catastrophes due to war, famine, etc.?
- Explore indications of physical/sexual/emotional abuse.

When you think about your parents' relationship, in your opinion, to what degree were they able to communicate in a loving, caring way?

To what extent were they considerate of each other's and their children's emotional needs?

Was one parent more dominant or demanding than the other? How did that play out? Can you give me a couple of examples so that I can understand this better?

Did you ever feel sorry for one or both of your parents?

Did you ever feel as if it was your responsibility to take care of/parent them?

What consequences were used for discipline or punishment in your family?

Did either of your parents lash out physically or verbally when upset, angry, or intoxicated? Who was this mostly directed at? How did you feel? How did you cope?

When you think back over your life, has anyone ever touched you or looked at you in an inappropriate way or which made you feel uncomfortable?

- Enquire about experiences of explicit or implicit rejection or criticism during childhood (family of origin, peers/friendship groups)
- Enquire about family illnesses during childhood (either the client, their friends, or family members). How was this responded to by family members? How families respond to illness is a rich source of information about EMS or coping modes the child might have formed. For example, parents' inability to respond and provide support to the child models helplessness in the face of adversity which might lead to the child developing a Vulnerability to Harm schema. If parents appeared to provide nurturance and support (e.g., from family, healthcare services) when the child was ill but were relatively distant when the child was healthy, the child might learn to behave sick and helpless as a coping strategy to get their needs for nurturance met.

Were physical illnesses taken more seriously than emotional struggles/difficulties in your family?

- Enquire about any significant losses or separations from a parent/family member/friend through divorce or death in childhood or adolescence. How did the child cope at the time? How much emotional support was available?
- Enquire about whether all siblings were treated equally or whether one of the siblings was given higher status? Were particular features/traits valued over others? For example, in some families there may have been one child who behaved and achieved according to parental expectations, whereas the child who was more extroverted, impulsive, or boisterous may have attracted disapproval.
- Did any of the siblings have disabilities or special needs that required significant parental attention? Alternatively, did any of the siblings develop physical or mental health problems that required a disproportionate amount of parental attention (e.g., cancer, drug and alcohol problems, anorexia nervosa)? How capable were the parents of setting limits on sibling behaviours that impacted other family members, or of seeking external help and support when required?
- Enquire about 'buffer' (protective) relationships; if relationships at home were strained, was there anyone else in the client's life on whom they could rely on for comfort, guidance, and support during childhood?
- Explore the extent to which the client and their family experienced a sense of belonging and community. How sociable did they perceive their parents to be (did they have 'family friendships', did the family belong to any local groups/communities, or were they relatively socially isolated)?
- Enquire about peer relationships and groupings. Did the client experience any close friendships during childhood and adolescence? If so, were these generally long lasting or short lived? Was the client able to maintain relationships outside school hours, or were social opportunities restricted? How much were these relationships based on emotional closeness (explore the nature of these relationships: was there a sense of emotional connection or were they relatively superficial in quality)? Did the client undergo any social exclusion, bullying, or teasing by siblings or peers?

- To what extent was the client influenced by cultural emphases based on individualistic values such as materialism, status, and financial success at the expense of health, happiness, and interconnection? What qualities did the parents value most during childhood? To what extent do they feel that they have those qualities most valued by parents? Does the client try to be more like either of their parents in any way?

How did your parents spend their time?

What aspects of life were most highly valued by your parents, grandparents, aunts, uncles (e.g., spending time with family, family holidays, work, buying nice things, appearance, having a nice house, etc.).

Were there any aspects of life where your parents felt insecure, or where you noticed they were competing with others (e.g., job status, possessions, school they send their kids to, fitness)?

To what extent do you think that appearances, status, and possessions were important to your parents?

What (if any) aspects of your parents' outlook did you respect or admire? Were there any of their values that you have 'inherited' but that maybe don't quite 'sit right' with you?

To what extent did your family participate as part of their local community? Did your family belong to any community groups or sports clubs? To what extent did your parents join in and get involved?

Connection to Self

Enquire about whether the client received sufficient nurturance, warmth, praise, empathy, and overt affection to develop the capacity to feel good about themselves and to think of themselves as a good person. Was the client cherished? If so, can they describe how this was expressed? Did they experience unconditional acceptance?

- Has the client had opportunities during childhood and adolescence to develop a coherent sense of self based on warm, nurturing attachment relationships?

To what extent did you feel others really knew you and understood the real you as a child (as opposed to feeling as if certain parts of you were unacceptable and needed to be shut off)?

Do you have a strong sense of who you are? Who are you? How do you describe your 'self'?

As you were growing up, did you ever doubt your own existence or feel like you weren't real?

As a child, did you ever notice feelings of derealisation or depersonalisation (as if you were a bystander in your own life, or weren't in your own body, or that certain body parts changed size or felt like they were disconnected from you in some way)?

As a child, did you ever have the feeling that others saw and accepted the 'whole of you', including your emotional needs, feelings, and opinions?

- To what extent was the client encouraged to develop their own interests, try new pursuits, and express themselves openly and without judgement?

What activities or pursuits give you a sense of well-being or happiness?

What do you care most about in life? What matters most to you?

- To what extent has the client had safe opportunities to learn to regulate their emotions (bottom-up), such as through healthy physical connection with others and body movements (dance, music, walking, running)? How have childhood experiences shaped the client's sense of agency and pleasure associated with the body? To what extent has there been unhealthy modelling of using the body in harmful ways in an attempt to self-regulate (e.g., self-harm)?

  In your family, did anyone use food or other external 'substances' (alcohol, drugs, self-harm) as a substitute for comfort, self-soothing?

  Did anyone use exercise or being 'super healthy' as a way of feeling good about themselves?

  What were your parents' attitudes towards their own bodies? In your opinion, did they treat their bodies with respect?

  How did they refer to others (in terms of body shape/size/appearance)? Did this affect the way you felt about yourself and your body in any way?

  Did you ever get involved in body activities (such as dance, running, playing an instrument, swimming, hiking, cycling, sailing) purely for pleasure without having to worry about it being a source of achievement or recognition, or worry about what others were thinking?

Connection to Nature

- Explore the extent to which clients have experienced opportunities to connect with nature and other living creatures. Use hypothetical questions to identify the extent to which the client feels connected to self and nature, for example:

  If you could find a place in your imagination where you feel truly calm, connected, and that you belong, where would it be?

  Is there anywhere in nature that you have experienced a feeling of safe and calm? Can you picture that now? What feelings does it bring up?

  Have opportunities been available for you to develop a sense of belonging and being 'part of' nature? For example, did your family spend much time in nature when you were a child (playing at the beach, hiking or cycling in the mountains, and so on)?

  If you had holidays, how did you choose where you went? What type of places did you visit (i.e., ascertain to what extent holidays were within man-made vs. natural environments)? If you were able to choose your ideal holiday destination in nature, where would it be?

  Did you have a pet? How did you feel towards your pet? How did your pet feel about you? If you didn't have a pet, what would your ideal pet have been and why? What needs could the pet have met that you didn't get from anywhere else?

Freedom of Self-Expression

- Was the client encouraged to express their emotions openly during childhood? Explore parental reactions to emotional events (e.g., loss, stress, conflict). Did family members openly discuss distressing issues and mutually seek emotional support? Did family members seek distraction from emotional issues (e.g., through staying busy, workaholism, alcohol, overeating)? Or were emotions expressed in an uncontained or histrionic manner?

- Who expressed anger, and how was it expressed within the family of origin? What might the client have learned about expression of anger and other emotions through these early experiences and observations?
- Inquire about how parents reacted to distress (their own and others'). How did parents react when the client demonstrated positive emotions (e.g., excitement) and negative emotions (e.g., anger, sadness) as they were growing up?
- Explore possible themes of parentification, whereby the client has learned to take responsibility for their parents' well-being. Sometimes this can be learned through explicit or implicit messages from the parents that their child 'should' be caring/responsible/close to the parent, but this pattern can sometimes develop more subtly. The client with a sensitive and/or highly attuned temperament may have learned to tune into parents' insecurities and stress and intuitively take action to nurture or care for them, whilst the parent remains unaware of this fact. Many clients have learned that if they ask for what they need, or express their feelings, it will overwhelm the parents who are already under pressure and struggling to cope. This may precipitate a pattern of 'shutting off' their own emotional needs and taking on the role of substitute spouse or carer for the parent, evolving into a pattern of enmeshment and, ultimately, emotional neglect. Use hypothetical questions to identify patterns of parentification or enmeshment within the family of origin:

When you were upset or distressed as a child, did you ever feel that you needed to protect others from your feelings? What did you fear might happen if you told others how you were really feeling or asked your parents for help?

Have you ever felt that one or both of your parents might struggle emotionally if you weren't there to support them?

Do your parents have anyone other than you in their life to support them with their difficulties and stress?

As a child, do you recall noticing when your parents were stressed or anxious and trying to make things better for them or to smooth things over? How did you do that?

If you were to go your own way and be completely independent of your parents, do you ever worry that you would be letting them down in some way? Do you ever get the message from anyone in your family that your independence makes them feel more insecure?

Do you ever feel guilty or like you are harming your parents if you form friendships with others?

Do you ever feel guilty if you prioritise your needs over taking care of your parents?

Do you feel that if you were to experience pleasure or happiness, that this would be hurtful or disrespectful to others in your family? Almost as if you are taking it from them?

Do you ever feel like you are an extension of one or both of your parents, like you don't have a right to be a separate person?

- Use hypothetical questions to identify patterns of emotional expression within the family of origin:

  If you felt excited for some reason as a child (e.g., a birthday, seeing a friend), who would you have shared your excitement with? What (if anything) might have held you back from expressing your excitement fully (e.g., fear of disapproval, being told off for making a noise, disturbing others, or being too loud)?

  Did you ever feel that you had to act happy and cheerful in order to boost others in your family?

  Sometimes children fear that happiness is a limited resource and that if they feel happy that it might threaten or hurt someone else. Did you ever have any fears around feeling happy or good about yourself?

  If you imagine yourself as a child telling your parents that you were happy and excited, how would you have felt about that? What feelings would come up for you? And how would you expect them to respond, based on how they were back then?

Play and Spontaneity

- Did the client experience opportunities to play, have fun, and be spontaneous during childhood? Did parents encourage the client to take time to relax and partake in enjoyable activities? Was the client encouraged to balance responsibilities and duties with time off for self-care and restoration? Was the client encouraged to develop an interest in activities that were purely for fun without any pressure to perform or meet certain standards?
- Enquire about how often (if ever) parents were playful, humorous, and engaged in fun activities. Did they spend time with the client during childhood, simply playing and using imaginative activities and ideas?
- Possible hypothetical questions:

  What kinds of games or activities did you like/would you have liked to have participated in as a child?

  If you had asked your parents to play these with you, how would they have responded?

  If their response was negative, what would they have preferred you to be doing with your time?

  If you had been involved in 'messy' activities as a child (e.g., painting, making cubby houses using household furniture, playdough), how would your parents have responded to this?

  If you made a joke or laughed out loud as a child, how would your parents respond to this?

Autonomy

- Did the child have adequate opportunities for the development of a sense of competence and achievement? Did they receive praise and encouragement? Were there any difficulties that may have contributed to a sense of failure or inadequacy (e.g., being compared negatively with siblings, relatives, friends; presence of a difficulty such as dyslexia; high levels of anxiety due to domestic problems)?

- Explore whether there was a natural development of independence, autonomy, and individuation throughout late childhood and adolescence. How did parents respond to the child as they reached developmental milestones (e.g., starting school, puberty, graduation, spending more time outside the home with friends)? Did the parents react supportively or were they threatened by these changes to their child's growth? Did parents allow space for the child to experience these events in their own way, or was there parental intrusiveness at these developmental junctures?

- To explore the potential presence of a dependency schema, explore possible overprotective or 'helicopter' parenting that may have contributed to schema development. Alternatively, this may be linked to an absence of the need for care, guidance, and protection being met in early childhood, whereby the child has been pushed to grow up and be independent too early (e.g., toilet trained by nine months, taking care of siblings at eighteen months, preparing their own food at two years, etc.), and has learned to cope either through becoming overly dependent as an adult (e.g., clinging within relationships, illness behaviours) or by becoming hyperautonomous (completely self-reliant, resists seeking help or support from others). If the client's need to be dependent was met with no response or even disdain/exasperation during childhood, then they will learn not to rely on others and not to ask for help (emotional and/or practical). Alternatively, if they don't have the opportunity to branch out into the world and return to a stable base without the parent becoming overly anxious and protective, then they learn not to trust their own capacity for independence. In an ideal situation, where the child's ever-changing needs for dependence and autonomy are met in an attuned way, the child learns healthy interdependence, whereby they can trust and rely on others to support them when needed, without fear that they will be viewed as a burden or 'too needy'. In this way there is often a strong overlap between a Dependence schema and other similar schemas, such as Emotional Deprivation and Abandonment schemas.

- Enquire about parents' capacity to be self-reliant and whether the client is influenced by parents' reliance or dependence on them for practical or emotional support, thereby limiting their own freedom and development of autonomy.

- Possible hypothetical questions to be used to explore possible issues linked to dependency/autonomy:

When you were a child, were there any invisible barriers to you growing up?

Did you feel like there was anything keeping you from growing up?

In some families there is confusion between dependence and love. Have you ever worried that if you are no longer dependent on your parents, you might not get the love you need? Can you think of any times in your life when this has happened (i.e., when becoming more independent has felt like a disconnection? e.g., temporary recovery from mental health problems, leaving home to attend university).

If you imagined telling your parents that you would like to move away, or that you couldn't contact them as frequently because you were spending more time with peers, how might they react? Would you have any concerns about conveying this message?

As a child, did you ever feel like others needed you to need them or be dependent on them, to give their life purpose or meaning? Do you still feel that now? If so, what do you fear might happen if you were to put up a boundary and take steps towards living your life your own way? What would you imagine that they would feel? What feelings come up for you when you imagine doing that?

Did you ever feel like you were too needy or dependent as a child? Where did you learn that? What happened that gave you that impression? Did anyone ever say anything, or was it more their facial expressions (e.g., exasperation) that conveyed this message? Can you give examples?

If you had asked for help as a young child, such as tying your shoes, making your packed lunch, or completing homework, what would have been a typical response from your parents?

How did your parents react when you reached puberty (e.g., changes in body shape and size, menstruation)? Did you sense it was a good thing or did it cause some level of anxiety or threat?

What happened (or would have happened) when you started spending more time with friends and less time at home? Did that change your relationship with your parents in any way? Did this lead to any feelings of insecurity in you or your parents? How did you feel about that?

Realistic Limits

- Explore the way in which clients and their siblings were disciplined as children. Was discipline consistent or unpredictable and chaotic? Was there a lack of appropriate limit/boundary setting or, alternatively, were consequences overly punitive?
- Enquire about how much freedom the client had during childhood: did they have too much or too little freedom?
- Enquire about whether either parent encouraged and supported the child to complete difficult or boring tasks (e.g., homework, household chores, tidying their room)? Were these followed up with fair consequences to ensure that the child followed through with normal responsibilities and commitments?
- Enquire as to what extent parents were able to set limits on the client and siblings during childhood, such as ensuring regular healthy meals, an appropriate sleep schedule, attending school, etcetera.
- Assess the extent to which parents were able to set limits on themselves and exert an appropriate level of self-control over their own behaviours and emotional reactions. Were parents unable to set limits on themselves or their children, such as through a lack of regular mealtimes, inadequate self-care and hygiene, and/or chaotic sleep schedules?
- Did either parent have difficulty controlling their temper and behaviours, either in the family home and/or in public? Enquire about uncontrolled rage outbursts, violence, road rage, and abusive behaviours. If so, what did the child learn about these emotions, and their own capacity to manage their own urges and impulses?
- Did either parent have a history of addictive behaviours, whereby they were unable to prevent themselves from falling into the same coping patterns (e.g., use of alcohol, overeating, drugs, gambling, compulsive exercise, internet/gaming addiction, workaholism, 'romantic love addiction')?
- Did the child have adequate support with learning to self-soothe in healthy ways (e.g., through talking about emotions, asking for affection and care, and using healthy forms of support such as being in nature, physical exercise)?

- Did the child experience their emotions as manageable, or as out of control and frightening? Did the child feel an urge to 'get rid' of these urges and emotions through acting them out (and/or suppressing them)?
- Did any siblings have trouble with out-of-control anger and/or controlling impulsive urges? How did that make the client feel at the time? How did the parents respond?
- Possible hypothetical questions:

If you can imagine that, as a child, you had told your mother/father about your out-of-control feelings and urges, how do you think they would have responded?

If you had told your parents about your strong compulsion to binge eat (or take drugs, gamble, etc.), how do you think they would have reacted? What stopped you from telling them about these urges?

If you showed your self-harm scars to your family, how would they have reacted? Would they have been more or less likely to give you the love and care you were needing?

If you left home for school (as a child) without having breakfast, how would your family members have reacted?

If you became openly angry and/or shouted as a child, how do you expect that others in your family might have responded to you?

If you can imagine that as a child you told your parents that you couldn't be bothered to complete your homework that was due in the following day, how do you think they might have responded?

As a child, did you ever test your parents to see how far you could take things before they would set limits on you (e.g., staying out late, taking drugs/alcohol, starving yourself, attacking siblings, missing school)?

Some children have never had the opportunity to learn to follow instructions. They can find it difficult to follow the rules at school and might act out in certain ways (e.g., consistently turning up late, non-attendance, rebelling against teacher instructions) – is this something that you ever experienced?

Since adolescence/adulthood, have you ever noticed any attraction to communities or environments with strict rules (e.g., military forces, police force, fundamentalist religious community or cults)? [Schema overcompensation.]

Alternatively, have you found it difficult to hold down a job due to not being able to follow the rules or expectations?

Have you ever been in trouble at work due to not following expectations? [Schema surrender.]

Index

Made in the USA
Middletown, DE
03 August 2023

36172423R00216